PAIN RELIEF - FROM ANALGESICS TO ALTERNATIVE THERAPIES

Edited by **Cecilia Maldonado**

Pain Relief - From Analgesics to Alternative Therapies
http://dx.doi.org/10.5772/63264
Edited by Cecilia Maldonado

Contributors

Bogdan Feliks Kania, Danuta Wronska, Mohamed Ibrahim Noordin, Karen Barros Parron Fernandes, Marcos Tadeu Parron Fernandes, Fernanda Bortolanza Hernandes, Thais Natália de Almeida, Vitor Pinheiro Sobottka, Regina Célia Poli-Frederico, Khawla Nuseir, Mohammed Al-Azzani, Manal Kassab, Abdur Rauf, Noor Jehan, Zarka Ahmad, Mohammad S. Mubarak, Shaip Krasniqi, Armond Daci, Silvia Ussai, Lauder, Huma Naz, Mohammad Saleem, Rehab Abdel-Rahman, Pawel Lizis, Wojciech Kobza, Grzegorz Mańko, Marcin Sitarz, Jarosław Pyka, Adriana Pajares, Norman Andino García, Mabel Bregliani, Alessandro Rizzardo, Christophe Mallet, Alain Eschalier, Laurence Daulhac, Dallas Schepers, Marta Vazquez, Pietro Fagiolino, Cecilia Maldonado

Published by InTech
Janeza Trdine 9, 51000 Rijeka, Croatia

Publishing Process Manager Martina Usljebrka
Technical Editor SPi Global
Cover InTech Design team

First published May, 2017
Printed in Croatia
Legal deposit, Croatia: National and University Library in Zagreb

Additional hard copies can be obtained from orders@intechopen.com

Pain Relief - From Analgesics to Alternative Therapies , Edited by Cecilia Maldonado
p. cm.
Print ISBN 978-953-51-3187-8
Online ISBN 978-953-51-3188-5

For EU product safety concerns:
IN TECH d.o.o., Prolaz Marije Krucifikse Kozulić 3, 51000 Rijeka, Croatia,
info@intechopen.com or visit our website at intechopen.com.

Meet the editor

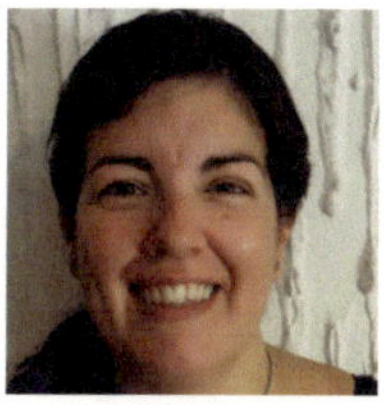

Cecilia Maldonado is an assistant professor at the Pharmaceutical Sciences Department in the Faculty of Chemistry, UdelaR, Uruguay, and a researcher at the University Hospital in the Therapeutic Drug Monitoring Service. She completed her PhD degree in Efflux Transporter and Its Relationship to Anticonvulsant Therapeutics. In the latest years, she worked with the Pain Interdisciplinary Unit in the University Hospital in the follow-up of patients with chronic pain and also investigated methadone pharmacokinetics. She has more than 20 papers in reputed journals and was awarded with the Grant for Professional Innovation from the International Pharmaceutical Federation (FIP) in 2013.

Contents

Preface

Since the beginning of times, pain treatment has been the motive of research giving birth to multiple groups of pharmacological families and therapies. Pain perception is a construction built over the biological phenomenon of signal transduction surrounded by different factors such as gender, age, and sociocultural status, among others. Therefore, it should be considered as a multidimensional process; and as such, a multidisciplinary solution is needed.

The concept of pain as the solely biological manifestation of defense is nowadays considered as a narrow-minded view of this topic. In this regard concepts such as newborns feel no pain or older people complain about everything therefore should not be paid attention when referring pain, are being left behind in the understanding that pain alleviation is a human right and everybody feeling pain should be helped for its relief.

At the very beginning, this book was solely intended to address analgesic drugs, but as chapter proposals arrived, the editorial team started to realize that any substance or technique that caused pain relief could be considered as an analgesic by the researchers. Therefore, this book started focusing on pain treatment rather than on analgesics; as a result, there is a rich variety of knowledge and expertise shared along the chapters.

This book comprises many aspects of pain treatment and the drugs involved in it. From old analgesics with new mechanisms of action for pain alleviation to analgesics potential for diminishing oxidative stress; from pharmacological therapies to electrical ones, going through alternative medicine; and from pain treatment in dentistry to chronic pain therapies, also boarding the treatment of migraine, different experts share their knowledge on the topic.

It has been a long journey in which all authors have made the greatest efforts to show in a comprehensive manner the results of their research and/or the state of the art in pain treatment. It is our wish that you find it useful in clinical practice as well as to be updated in the latest investigation related to pain relief.

Acknowledgments

I am grateful to Drs. Irene Retamoso, Andrea Graña, and María José Montes for their support and for all the knowledge shared during the time together in the Interdisciplinary Pain Management Service of the University Hospital "Dr. Manuel Quintela," Montevideo Uruguay.

Dr. Cecilia Maldonado
Pharmaceutical Sciences Department, UdelaR,
Montevideo, Uruguay

Chapter 1

Introductory Chapter

Cecilia Maldonado

Additional information is available at the end of the chapter

http://dx.doi.org/10.5772/intechopen.68903

1. Pain

Pain is one of the most common ailments which drive patients to a clinic, and pain alleviation is a key factor in the understanding of the well-being. There is a heightened awareness of pain as the "fifth vital sign," therefore it should be monitored as cautiously as blood pressure, temperature, respiratory rate, and pulse. This also entails a change in paradigm, which means pain treatment has shifted from decisions taken by an individual physician with an unspecified follow-up to more systematic approach by multidisciplinary teams [1, 2].

Pain is defined by WHO as "an unpleasant sensory and emotional experience associated with actual or potential tissue damage, or described in terms of such damage." The inclusion of the word "emotional" is crucial for the understanding of the implications of pain perception by a subject. The obvious consequence of this is that that pain perception is unique to each individual, as well as pain threshold is different in subjects. Cultural aspects should also be considered as it is nowadays preconized that no one should experience pain, not even when giving birth. Pain is culturally determined and cannot be defined so coarsely when it has so many influencing factors on how it is apprehended and expressed, being culture one of the most efficacious ones [3–6]. The clinician should then make a great effort to conceptualize pain in the search for pain alleviation because pain relieving is one of the main goals in practice.

Even though it is an ailment common to many diseases and medical procedures and in many cases, an illness in itself, it is not common to find a specialization on pain in medical schools. In general, pain management or pain medicine should entail, though not always does, a multidisciplinary approach for easing the suffering and improving the quality of life of those patients suffering from it [2, 7–9].

Although it may not be correct, it is possible to distinguish between acute and chronic pain. The first one has gained more attention because the success in its treatment, due to advances in pharmacology, and also because it is generally easily associated with a biomedical pathological cause. It is also in this kind of pain that neurophysiological explanations are fundamental for its understanding [10].

In acute pain, a pharmacological approach is usually successful in the treatment because in general a biological approximation to the matter is acceptable. Collectively, non-steroidal anti-inflammatory agents (NSAIDs) and acetaminophen (paracetamol) are the most commonly used pain medications, followed by opioids generally used in moderate to severe pain [11, 12].

The definition aforementioned is not adequate for chronic pain because chronic pain does not only entail a biological state but also a psychological one, which in many cases is able to control patients' lives. An ordinary approximation to chronic pain would give us a false impression that it can be successfully treated by the ample arsenal of drugs available; however, in many aspects, chronic pain is still an enigma for medicine. Chronic pain may be defined then as a state of sensitized perception of pain that exceeds the simple sensorial experience. Medicine treats injury and pathology to support and speed healing and treats distressing symptoms such as pain to relieve suffering during treatment and healing. When a painful injury or pathology is resistant to treatment, when pain persists after the injury or pathology has healed, and when medical science cannot identify the cause of pain, the task faced is much more difficult. The obvious consequence of this is that treatment approaches to chronic pain not only include pharmacologic measures, such as analgesics, tricyclic antidepressants, and anticonvulsants but also interventional procedures, physical therapy, and psychological measures [10, 13–16]. As a consequence of this, the typical chronic pain management team includes anesthesiologists, occupational therapists, physiotherapists, clinical psychologists, and pain nurses. Together the multidisciplinary team can help create a package of care suitable to the patient. While acute pain usually resolves once the underlying trauma or pathology has healed and is treated by one practitioner, effective management of chronic pain frequently requires the coordinated efforts of multiple disciplines [14].

2. Pain treatment

In the last decades, the understanding of the multiple mechanisms and molecules that underlie pain perception have turned its treatment into a puzzle formed by therapies that involve not only the common substances considered as analgesics (NSAIDS and opioids) but also a wide array of other drugs such as anticonvulsants and antidepressant and not less important manual techniques, together with psychological follow-up, which has also proved to be successful in containing patients emotionally [10, 12–14]. The understanding of the different routes involved in this complex phenomenon has opened its therapy not only to drugs, not previously considered as analgesics, but also to the development of pharmaceutical forms able to alleviate pain for long periods of time as well as electrical techniques for the interruption of pain signal transduction [13, 14, 17].

Even though medicines seem to be the most common resource for pain relief, and despite all the advances in pain understanding, many people still restore to nontraditional or alternative medicine, some forced by the high costs of health care and others pushed by the inefficacy of conventional treatments [18].

2.1. Analgesics

The word analgesic derives from Greek an- (ἀν-, "without"), álgos (ἄλγος, "pain"), and -ikos (-ικος, forming adjectives). Such drugs were usually known as anodynes before the twentieth century.

Both broader classes of analgesics have a natural origin. Salicylic acid extracted from the bark of Willow tree gave birth to NSAIDs, whereas *Papaver somniferum* is the origin of opioids [19, 20].

The mechanism of action shown by acetylsalicylic acid was at first generalized to all NSAIDs; however, nowadays this group comprises diverse classes of structures which have demonstrated different potential as anti-inflammatory, antipyretic, and analgesic drugs. In the last century, acetaminophen has gained field in treatment of mild pain, but it is still nowadays studied regarding its mechanism of action as it seems not to be like any other kind of analgesic [21].

The long use of these substances has allowed a thorough study of their efficacy as well as their safety profile; however, in many countries NSAIDs being sold as over-the-counter drugs, give the false impression of innocuous products when in fact they are not [22, 23].

NSAIDs differ from acetaminophen in that they possess anti-inflammatory properties and are associated with a different side effect profile that includes bleeding, gastrointestinal ulceration, renal dysfunction, and an elevated risk of adverse cardiovascular events. On the other hand, paracetamol, though a widespread option for mild pain, rises concerns regarding its safety in people with impaired hepatic function, alcoholics, etc. [24–26].

Morphine derivatives are in general more cautiously used, and in the last decades, attitude toward opioids has shifted from willingness to fear of their use especially because of their potential for addiction which leads to the prescription of lower than effective doses.

In many settings, morphine is still the standard of care in active cancer because of its short half-life, which allows a more flexible administration regimen. The availability of multiple pharmaceutical dosage forms and, last but not least, economic reasons have maintained morphine as a current option [27–29]. In contrast, the long-term administration of an opioid for the treatment of chronic noncancer pain continues to be controversial accompanied by the folk knowledge that sustains the use of opioids in terminal illnesses [30–32]. In this setting, opioids, such as tramadol, methadone, and oxycodone, have gained field to morphine because of either their more advantageous pharmacokinetics parameters or the addition of adjunctive mechanisms of action (serotonin, norepinephrine reuptake inhibition, and NMDA antagonism).

Even though opioids are the first-line approach for moderate or severe pain in populations with active cancer, the comprehensive management of pain in this kind of patient also requires expertise in the use of the nonopioid analgesics, such as acetaminophen (paracetamol), nonsteroidal anti-inflammatory agents (NSAIDs), and drugs referred to as "adjuvant" analgesics or coanalgesics [33].

The knowledge that serotonin and norepinephrine play an important role in pain has influenced the incorporation of serotonin-norepinephrine reuptake inhibitor (SNRI) drugs in the wide array of drugs for pain alleviation. SNRIs are commonly used in conjunction with opioids (especially tapentadol and tramadol) with greater success in pain relief. This is the case of chronic pain syndromes, which usually require the use of this "adjuvant analgesics." The treatment of neuropatic pain has changed with time. At the beginning it included tricyclic antidepressants and anticonvulsants such as carbamazepine. Nowadays, the arsenal has spread with the use of gabapentinoids and SNRI antidepressants, such as duloxetine which in recent years has acquired approved indications for pain. For migraine pain, anticonvulsants such as valproic acid and topiramate are also used [34, 35]. And last but not least the T-type calcium channel blockers have also been included in pain treatment protocols in animals and human models [36–39].

2.2. Other targets and techniques for pain alleviation

When Western medicines seem not to be effective, many people restore to nontraditional or alternative medicine. There is some evidence that some treatments using alternative medicine can relieve some types of pain more effectively than placebo [40, 41]. Medicinal plants (MPs) have been used for centuries by many cultures to treat pain and this knowledge has been embraced by the pharmaceutical industry which has used it to synthesize and elaborate analgesics commonly used in traditional Western treatments. The scientific verification process of this tradition is ongoing. The natural origin of MPs may lead to the false impression of innocuity and ample safety [42, 43], but despite presenting a wide therapeutic range, MPs are not exempt of adverse effects and interactions [44]; phytovigilance should be performed as for conventional medicines and should be sustained on a scientific basis regarding their toxicity and its allergenic potential [44]. Despite all this evidence, MPs use should not be discouraged, because for certain population, they are not only the adequate option but may be the only one available or affordable.

As it has been stated that the two main systems addressed in pain treatment are the routes involving COXs enzymes and opioids receptors and lately the inhibition of monoamines reuptake. Seeking for other options, lately, the endocannabinoid/vanilloid systems have also been studied regarding their effect on pain alleviation [45–47]. Although cannabis has proved to be useful in pain alleviation, there are two drawbacks for this option. First, cannabis is still a prohibited plant in many countries and second, as with many other plants, it is troublesome to identify the substance responsible for the action. To make matters worse, what raises concerns in this case is that tetrahydrocannabinol (THC) which is responsible for pain alleviation is also responsible for the psychoactive effects of marijuana. THC is not the only natural occurring substances capable of agonizing the endocannabinoid receptors and efforts are being made to find synthetic derivatives with a safer profile. The entourage effect is also a problem when extracting substances from biological matrixes, as sometimes the final effect of a treatment depends on a group of substances and not just an isolated one.

Local anesthetics have also proven to be a useful tool in acute and chronic pain relief; lidocaine presents good results in this regard because of the rapid alleviation obtained after administration, though cardiovascular adverse effects should also be taken into consideration [48, 49].

In newborns, sweet solutions have also presented analgesic properties showing promising results at very low cost and placing babies at minimum risk of side effects. There is also ongoing research over different forms of administration including patient-controlled analgesia, different pharmaceutical forms for a more effective pain control as well as electrical techniques for disrupting pain signal.

3. Conclusion

It has been clearly stated that pain treatment is a challenge difficult to face. Health care teams have to articulate the resources available and patients' needs in a particular scenario where previous experiences are sometimes difficult to extrapolate. This book intends to give those involved in pain management a proper idea of the tools available for pain relief, comprising pharmacological ones and adjuvant techniques, as well as presenting late research on analgesics, their benefits and security profile.

Acknowledgements

The author would like to thanks Drs. Irene Retamoso, Andrea Graña, and María José Montes for their support and for all the knowledge shared during the time together in the Interdisciplinary Pain Management Service of the University Hospital Dr. Manuel Quintela, Montevideo Uruguay.

Author details

Cecilia Maldonado

Address all correspondence to: cmaldonado@fq.edu.uy

Pharmaceutical Sciences Department, Faculty of Chemistry, UdelaR, Montevideo, Uruguay

References

[1] Fishman SM. Pain as the fifth vital sign how can I tell when back pain is serious? Journal of Pain & Palliative Care Pharmacotherapy. 2009;**19**(4):77-79

[2] Kaiser U, Arnold B, Pfingster M, et al. Multidisciplinary pain management programs. Journal of Pain Research. 2013;**6**:355-358

[3] Lovering S. Cultural attitudes and beliefs about pain. Journal of Transcultural Nursing. 2006;**17**(4):389-395

[4] Zborowski M. Cultural components in response to pain. Journal of Social Issues.1952;**8**(4): 16-30

[5] Diller A. Cross-cultural pain semantics. Pain. 1980;**9**(1):9-20

[6] Callister LC. Cultural influences on pain perceptions and behaviors. Home Health Care Management and Practice. 2003;**15**(3):207-211

[7] Jensen MP, Turner JA, Romano JM. Changes in beliefs, catastrophizing, and coping are associated with improvement in multidisciplinary pain treatment. Journal of Consulting and Clinical Psychology. 2001;**69**(4):655-662

[8] Jensen MP, Turner JA, Romano JA. Changes after multidisciplinary pain treatment in patient pain beliefs and coping are associated with concurrent changes in patient functioning. Journal of Pain Research. 2013;**6**:355-358

[9] DeBar LL, Kindler L, Keefe JF, et al. A primary care-based interdisciplinary team approach to the treatment of chronic pain utilizing a pragmatic clinical trials framework. Translational Behavioral Medicine. 2012;**2**(4):523-530

[10] Grichnik KP, Ferrante FM. The difference between acute and chronic pain. Mount Sinai Journal of Medicine. 1991;**58**(3):217-220

[11] Blondell RP, Azadfard M, Wisniewski A. Pharmacotherapy for acute pain. American Family Physician. 2013;**87**(11):766-772

[12] De Andres J, Fabregat-Cid G, Asensio-Samper JM, et al. Management of acute pain in patients on treatment with opioids. Pain Management. 2015;**5**(3):167-173

[13] Whitten CE, Donovan M, Cristobal K. Treating chronic pain: New knowledge, more choices. The Permanente Journal. 2005;**9**(4):9-18

[14] Chang KL, Fillingim R, Hurley RW, et al. Chronic pain management: Nonpharmacological therapies for chronic pain. FP Essentials. 2015;**432**:21-26

[15] Cherkin DC, Deyo RA, Battié M, et al. Comparison of physical therapy, chiropractic manipulation, and provision of an educational booklet for the treatment of patients with low back pain. The New England Journal of Medicine. 1998;**339**:1021-1029

[16] Lee BH, Scharff L, Sethna NF, et al. Physical therapy and cognitive-behavioral treatment for complex regional pain syndrome. Journal of Pediatrics. 2002;**141**(1):135-140

[17] Jones I, Johnson MI. Transcutaneous electrical nerve stimulation. Critical Care Pain. 2009;**9**(4):130-135

[18] Maroon JC, Bost W, Marron A. Natural anti-inflammatory agents for pain relief. Surgical Neurology International. 2010;**1**:80

[19] Mahdi JG. Medicinal potential of willow: A chemical perspective of aspirin discovery. Journal of Saudi Chemical Society. 2010;**14**(3):317-322

[20] Calixto JB, Beirith A, Ferreira J, et al. Naturally occurring antinociceptive substances from plants. Phytotherapy Research. 2000;**14**:401-418

[21] Zhang W, Jones A, Doherty A. Does paracetamol (acetaminophen) reduce the pain of osteoarthritis? A meta-analysis of randomised controlled trials. Annals of the Rheumatic Diseases. 2004;**63**:901-907

[22] Sostres C, Gargallo CJ, Arroyo MT, et al. Adverse effects of non-steroidal anti-inflammatory drugs (NSAIDS, aspirin and coxibs) on upper gastrointestinal tract. Best Practice & Research: Clinical Gastroenterology. 2010;**24**(2):121-132

[23] Layton D, Souverein PC, Heerdink ER, et al. Evaluation of risk profiles for gastrointestinal and cardiovascular adverse effects in nonselective NSAID and cox-2 inhibitor users a cohort study using pharmacy dispensing data in the Netherlands. Drug Safety. 2008;**31**(2):143-158

[24] Bearden W. Common adverse events and interactions with OTC pain medications. US Pharmacist. 2008;**33**(5):44-56

[25] Pirmohamed M, Kitteringham NR, Park BK. The role of active metabolites in drug toxicity. Drug Safety. 1994;**11**:114-144

[26] Pirmohamed M, Breckenridge A, Kitteringham NR, et al. Adverse drug reactions. British Medical Journal. 1998;**316**:1295-1298

[27] Hanks GW, Conno F, Cherny N, et al. Expert working group of the research network of the European association for palliative care. Morphine and alternative opioids in cancer pain: The EAPC recommendations. British Journal of Cancer. 2001;**84**(5):587-593

[28] Mercadante S. Intravenous morphine for management of cancer pain. The Lancet Oncology. 2010;**11**(5):484-489

[29] Mercadante S, Villari P, Ferrera P, et al. Safety and effectiveness of intravenous morphine for episodic (breakthrough) pain using a fixed ratio with the oral daily morphine dose. Journal of Pain and Symptom Management. 2004;**27**:352-359

[30] Rosenblum A, Marsch LA, Joseph H, et al. Opioids and the treatment of chronic pain: Controversies, current status, and future directions. Experimental and Clinical Psychopharmacology. 2008;**16**(5):405-416

[31] Ballantyne JC, Mao J. Opioid therapy for chronic pain. The New England Journal of Medicine. 2003;**349**:1943-1953

[32] Furlan AD, Sandoval JA, Mailis-Gagnon A, et al. Opioids for chronic non-cancer pain: A meta-analysis of effectiveness and side effects. Canadian Medical Association Journal. 2006;**174**(11):1589-1594

[33] McNicol E, Strassels SA, Goudas L, et al. NSAIDs and paracetamol alone or combined with opioids, for cancer pain. The Cochrane Database of Systematic Reviews. 2005;**25**(1):CD005180. DOI: 10.1002/14651858.CD005180

[34] Sindrup SH, Otto M, Finnerup NB, et al. Mini review antidepressants in the treatment of neuropathic pain. Basic & Clinical Pharmacology & Toxicology. 2005;**96**:399-409

[35] McQuay H, Carroll D, Rjadad A, et al. Anticonvulsant drugs for management of pain: A systematic review. British Medical Journal. 1995;**311**:1047-1052

[36] Perret D, Luo D. Targeting voltage-gated calcium channels for neuropathic pain management. Neurotherapeutics. 2009;**6**(4):679-692.

[37] Snutch TP. Targeting chronic and neuropathic pain: The n-type calcium channel comes of age. NeuroRx. 2005;**2**(4):662-670

[38] Zamponi GW, Lewis RJ, Todorovic SM, et al. Role of voltage-gated calcium channels in ascending pain pathways. Brain Research Reviews. 2009;**60**(1):84-89

[39] Cox B. Calcium channel blockers and pain therapy. Current Review of Pain. 2000;**4**(6): 488-498

[40] Kakatum N, Jaiarree N, Makchucit S, et al. Antioxidant and anti-inflammatory activities of Thai medicinal plants in Sahasthara remedy for muscle pain treatment. Journal of the Medical Association of Thailand. 2012;**95**(1):120-126

[41] Stolz ED, Müller LG, Trojan-Rodrigues M, et al. Survey of plants popularly used for pain relief in Rio Grande do Sul. Revista Brasileira de Farmacognosia. 2014;**24**(2):185-196

[42] Williamson E, Driver S, Baxter K, editors. Stockley's Herbal Medicines Interactions. London: Pharmaceutical Press; 2009

[43] Kupiec T, Raj V. Fatal seizures due to potential herb-drug interactions with *Ginkgo biloba*. Journal of Analytical Toxicology. 2005;**29**:755-758

[44] Russo EB. Cannabinoids in the management of difficult to treat pain. Therapeutics and Clinical Risk Management. 2008;**4**(1):245-259

[45] Grant I, Atkinson JH, Gouaux B. Medical marijuana: Clearing away the smoke. The Open Neurology Journal. 2012;**6**:18-25

[46] Manzanares J, Julian MD, Carrascosa A. Role of the cannabinoid system in pain control and therapeutic implications for the management of acute and chronic pain episodes. Current Neuropharmacology. 2006;**4**(3):239-257

[47] Carroll I, Gaeta R, Mackey S. Multivariate analysis of chronic pain patients undergoing lidocaine infusions: Increasing pain severity and advancing age predict likelihood of clinically meaningful analgesia. The Clinical Journal of Pain. 2007;**23**(8):702-706

[48] Kosharsky B, Almonte W, Shaparin N, et al. Intravenous infusions in chronic pain management. Pain Physician. 2013;**16**(3):231-249

[49] Petersen P, Kastrup J, Zeeberg I, et al. Chronic pain treatment with intravenous lidocaine. Neurological Research. 1986;**8**(3):189-190

Section 1

Pharmacotherapy of Pain Relief

Advance Delivery System Dosage Form for Analgesic, Their Rationale, and Specialty

Mohamed Ibrahim Noordin

Additional information is available at the end of the chapter

http://dx.doi.org/10.5772/68096

Abstract

Drugs including analgesics need a delivery system to deliver it to the site of action upon administration. Delivery can be achieved using various types of dosage forms including tablets, capsules, creams, ointments, liquids, aerosols, injections, and suppositories. Conventional drug delivery systems provide immediate release of the analgesics without controlling the rate of release. A number of doses must be given daily in order to achieve and maintain effective plasma concentrations. Frequent administration causes fluctuations in plasma levels of the drug. The drug plasma levels could fall below the minimum effective concentration and can also exceed the minimum toxic concentration. The purposes behind controlling the drug delivery for analgesic are to achieve more effective therapies while eliminating the potential for both under and overdosing. The need for fewer administrations for "no pain" maintenance and with optimal use of the drug in question is to avoid adverse effect, and to increased patient compliance. Modified-release analgesics have enabled patients to better maintain pain control by convenient dosing intervals and sustained blood concentrations. The differences between available modified-release products are half-life, cost, and formulation and drug-release properties.

Keywords: analgesic, pain management, modified drug delivery system, specialty product and polymer

1. Introduction

Analgesics are medicines that relieve pain or in other words they are drugs that are used to provide pain relief. When we browse the topic on analgesics we will also come across the term narcotic as first analgesics as they were narcotics, and their derivatives and analogs were chemically based on the morphine molecule [1]. Additionally, analgesics may include nonsteroidal anti-inflammatory drugs (NSAIDs) and paracetamol (acetaminophen). Practically, the term may also include others like tricyclic antidepressants and substances such as gabapentin, although they are not commonly classified as analgesics [1]. It should be well differentiated that usually analgesics give symptomatic relief, but have no effect on the body condition, although NSAIDs are beneficial in both reducing pain and inflammation.

2. Pain

Why god created pain? To the author, the answer to this question explains the term "productive pain" which has been described in literatures as a warning on the occurring of injury in the body. This pain will guide the person to seek treatment, and this pain will also facilitate diagnosis. "Nonproductive" pain by definition serves no purpose either as a warning or diagnostic tool. It is important for us to understand pain pathophysiology for management purpose.

Pain syndromes may be different, but their sensory pathways are the same. It starts from the affected organ and the message flow to the brain for interpretation. The pharmacological path of analgesics' action is by working at the level of the nerves, they work by either blocking the signal originating from the peripheral nervous system, or can work centrally by distorting the interpretation by the central nervous system.

Practitioners' selection of an appropriate analgesic is first based on the type of pain and severity and then the knowledge of risk and extra benefit and indirectly considering existing risk-benefit of a particular drug. The decision will also depend on the knowledge on the classes of drugs, and their adverse effect. Text books have divided pain into two classes, acute and chronic. In selecting the analgesic to be used, severity and predicted survival of patient must also be considered as a selection criteria [2].

2.1. Acute pain

Acute pain duration is self-limiting and this includes postoperative pain, pain of injury, and childbirth. This type of pain is foreseen to be short in duration so the treatment using narcotic pain killer is considered to be safe as there will not be long-term addiction problem on using narcotics. Using NSAIDs will also be beneficial as it allows fluctuation of dose but with limiting concern on the risk of ulcers. For both categories of painkillers, their doses may be adjusted based on observation of healing rate, changing doses from high to low doses, and from narcotic analgesics to nonnarcotics as required. In severe pain, it is the rule of thumb that patients should not be subject to the return of pain so painkiller needs to be dosed adequately to ensure that pain is at least tolerable to avoid the occurrence of anxiety, usually after the return of pain [3]. Generally, in pain management, painkiller should never be dosed on as needed basis, but should be administered often enough to assure effective plasma level (this could be warrantied with the use of a sustained release preparation).

2.2. Chronic pain

Chronic pain is defined as pain lasting over 3 months and severe enough to have effect on body function. This condition is more difficult to treat, as the expected side effects of the drug are more difficult to manage because of the long-term exposure to the drug. There will be addiction potential for those who are on narcotic analgesics which can exacerbate to respiratory depression and constipation. For those using NSAIDs, the risk of gastric ulcers is evident. Drugs with narcotic agonist-antagonist properties such as buprenorphine, nalbuphine, pentazocine, or the COX-2 inhibitors, such as celecoxib and rofecoxib, which reduces the common side effect, are still not recommended for long-term management of severe pain. Usually, practitioners following the guidelines for chronic pain management will recommend a combination of drug therapy to suite the lifestyle and other treatment modalities [2]. Modification of the delivery system of the drug for the purpose of long-term treatment is also beneficial [4].

3. Group of analgesic drug

3.1. Narcotic analgesics

Narcotic analgesics are all derived from opium. They include morphine, codeine, and a number of semisynthetics including meperidine (Demerol), propoxyphene (Darvon) tramadol, and a few others. Different narcotic analgesics may vary in their potency, but all of them are effective in the treatment of visceral pain. Generally, their adverse effects are very much dose-related as they are all addictive in nature [5]. These category of drug are regulated by the authorities as they are open for abuse, usually they are controlled under the nation's laws.

3.2. NSAIDs

NSAIDs are available as effective analgesics even at low doses where there is no antiinflamatory effect. They are in the form of various chemical types although they have demonstrated similar pharmacological effect in reducing pain. They may even possess similar side effects. They are mostly provided in the form of oral dosage although some may be in the form of injection [6].

Paracetamol, or acetaminophen as Americans call it, is a nonnarcotic analgesic with no antiinflammatory properties. It is the most popular analgesic which is appropriate for mild to moderate pain. It is well tolerated in normal recommended doses but it may have significant liver toxicity at high doses. Clinically, paracetamol has been considered the first choice for mild pain as it is considered to be very safe at therapeutic doses.

4. Various dosage form of analgesic and their mode of actions and limitations

4.1. Conventional dosage forms of analgesics

Conventional dosage forms of analgesic are the same as any conventional dosage form of general pharmaceuticals. Dosage which is synonymous with unit doses, means pharmaceutical drug products in the form found commercially in the market with a specific mixture of active ingredients and inactive excipients in specific form or configuration. Dosage forms come in several types, depending on the route of administration. The general forms include liquid, solid, and semisolid forms. Specifically, conventional dosage forms are solutions or suspensions for injection, pill, tablet, capsule, and syrup. Clearly, the administrative route of the drug is dependent on the dosage form of the substance. An oral solid dosage form is the solid form of a dose of a chemical compound used as a drug or medication intended for oral consumption. More than one dosage forms may exist for a single particular drug. This is due to the fact that different clinical conditions may need different routes of administration [8]. For example, where there is a condition of nausea or vomiting, it may be difficult to use an oral dosage form. Such condition may warrant an alternative route such as injection or rectal route. Dedicated specific route may be a requirement for certain kinds of drugs, as there may be issues with various factors like chemical stability or pharmacokinetics. A good example is the analgesic paracetamol, it exist in a number of dosage form, that is, tablet, capsule, syrup, suppository, and injection (**Table 1**).

	Type of pain killer in the market	Common dosage form available
1.	Paracetamol (acetaminophen)	Tablets, solution, suspension, suppository, injection
2.	Paracetamol with codiene	Tablets, solution, suspension
3.	Celecoxib	Capsules
4.	Diclofenac	Tablets, capsules, gel (local application)
5.	Fentanyl	Tablets, capsules, *transdermal patch
6.	Hydrocodone	Tablets, elixer
7.	Hydrocodone with paracetamol	Tablets, elixer
8.	Hydromorphone	Tablets, injection, suppositories, liquid
9.	Ibuprofen	Tablets, solution, suspension
10.	Meloxicam	Tablets, oral suspension
11.	Methadone	Tablets, oral solution, oral concentrate, injection
12.	**Methylprednisolone	Tablets, injection
13.	Milnacipran	Tablets, injection

	Type of pain killer in the market	Common dosage form available
14.	Morphine	Tablets, injection
15.	Naproxen	Tablets, *delayed-release enteric coated tablets, suspension
16.	Oxycodone	Tablets, oral concentrate, oral solution
17.	Oxycodone with paracetamol	Tablets
18.	**Prednisone	Tablets, solution
19.	Sumatriptan	Injection, tablets, *nasal spray

*Analgesic specialty products.
**Steroids as adjuvant to analgesic, OK.

Table 1. Some of the analgesic and their dosage form available in the market.

5. Various new dosage forms, making their way to the market

5.1. Research in the development of new delivery system with existing analgesic

Development of modified release painkiller is a popular research. This type of research looks into the development of techniques and evaluation of the modified forms used in the management of chronic pain in comparison with existing dosage form [7]. The realization on the importance of pain management and the treatment of pain has initiated more research in this area among healthcare researchers. Modified-release products have enabled patients to better maintain pain control due to convenient dosing intervals and sustained blood concentrations. With the above statements, it is evidenced that development of modified release is very much needed for pain management drug, so as to be very effective and to prolong the effect for more effective pain management [7].

All drugs need a delivery system to deliver it to the site of action upon administration. Delivery of the drugs can be achieved using various types of dosage forms including tablets, capsules, creams, ointments, liquids, aerosols, injections, and suppositories. These conventional drug delivery systems provide immediate release of the drug without controlling the rate or drug release. A number of doses given daily in order to achieve and maintain therapeutic level to achieve effective plasma concentrations cause fluctuations in plasma levels of the drug [8–10] and drug plasma levels could fall below the minimum effective concentration and can also exceed the minimum toxic concentration (**Figure 1**).

5.2. The various types of modified release preparation possible for analgesics delivery

The purpose behind controlling the drug delivery for analgesic are to achieve more effective therapies while eliminating the potential for both under- and overdosing of analgesic.

Maintenance of analgesic levels within a desired range to combat pain is indirectly combating stress to the patient. The need for fewer administrations of analgesic or optimal use of

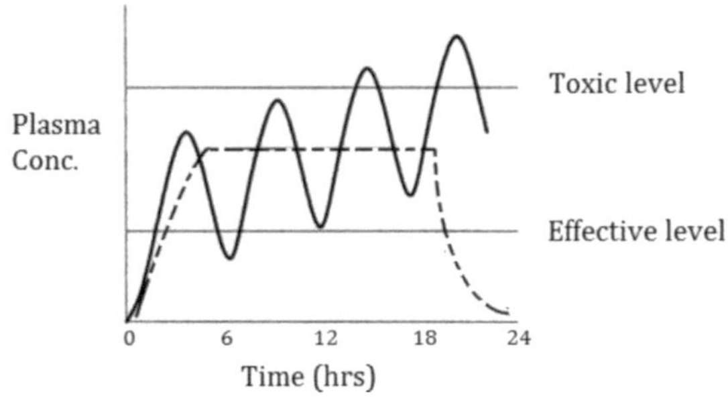

Figure 1. The conventional four times daily oral doses of diclofenac sodium (25 mg) plasma level compared to a daily doses sustained release formulation (100 mg) plasma level.

analgesic toward "no pain" maintenance is to avoid adverse side effect and indirectly to increase patient compliance in their pain management [8].

5.2.1. The polymeric delivery system: polymers in controlled drug delivery

The use of various polymers in controlled drug delivery is very popular among formulation researchers. These polymers can be natural or synthetic in nature. Different polymer is combined with a drug in such a way that the active agent is released from the material in a predesigned manner. The release of the active agent may be constant over a long period or it may be cyclic over a long period or it may be triggered by the environment or other external events [9].

Polymer can be used to encapsulate drug molecules for the purpose of sustaining the release and extending the availability of the drug so that dosage administration frequency can be reduced while maintaining the plasma level steady state. A good example would be the sustenance of release preparation of diclofenac sodium for oral administration [8].

Polymer can also be used in protecting the drug from the environment in order to target the delivery of the drug to certain side of the body. A very simple targeting is the delivery of weak base drug to the small intestine where most of this type of drug is acid labile. So the polymer is used as a protective shield. This can be a pH-sensitive polymer where in acidic environment it is very stable and will disintegrate in basic environment.

Characteristics of polymer may be engineered to the advantage in the development of a drug delivery system. A mucoadhesive polymer which can stick to the mucosa can be used to encapsulate drug and attach to the mucosa and sustain the release of the drug it encapsulates. A biodegradable polymer can be used to encapsulate drug for slow release as the polymer degrades. A pH-sensitive polymer can be used to target the release of drug either in acidic or basic environment. Combining all these characteristic, a researcher can even deliver a drug which currently can only be delivered by parenteral route, using the enthrall route. Logically, the drug can have an outer encapsulation with a pH-sensitive polymer which can save it from the acidic environment in the stomach and can have a mucoadhesive polymer inner encapsulation for it to stick to the small intestine lining and to release the drug direct across the membrane into the blood.

http://dx.doi.org/10.5772/68096

The vast uses of polymer in the gastrointestinal, enthrall, or oral drug delivery system do not limit the same polymer to be used in other route of dosage administration. Several polymers in the form of nano size particles are used to deliver drug as an intravenous dosage form [11]. Researchers are also looking into various polymers which can act as a depot for big dose administration of drug through implantation in the subcutaneous area for cases of difficult patient compliance such as delivery of antipsychotics and cancer drugs.

Some of the synthetic materials that are currently being used or studied for controlled drug delivery are as depicted in **Table 2**.

Polymer are sometimes crudely extracted from natural resources be it from animals or from plants. Such natural materials are depicted in **Table 3**.

Polymer	Polymer structure
Poly(2-hydroxy ethyl methacrylate). **$(C_6H_{10}O_3)_n$**	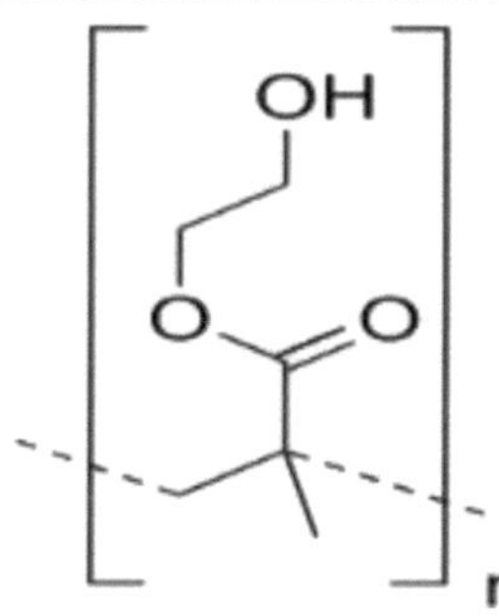
Poly(N-vinyl pyrrolidone). **$(C_6H_9NO)_n$**	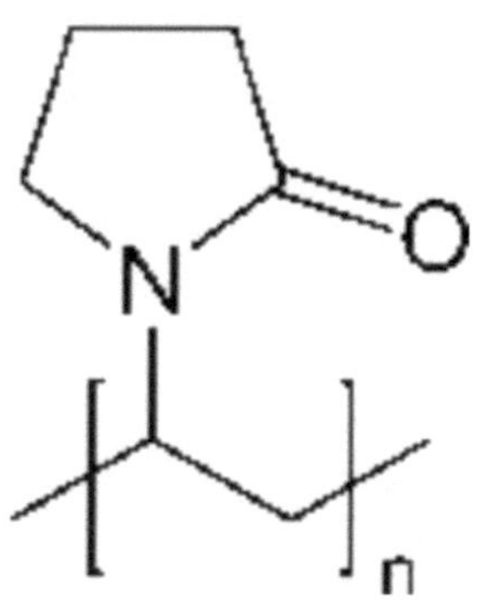
Poly(methyl methacrylate). **$(C_5O_2H_8)_n$**	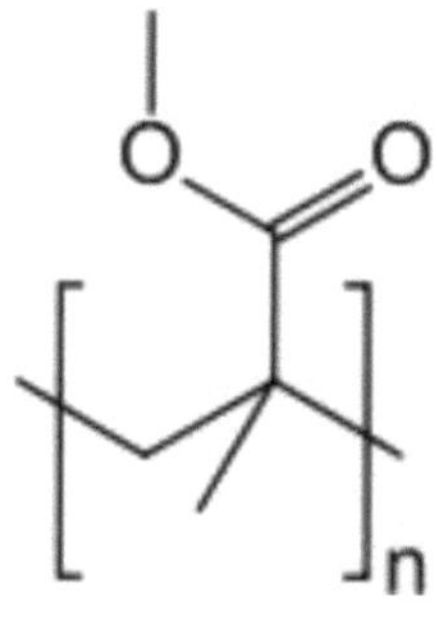

Polymer	Polymer structure
Poly(vinyl alcohol). **$(C_2H_4O)x$**	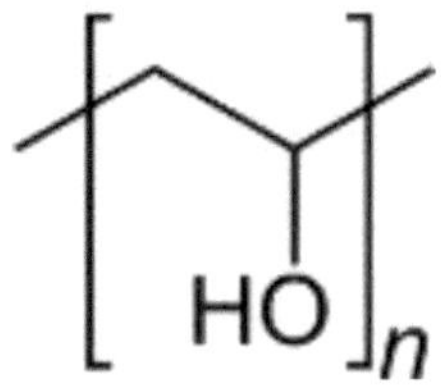
Poly(acrylic acid). **$(C_3H_4O_2)_n$**	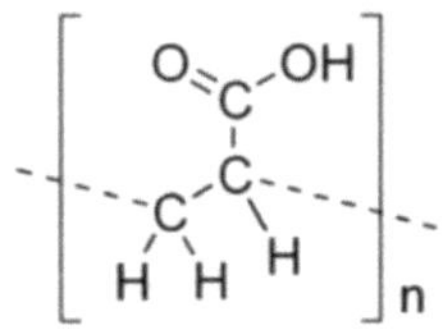
Polyacrylamide. **$(C_3H_5NO)_n$**	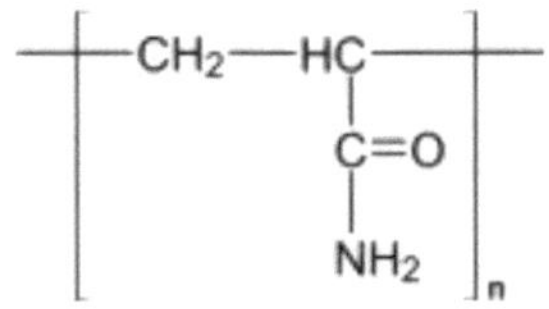
Poly(ethylene-co-vinyl acetate). **$(C_2H_4)_n(C_4H_6O_2)_m$**	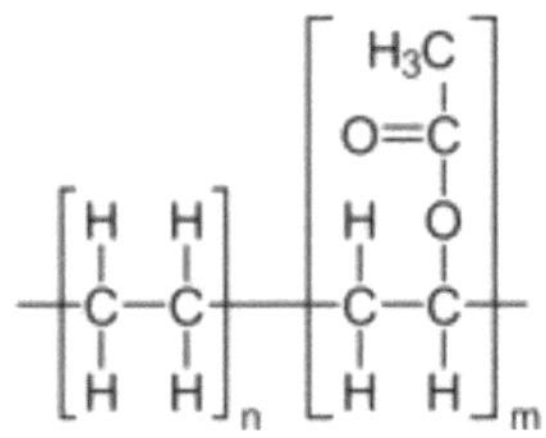
Poly(ethylene glycol). **$C_{2n}H_{4n+2}O_{n+1}$**	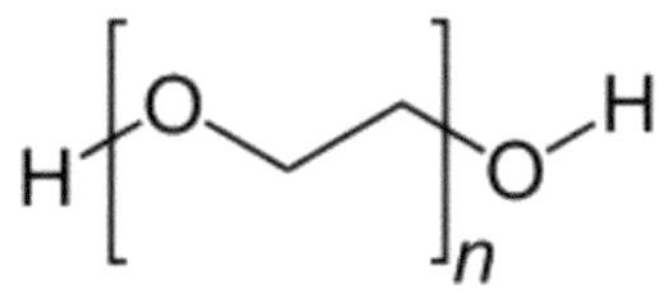
Poly(methacrylic acid). **$(C_4H_6O_2)_n$**	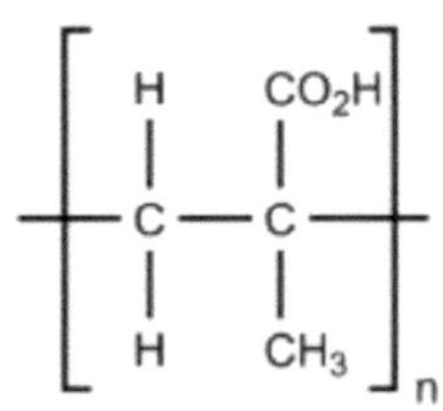

Table 2. Example of synthetic polymer available in the market.

5.3. Controlled-release mechanisms in the case of using polymer as a drug delivery system

There are three primary mechanisms by which active agents can be released from a delivery system: diffusion, degradation, and swelling followed by diffusion. Any or all of these mechanisms may occur in a given release system [12]. We can easily understand this mechanism through **Figures 2–8**.

Material	Illustration	Structure (if available)
Gelatin	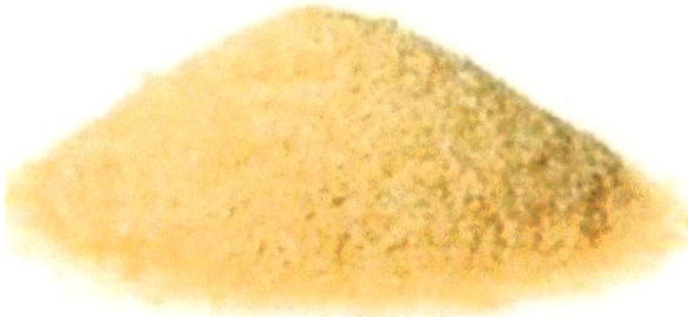	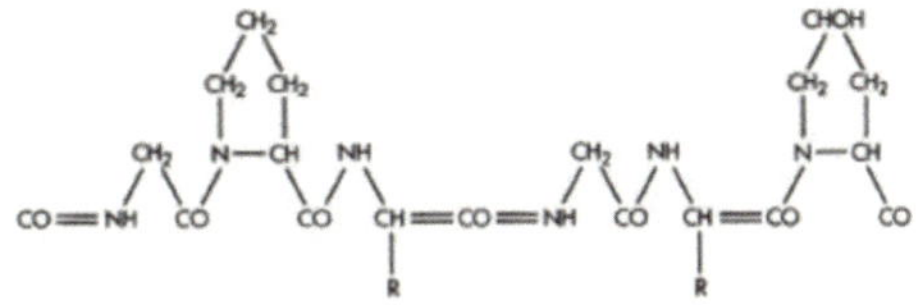
Carrageenan	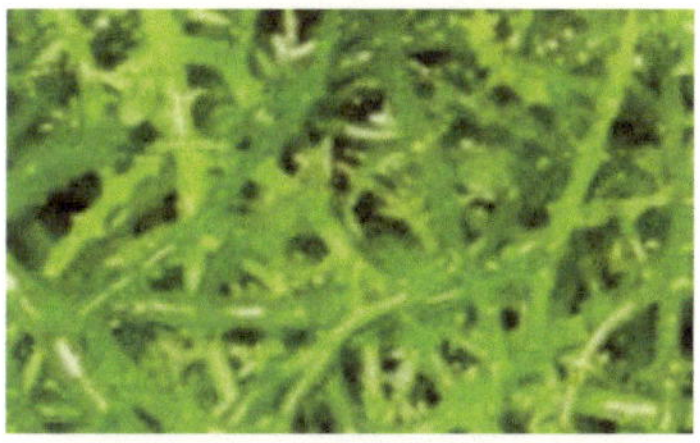	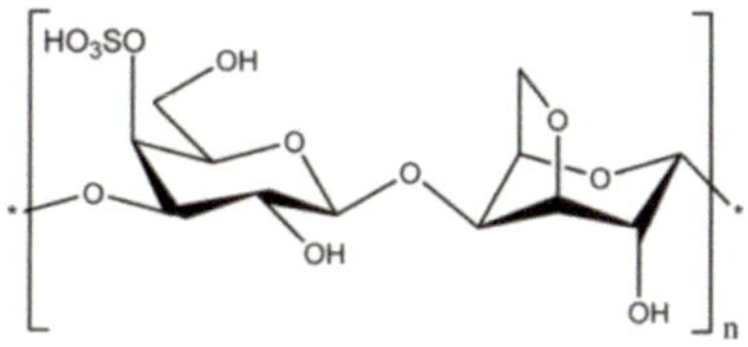
Chitosan	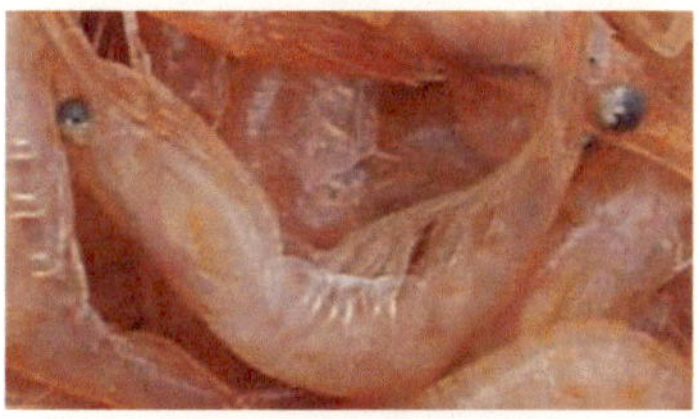	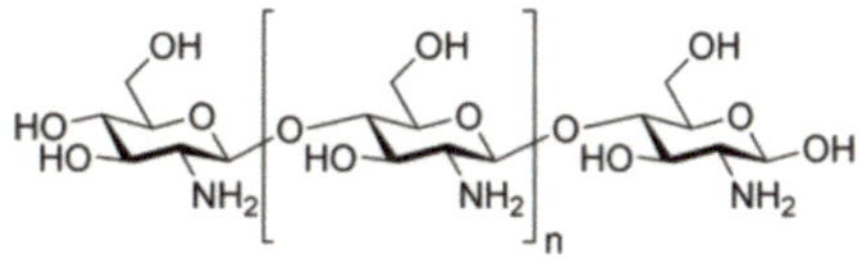
Arabic gum	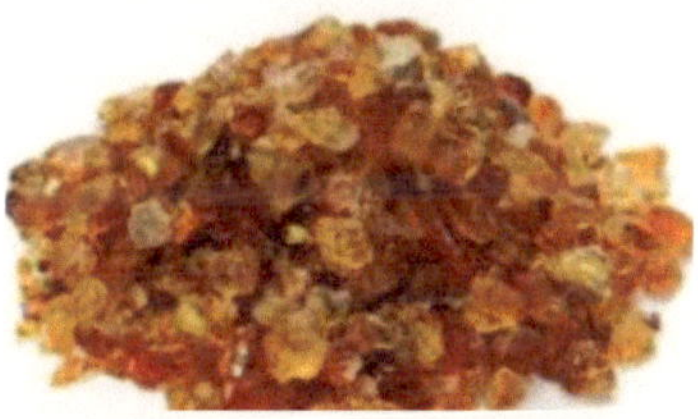	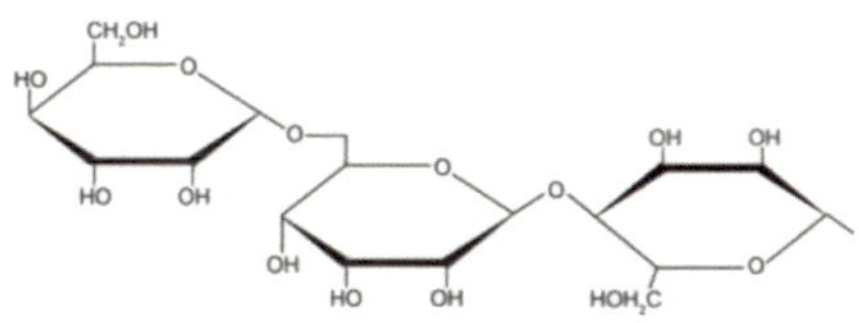
Tamarind seed gum	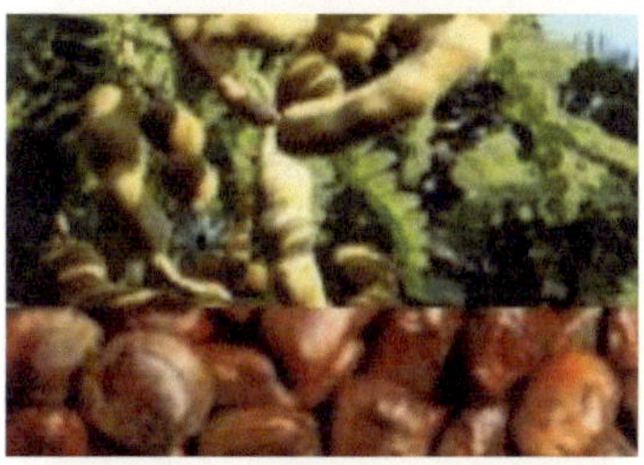	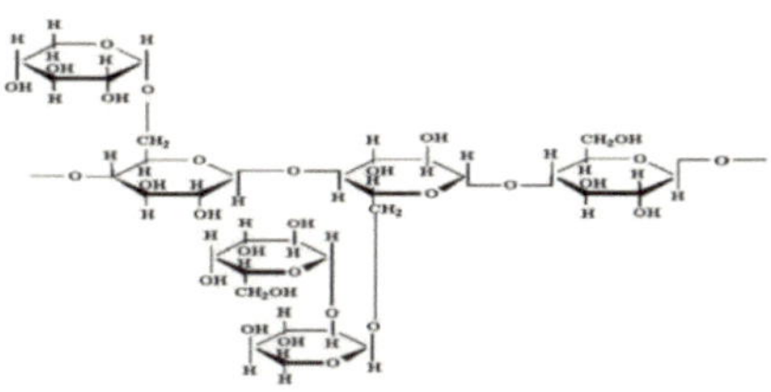
Hibiscus esculentus gum	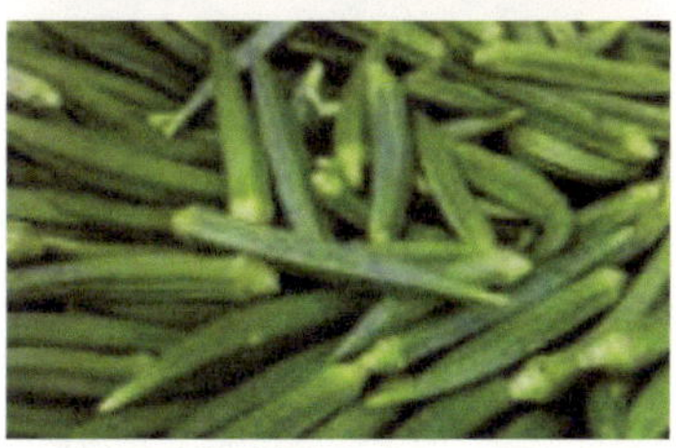	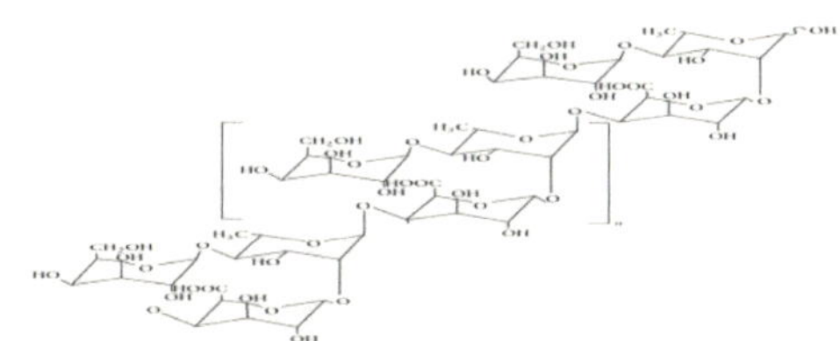

Table 3. Example of natural polymer used in drug delivery research.

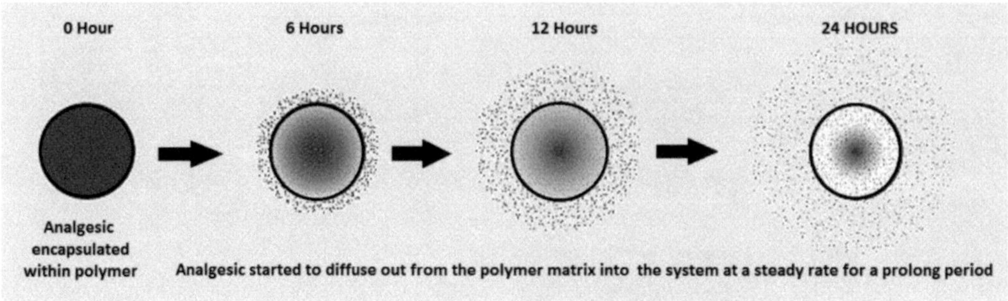

Figure 2. Analgesic diffusing out from a matrix of polymer in a sustain release model.

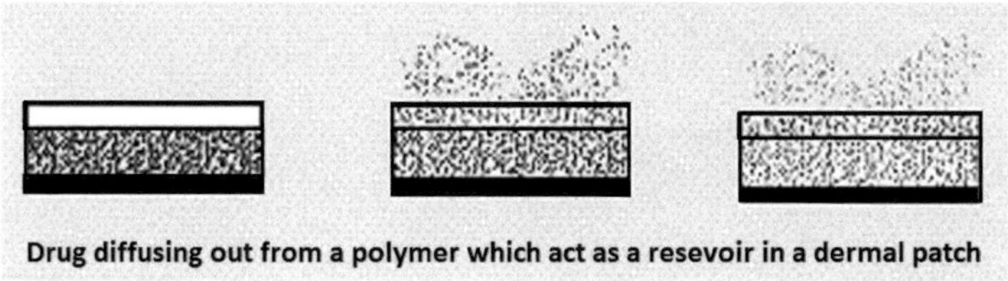

Figure 3. A dermal patch model illustrating the diffusion analgesic from a dermal path polymer matrix.

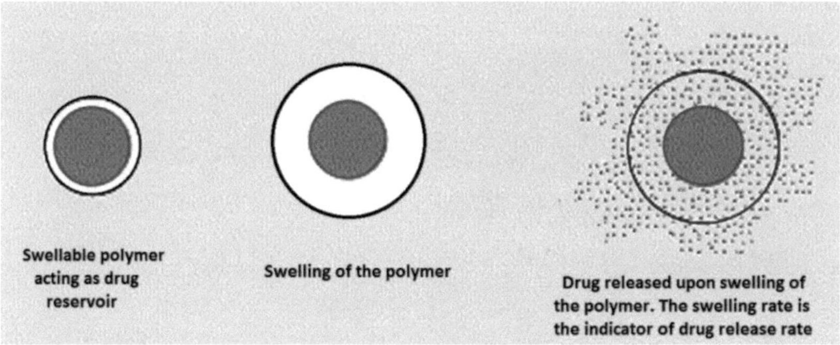

Figure 4. Analgesic delivery system by swelling of polymer acting as drug reservoir.

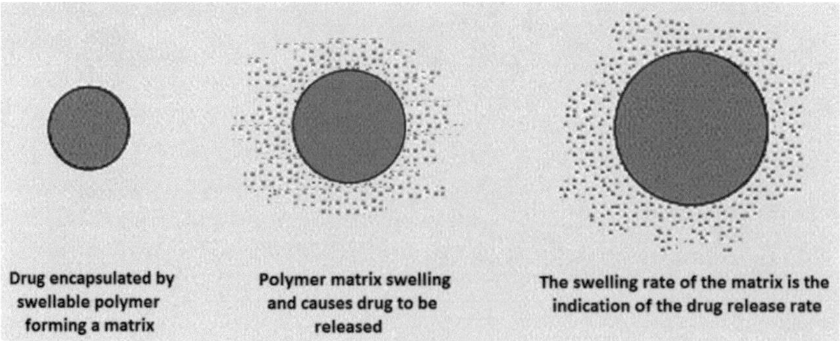

Figure 5. Analgesic delivery system by swelling of the polymer matrix encapsulating the drug.

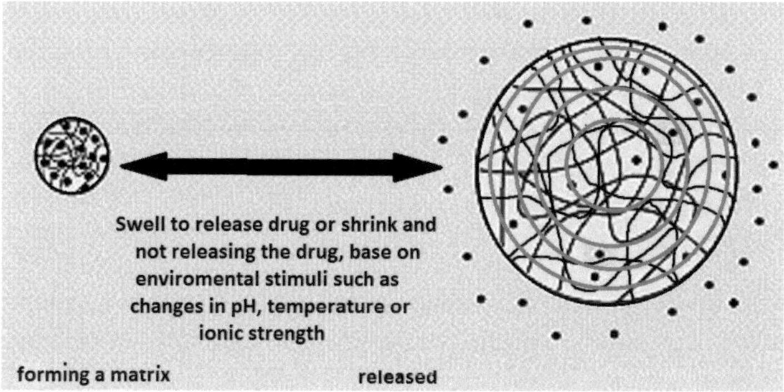

Figure 6. Drug delivery from environmental sensitive release system.

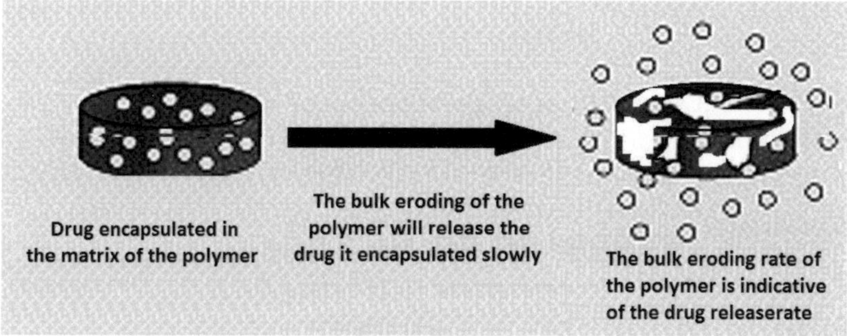

Figure 7. Bulk eroding biodegradable polymeric delivery system.

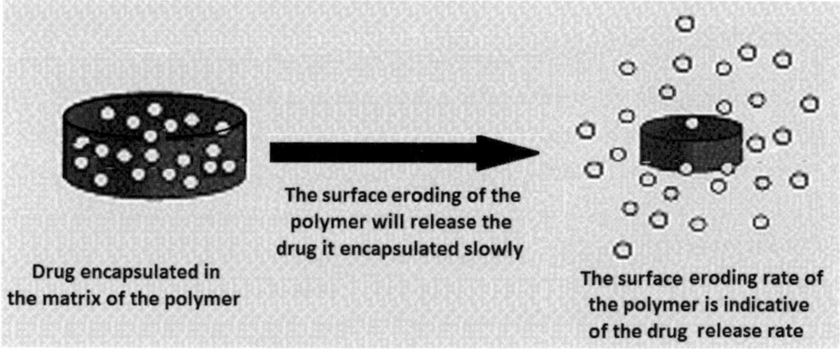

Figure 8. Surface eroding biodegradable polymeric delivery system.

6. Transdermal drug delivery

Transdermal delivery patch usually consists of a reservoir of drug on a protective backing layer, a rate-limiting release membrane, and an adhesive layer to attach the patch to the skin. The physicochemical of the drug suitable for transdermal delivery includes low molecular weight (<500 daltons), big molecules will have difficulty in penetrating the stratum corneum of the skin, high potency drug, water solubility (to facilitate movement of the drug out of the reservoir and to allow passage through the epidermal and dermal layers of the skin), and lipid solubility (to permit penetration of the stratum corneum of the skin). Fentanyl, a synthetic opioid agonist, is delivered by transdermal patch. For transdermal drug delivery, the penetration of the drug through the skin constitutes an additional series of diffusional and active transport steps [13].

The skin functions to maintain homeostasis of the body through temperature regulation, protection of underlying tissues, control water loss, rich sensory receptors, synthesizing of certain body chemicals, and excretion of wastes by sweating. The skin is made up of an outer epidermis and a dermis, followed by underlying tissue of subcutaneous layer (**Figure 9**). The epidermis is made up of stratified squamous epithelium and lacks blood vessels and it forms good barrier to protect the underlying tissue and blood capillaries. This becomes an important issue in the development of transdermal dosage forms so as to deliver the drug across the stratified layers [14].

Drug in the transdermal dosage form are generally poorly absorbed, but in the positive manner this will form a dosage form with a very controlled depot effect. It is an ideal dosage form for analgesics but the common problem is that the drug may cause focal irritation. Currently, in the market transdermal drug delivery for systemic effects is limited to very few drugs, those having low molecular weights and high lipophilicity. Transdermal drug delivery system may be optimized for controlled release of the drug for a steady plasma profile. This will reduced systemic side effects and may also improve efficacy of the analgesic drug. It is user-friendly, convenient, painless, and offer prolong dosing and all this will contribute to improved compliance [15]. Examples of such dosage forms available in the market are the morphine and sufentanil patches.

Normally, transdermal system in a patch form is made up of an outer covering which forms the barrier, a drug reservoir, a control membrane to control the release of the drug, a contact adhesive applied to some or all parts of the system to make it stick to the skin surface, and a covering protective layer that is removed before the patch is applied (**Figure 10a**). The drug reservoir is sometimes replaced with a matrix of polymer where the drug is encapsulated (**Figure 10b**).

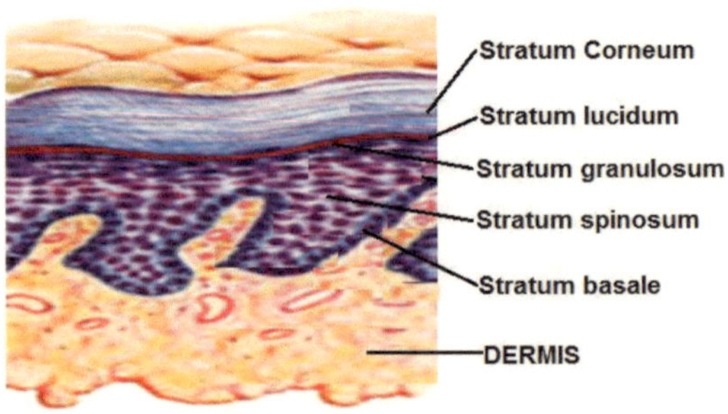

Figure 9. The barriers in epidermis which limit the penetration drug through the skin.

Researchers can be creative in the development of transdermal delivery system for analgesics. The followings are a few creative ideas on delivery of drug using various dermal patches with each having its own technique of engineering.

6.1. Iontophoresis

An active state of transdermal technologies uses low voltage electrical current to drive charged drugs through the skin. This will enable charged particles of drugs to move across the stratum corneum. Each iontophoresis patch is a device consisting of a housing which contains the battery and related electronics, two polymeric reservoirs for anode and cathode, and skin adhesive. Only one of the polymeric reservoirs contains the drug. The other may contain only pharmacologically inactive ingredients. **Figure 11** depicts the iontophoresis system. The choices on whether the anode or the cathode contains the drug are dependent on the drug charge.

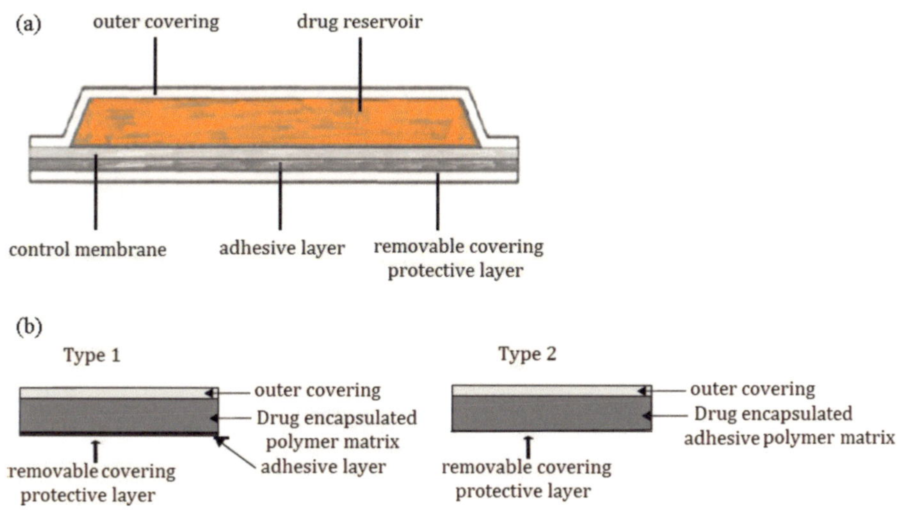

Figure 10. (a) The structure of a reservoir dermal patch. (b) Two types of structures for matrix dermal patch.

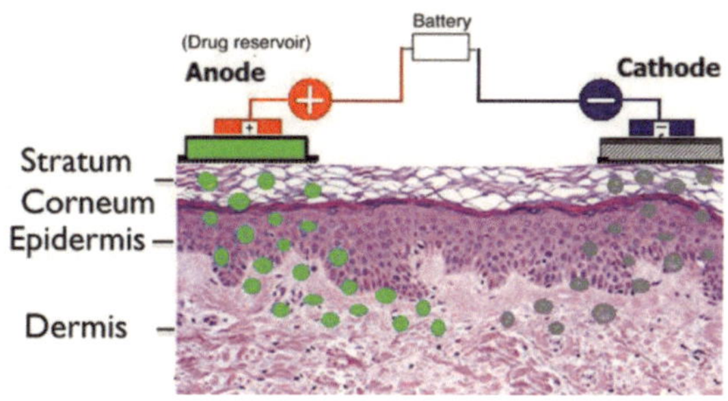

Figure 11. Iontophoresis patch illustration.

The technique of iontophoresis has the potential to be expanded to deliver proteins and peptides. The current can be literally switched on and off and modified, also iontophoretic delivery enables rapid onset and offset, and drug delivery is highly controllable and programmable.

6.2. Electroporation

This transdermal drug delivery technique uses short electrical pulses of high voltage to create transient aqueous pores in the skin, in a variety of forms, temporarily to disrupt the stratum corneum and to allow drug in the reservoir or the polymeric matrix to cross the stratum corneum and then penetrate the blood vessel (**Figure 12**).

6.3. Sonophoresis

This transdermal drug delivery technique uses low-frequency ultrasonic energy (15-second burst of ultrasound at 55 kHz) to disrupt the stratum corneum and to allow drug in the reservoir or the polymeric matrix to cross the stratum corneum and then penetrate the blood vessel. Similar to the electroporation effect, the sound waves create cavitation bubbles in the tissue that disrupt the lipid bilayers of the cells of the stratum corneum creating microchannels. The ultrasound poration can increase the transport properties of the stratum corneum by 100-fold. **Figure 13** illustrates the effect of sonophoresis.

6.4. Microneedle dermal patch

This transdermal patch technique makes use of microneedles, which are microscopic, just a few hundred microns in size. They can pierce the skin in a minimally invasive manner

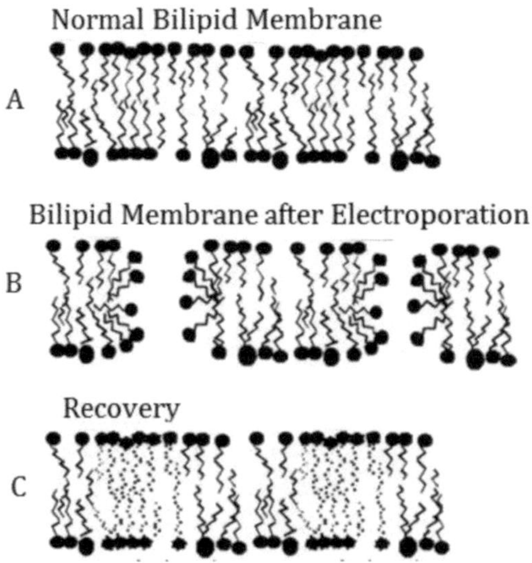

Figure 12. Temporary disruption of the bilipid membrane after electroporation. A: Normal arrangement of the bilipid membrane B: Bilipid membrane after electroporation C: Recovery of the Bilipid membrane after an interval.

without causing pain or injury [16]. A lot of research in the literature shows that this piercing effect increases transdermal flux of large molecular weight compounds by many folds. There are two ways of utilizing the microneedles, one of the ways in which drug delivery is achieved is to coat the drug onto microneedle shafts and insert them into the skin where they deposit the drug. The second way is upon piercing skin they create microconduits across stratum corneum and this will provide a direct route for transport of drugs into the skin from the patch reservoir (**Figure 14**).

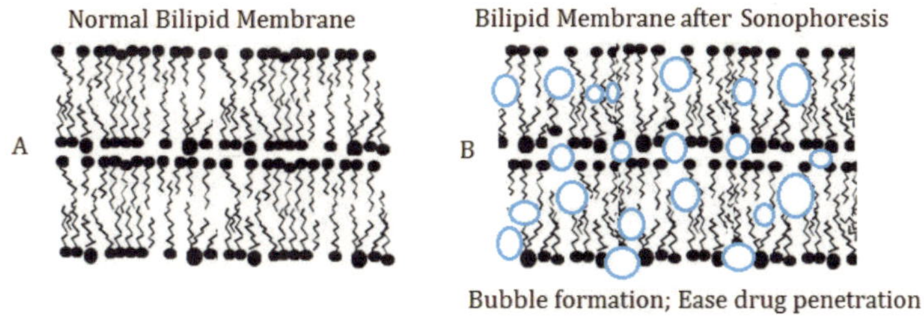

Figure 13. Bubble formation after sonoporesis process, forming channel for drug penetration. A: Normal arrangement of the bilipid membrane B: Formation of bubbles in Bilipid membrane after sonoporesis.

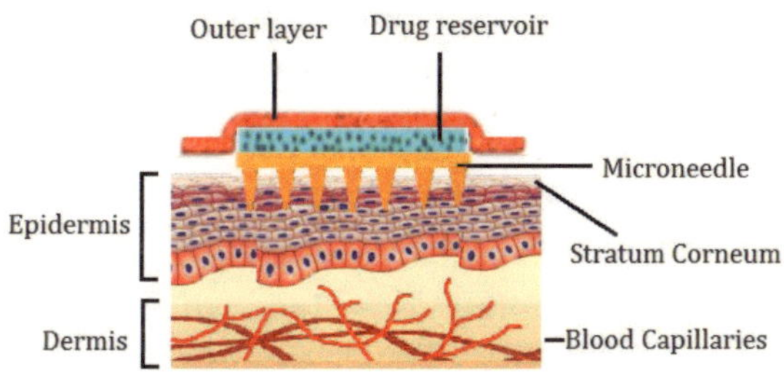

Figure 14. Illustration of microneedle transdermal patch with drug reservoir.

7. Nanoparticle delivery systems

Nanoparticle systems as drug carriers may also play a very important role in the delivery of analgesics. The advantages of nanoparticles used as drug carriers include fast action of the nano formulation, high product stability, good loading capacity, both hydrophilic and hydrophobic substances can be given together in the same formulation, and various routes of administration can be utilized [11]. Analgesics in nanoparticulate systems would be transported and released in a controlled manner at the target area, depending on the environmental conditions. Analgesic nanoparticulate can have the following advantages: reducing the dose of the drug, some specialty formulation may allow analgesic drugs that normally do not cross the blood brain barrier to penetrate into the brain where this can reduce the peripheral side effects by lowering the amount needed to act directly on the central nervous system. The development of the analgesic-loaded nanoparticulate systems may represent a future challenge to achieve promising agents for regional drug delivery in pain management strategy.

Nanoparticles can also be solid or soft colloidal matrix-like polymeric particles or lipids. They can be drug carrier system such as liposomes. Other drug delivery systems are based on using nanoparticles composed of biodegradable polymers, this has been explained in the earlier subsection on polymeric drug delivery system [17]. These microparticles may consist of polymeric nanospheres in an oily reservoir or aqueous medium. It was shown in research that a numbers of analgesic drugs such as ibuprofen, flurbiprofen, and acetyl salicylic acid have been successfully delivered by entrapping in nanoparticles [18].

8. Multiphase liposomal drug delivery system

Liposome is a drug delivery system suitable for various routes of drug administration, i.e., oral, rectal, parenteral, and particularly local administration to the skin, eye, and mucous membranes [19]. Liposomes are microscopic phospholipid-bilayered vesicles and they have the advantage in which they can be used to entrap both hydrophilic and lipophilic drug for delivery. **Figure 15** illustrates the formation of liposome for drug delivery. Liposomes are generally administered by intravenous route but they are also developed for transdermal or subcutaneous implantation.

8.1. The concept of LipoSpray

Using the liposomal concept "LipoSpray" is an innovative idea in delivering an analgesic in the form of liposomal suspension. The suspension is sprayed into the mouth and under the tongue. Liposomes penetrate the mucosal tissue of the mouth, and the drug is released from the liposome into the bloodstream, distributing the drug throughout the body in minutes.

This path bypasses the gastrointestinal (GI) track and bypasses the first-pass effect of the liver. The analgesic in question would have a fast effect in pain management.

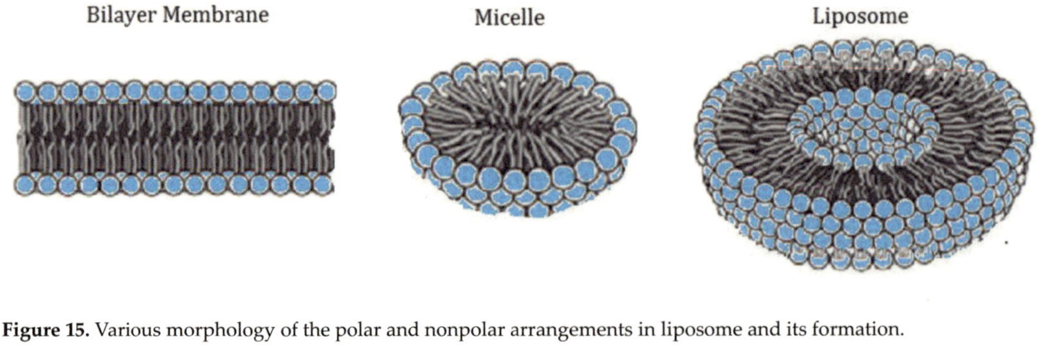

Figure 15. Various morphology of the polar and nonpolar arrangements in liposome and its formation.

9. Basic research methodology in development of new drug delivery systems in delivering analgesics

This subchapter illustrates an example of research steps in the development of a drug delivery system using nano technology. The steps illustrated in this section may be applicable to certain extent in research toward the development of an analgesic drug special delivery system. The techniques are not exhaustive and are just an example to guide the researchers.

9.1. Getting the delivery material (e.g., polymerization reaction to get the polymer)

At the beginning of the investigation, efforts should focus on the preparation of a polymeric system. There are two different types of polymerization reactions: addition polymerization and condensation polymerization. Addition polymerization involves the use of a radical generating initiator which triggers polymerization reaction of monomers. Condensation polymerization involves reaction of monomers containing reactive functional groups to form a polymer.

The FTIR and ^{1}HNMR spectra need to be used to confirm the formation of the desired polymer. Further attempts to synthesize larger amount of the polymer for characterization studies need to be done.

One important characterization is the determination of molecular weight. Gel permeation chromatography (GPC) can be used to analyze molecular weight of the polymer. A solution of 1 mg/1 ml of the polymer in tetrahydrofurane needs to be prepared and analyzed by GPC.

9.2. Determination of polymer stability

Another important criterion is to determine the *in vitro* degradation of the polymer so as to ensure its stability as required. The *in vitro* degradation study can be carried out through preparing polymeric devices and placing them in phosphate buffer solution for different periods of time, and analyzing their wet and dry weight loss [20].

Scanning electron micrographs of sample need to be taken by scanning electron microscope (SEM) to observe the erosion characteristics of the polymer. SEM is a technique for the preparation of high resolution images from surface of different compounds. Electrons are used for imaging in scanning electron microscopes.

The differential scanning calorimetry (DSC) is also a requirement in the determination of the thermal stability of the polymeric system [21].

9.3. Cytotoxicity issues

If the polymer being optimized is a new polymer then it is important to establish the cytotoxicity of the synthesized polymer to evaluate whether the polymer is appropriate for application in drug delivery systems or not. In other words, the synthesized polymer should be nontoxic to normal body cells and tissues, and cause minimum side effects at the site of action. There are different types of tests and assays for the evaluation of cytotoxicity of polymers, as well as drugs. Cell-based assays are the most widely used methods for assessing cell toxicity effects of different polymers or drugs on a particular cell line.

9.4. Preparation of drug-loaded polymeric system

Thin film hydration method can be one of the methods for the preparation of the drug-loaded polymeric system. An example is by using a solution of 2 mg/ml of polymer in ethanol (10 ml) and mixed with a solution of 5 mg/ml model drug in ethanol (1 ml). After stirring for 15 minutes at room temperature, the solvent needs to be evaporated by rotary evaporator. The precipitant is then mixed with 20 ml distilled water. The mixture is then centrifuged at 6000 rpm for 10 minutes. The supernatant is then taken for further analysis for entrapment characteristics of the drug in the polymer.

9.5. Determination of entrapment efficiency

In order to obtain the entrapment efficiency, the concentration of the free drug is to be determined upon preparation of the entrapment, 1 ml of the supernatant is taken and diluted with 3 ml water, and the concentration of the drug is determined by high performance liquid chromatography (HPLC). Entrapment efficiency is calculated by the following equation:

$$\mathrm{EE}(\%) = \frac{\text{total drug} - \text{free drug}}{\text{total drug}} \times 100 \quad (1)$$

9.6. Determination of polydispersity

The polydispersity index (PDI) is a reflection of the heterogeneity and a measure of the distribution of molecular mass in a given polymer sample. PDI is calculated as the weight average molecular weight, divided by the number of average molecular weight. It indicates the distribution of individual molecular masses in a batch of polymers. PDI value of 1 reflects that the polymer is of the same size and indicates uniformity of the chain length. The following equation denotes the PDI:

$$\mathrm{PDI} = M_{\mathrm{w}}/M_{\mathrm{n}} \quad (2)$$

where M_{w} is the weight average molecular weight and M_{n} is the number average molecular weight.

9.7. Determination of size, size distribution, and zeta potential of nanoparticles

Scanning electron microscopy (SEM) and dynamic light scattering (DLS) can be used to determine the size of nanoparticle. DLS is used for determining the size distribution and zeta potential of nanoparticles as well. Dynamic light scattering, which is also known as photon correlation spectroscopy, is one of the most widely used methods for the determination of size, size distribution, and zeta potential of nanoparticles. This instrument works through radiation of a light beam into a particulate system with Brownian motion.

9.8. Determination of the thermal characteristic of the delivery system

Differential scanning calorimetry (DSC) technique is the most common thermal analysis equipment used in the determination of material in the delivery system. This primary technique directly assesses the uptake of heat energy during the fluctuation of temperature in order to specify any connection among temperature and physical properties of samples. Calorimetry is a suitable thermal analysis technique for qualifying the purity, the melting point, and the polymorphic forms of samples [21].

9.9. *In vitro* drug release study

Drug release from the polymeric system shall be studied to prove good delivery as stipulated. Commonly, the *in vitro* dissolution of the drug from the formulation is done following the available compendium method where standard dissolution apparatus are recommended. Other methods include using dialysis method where the formulation prepared is placed in the dialysis bag. The dialysis bags are then placed in a bath shaker at the temperature of 37°C and rotated at the rate of 100 rpm. Samples were collected at different time intervals and analyzed.

9.10. *In vivo* animal study

This is one of the stages for preclinical study on the new formulation which can also be a new type of polymer or material used [19]. The safety and efficacy of this formulation need to be established. Before starting the study, the animal ethic committee needs to be consulted to get approval to start the study. Most of the studies are to prove that the pharmacokinetics of the drug delivered is appropriate as stipulated. The ADME (Absorption, Distribution, Metabolism, and Excretion) of the drug delivered by the system is important at this stage, especially the absorption and distribution.

For the technique in determining the absorption and the distribution of the active in a formulation, a researcher may in his or her study use optical *in vivo* imaging technique for monitoring the distribution of the drug in question the proposed delivery system in comparison with the conventional dosage form available. This technique is able to image the whole body of small animals and body cells. This technique includes both fluorescence *in vivo* imaging and fluorescence microscopy, and a low-light camera and proper filters were also used to collect fluorescence excitation and emission light from samples. In fluorescence microscopy, the objects of imaging are cells, slides, or culture dishes, while the whole body of small animals is pictured with optical *in vivo* imaging system. However, *in vivo* imaging is technically a more challenging process, as the animal tissues are opaque or/and thick, therefore, they absorb scatters photons and generate strong autofluorescence. Furthermore, it is essential to apply an appropriate imaging probe, which provides biologically stable distribution and preferential accumulation at the intended target site. Loading near-infrared (NIR) fluorophores with drug delivery agents would be a great opportunity to follow medicine distribution with optical *in vivo* imaging system without using specific conjugated antibodies. Near-infrared excitable fluorescent agents (NIR) provided deep tissue penetration and low tissue autofluorescence.

Researcher performing the animal study should also take the opportunity to do plasma level drug monitoring, urine metabolite level, and histological studies on heart, lungs, kidneys, spleen, and the liver.

9.11. The human bioavailability study

This is a regulatory requirement as to prove that the new system will make the drug available as the conventional system. It indirectly also determines if the drug pharmacokinetic parameters in human are the same as for the original available formulation. This is different from bioequivalence, which is used to evaluate the predictable *in vivo* biological equivalence of two proprietary preparations of a drug. Two pharmaceutical products are bioequivalent if they are pharmaceutically equivalent and their bioavailabilities after administration in the same dose are similar to such a degree that their effects, with respect to both efficacy and safety.

Bioavailability measures the extent of a drug reaching the systemic circulation and is therefore available for action at the expected site. For most drugs that are taken orally, the drug is released in the gastrointestinal (GI) tract and arrives at their site of action via the systemic circulation. Plasma concentrations of the drug or its metabolite would provide a marker for the concentration at the site of action and a valid measure of bioavailability. The researcher needs to build a plasma blood concentration time curve to prove the release of the drug from the preparation and its absorption from the GI tract, but also other factors including presystemic metabolism, distribution, and elimination. Bioavailability is proven through the area under the blood drug concentration versus time curve (AUC), the maximum blood concentration (C_{max}) and the time to reach maximum concentration (T_{max}). Clearly, bioavailability studies of the new delivery systems compared to the conventional ones need to be done so as to be assured that the new delivery system is not inferior compared to the existing systems.

10. Concluding statements

Drug delivery system represents a vast, vital area of research and development of new analgesic product. It is pertinent for analgesic as pain management needs the painkiller to be fast in action, prolong action, and reduce adverse or side effect. So development of specialty product using advance drug release system is the answer to the betterment of pain management and the research on this area is not exhaustive. In this chapter, we have discussed the available conventional dosage forms and gave examples. We also based our discussions on ideas in research and development of various advance new delivery system such as polymeric delivery system, sustain release system, transdermal delivery system, and liposome.

Author details

Mohamed Ibrahim Noordin

Address all correspondence to: ibrahimn@um.edu.my

1 Malaysian Institute of Pharmaceuticals and Nutraceuticals (IPharm), National Institutes of Biotechnology Malaysia, Ministry of Science, Technology and Innovation, Penang, Malaysia

2 Department of Pharmacy, University of Malaya, Kuala Lumpur, Malaysia

References

[1] Mark HB et al, editors. The Merck Manual of Medical Information. 2nd Home ed. Whitehouse Station, NJ: Merck; 2003

[2] Kehlet H. Postoperative pain. In: Wilmore DW, Brennan M, Harken A, et al, editors. Care of the Surgical Patient. New York: Scientific American Inc; 1988. pp. 121-133

[3] Ventafridda V, Stjernsward J. Pain control and the World Health Organization analgesic ladder. The Journal of America Medical Association. 1996;**275**(11):835-836

[4] Bansal SS, Joshi A, Bansal AK. New dosage formulations for targeted delivery of cyclo-oxygenase-2 inhibitors: Focus on use in the elderly. Drugs & Aging. 2007;**24**(6):441-451

[5] Khan MI, Walsh D, Brito-Dellan N. Opioid and adjuvant analgesics: Compared and contrasted. The America Journal of Hospice Palliative Care. 2011;**28**(5):378-383

[6] Jenkins CA, Bruera E. Nonsteroidal anti-inflammatory drugs as adjuvant analgesics in cancer patients. Palliative Medicine. 1999;**13**(3):183-196

[7] Hersh EV. New formulations of old analgesics. Clinical Therapeutics. 2015;**38**:424-425

[8] Marzo A, Dal Bo L, Verga F, Monti NC, Abbondati G, Tettamanti RA, Crivelli F, Uhr MR, Ismaili S. Pharmacokinetics of diclofenac after oral administration of its potassium salt in sachet and tablet formulations. Arznein-Forsch/Drug Research. 2000;**50**(1):43-47

[9] Kim T, Kim J, Kim S. Extended release formulation of morphine for subcutaneous administration. Cancer Chemotherapy and Pharmacology. 1993;**33**:187-190

[10] Lötsch J, Kettenmann B, Renner B, Drover D, Brune K, Geisslinger G, Kobal G. Population pharmacokinetics of fast release oral diclofenac in healthy volunteers: Relation to pharmacodynamics in an experimental pain model. Pharmaceutical Research. 2000;**17**(1):77-84

[11] D'Souza, S. A review of in vitro drug release test methods for nano-sized dosage forms. Advances in Pharmaceutics. 2014; Vol. **2014**:1–12

[12] Rowe, Raymond C; Sheskey, Paul J; Owen, Siân C; American Pharmacists Association.5th ed. / edited by Raymond C. Rowe, Paul J. Sheskey, Siân C. Owen. London ; Chicago: Washington, DC : Pharmaceutical Press ; American Pharmacists Association, 2006.

[13] Keleb E, Sharma RK, Mosa EB, Aljahwi AZ. Transdermal drug delivery system - design and evaluation. International Journal of Advances in Pharmaceutical Sciences. 2010;**1**:201-211

[14] Tortara GS, Grabowski SK. Principles of Anatomy and Physiology. 9th ed. New York, Chichester: Wiley; 2000. pp. 140-194

[15] Barry B. Transdermal drug delivery. Aulton ME (2002) 'Pharmaceutics' The Science of Dosage Form Design, 2nd ed., Churchill Livingstone, Spain, pp. 499-533

[16] Kumar JA, Pullakandam N, Prabu SL, Gopal V. Transdermal drug delivery system: An overview. International Journal of Pharmaceutical Sciences Review and Research. 2010;**3**(2):49-54

[17] Peniche C, Arguelles-Monal W, Peniche H. et al. Chitosan: An attractive biocompatible polymer for microencapsulation. Macromolecular Bioscience. 2003;**3**:511-520

[18] Gupta M, Majumdar DK. Effect of concentration, pH and preservatives on *in vitro* transcorneal permeation of ibuprofen and flurbiprofen from non-buffered aqueous drops. Indian Journal of Experimental Biology. 1997;**35**:844-849

[19] Smith LJ, Valenzuela JR, Krugner-Higby LA. et al. A single dose of liposome encapsulated hydromorphone provides extended analgesia in a rat model of neuropathic pain. Comparative Medicine. December, 2006;**56**(6):487-492

[20] Crompton TR. Polymer Reference Book. 1st ed. Smithers Rapra Publishing, USA; 2006

[21] Gill P, Moghadam TT, Ranjbar B. Differential scanning calorimetry techniques: Applications in biology and nanoscience. Journal of Biomolecular Techniques. 2010;**21**(4):167

Chapter 3

Pharmacotherapy of Chronic Pain

Marta Vázquez and Pietro Fagiolino

Additional information is available at the end of the chapter

http://dx.doi.org/10.5772/66444

Abstract

In the past two decades, many preclinical works have been carried out assisting in our understanding of the underlying pathophysiological mechanisms that cause chronic pain. Chronic pain involves multiple pathophysiological mechanisms with peripheral and central components. This research in basic and clinical research has greatly expanded the options for analgesic pharmacotherapy. This chapter gives information regarding the major classes of medication used to assist in the management of chronic pain, including nonopioids analgesics such as NSAIDs and acetaminophen, opioids analgesics, antidepressants and anticonvulsants and an emerging area as the field of cannabinoids is. Importantly, chronic pain treatment encompasses multiple agents to take advantage of synergistic mechanism of actions, but drug-drug interactions have to be taken into account in order to avoid lack of efficacy or toxicity.

Keywords: nonopioid and opioids analgesics, antidepressants, anticonvulsants, cannabis, interactions, chronic pain

1. Introduction

Chronic pain is one of the most prevalent and disabling conditions in the clinical setting with both physical and psychological symptoms [1]. In the past three decades, there has been a better understanding of the underlying pathophysiological mechanisms that cause chronic pain, yet it still remains a significant problem. Multiple levels of the nervous system with multiple neurotransmitters are involved in pain transmission. Therefore, it is not so easy to plan effective pharmacological therapy for chronic pain and pain treatment often involves the use of one or a combination of agents with analgesic action [2]. Chronic pain may be nociceptive or neuropathic. Nociceptive pain usually is treated with anti-inflammatory or analgesic medications. Neuropathic pain typically is treated with medications that influence neurotransmitters (e.g., antidepressants, antiepileptic drugs), and treatment with opioids is reserved for patients with refractory neuropathic pain. There are no truly effective medicines for certain types of pain; thus, a better understanding of the existing ones [opioids: methadone and tramadol; antidepressants: tricyclic antidepressants (TCAs), selective serotonin reuptake inhibitors (SSRIs), serotonin-noradrenalin reuptake inhibitors (SNRIs); anticonvulsants: gabapentin and pregabalin] or the search for new or perhaps the oldest form of medicine (cannabis) is needed.

The usual approach is to start with a nonopioid analgesic such as a nonsteroidal anti-inflammatory drug (NSAID) or acetaminophen for mild-to-moderate pain. If this is inadequate, the next step may be to add an antidepressant. If there is a component of neuropathic pain, then a trial of one of the anticonvulsant analgesic agents could be the option. If these steps are inadequate, then an opioid analgesic may be added. In an individual patient, one or several mechanisms may be at play in the etiology of the pain and more than one agent may be necessary for pain control; thus, it may be appropriate to use a combination of agents with different mechanisms of action in an effort to obtain adequate pain control [3].

This chapter focuses on pharmacotherapeutic options for patients with chronic, no cancer pain and possible drug-drug interactions that can result from a combined therapy.

2. NSAIDs and acetaminophen

Nonselective NSAIDs act inhibiting both the COX-1 and the COX-2 enzymes, leading this mechanism of action to both the therapeutic and toxic effects associated with their use. They are extensively prescribed to treat acute and chronically painful conditions. Complications with the use of these agents range from minor gastric complaints (nausea, abdominal pain, etc) to serious complications (gastric ulcers, bleeding, etc). These drugs inhibit platelet aggregation and increase bleeding time. The introduction of COX-2 selective NSAIDs in the market did not lead to a more effective and safer therapy, and cardiovascular complications associated with these agents culminated in the withdrawal of rofecoxib and valdecoxib from the market in 2004 [3, 4].

Both COX-2 selective and nonselective NSAIDs can also cause adverse renal outcomes in chronic use [3, 5]. So, risks associated with prolonged NSAIDs use must be addressed, as well as the benefits, on a patient-by-patient basis.

A weak acid drugs NSAIDs are, a plasma-gastrointestinal tract recirculation process through pancreatic/intestinal juices must be expected, although a systematic overview of the literature made no mention of this phenomenon. Due to the high concentration of sodium bicarbonate, pancreatic juice pH is above 8. This fact makes the transfer of an acidic drug from blood to the pancreatic lumen possible. Once in the duodenum, the accumulated drug in the pancreatic juice is available for reabsorption, resulting in a perceptible multiple peak plasma concentration-time profile. This phenomenon was evidenced by our group in a study carried out in healthy volunteers after ketoprofen administration [6]. In this work, no evidence of secondary peaks was obtained, probably because of the small amount of drug in blood, but once the reabsorption of ketoprofen took place, after the ingestion of food, significant R- to S-isomers conversion could be detected. This reveals the importance of drug recirculation at the duodenum level, contributing in some way to the duodenum irritation that arylacetic and arylpropionic acids produce.

Acetaminophen has antipyretic activity and peripheral anti-inflammatory effects but lacks antiplatelet effect. Although it is a weaker analgesic in comparison with NSAIDs, it can be considered as first-line option among nonopioids due to a more favorable safety profile [3]. The main concern is that of hepatic impairment at high doses. For chronic pain that is responsive to acetaminophen, daily doses should not exceed 4 g [3, 7]. Acetaminophen blood intestine recirculation was also observed in a study carried out by our group [8]. In this case, it was detected by simultaneous drug monitoring in saliva and plasma. The mechanism of this cycling was through biliary secretion of acetaminophen and its glucuronide metabolite.

3. Opioids

There has been a dramatic change in the way pain specialists view the use of opioid drugs for the management of chronic, no cancer pain. There is growing recognition that some patients can be provided opioid drugs for prolonged periods without evidence of tolerance and toxicity. Serious adverse effects are rare, and addiction is rare, particularly, if there is no history of chemical dependency.

3.1. Conventional opioids

The conventional opioids most commonly used for chronic pain management are morphine, oxycodone and codeine. These agents are all primarily μ-opioid receptor agonists. Opioid analgesia is mediated not only via its central effects but also via its peripheral action. For individuals with moderate-to-severe pain, a stronger opioid (such as morphine or oxycodone) should be chosen in the first place, and codeine is not recommended.

It is important to take into account that codeine depends on conversion to morphine for its analgesic effect. As O-demethylation of codeine to morphine is dependent on cytochrome CYP2D6 isoenzyme, which is known to exhibit genetic polymorphism, there is significant variation in the metabolism of codeine [9, 10]. Moreover, if another drug inhibits that isoenzyme, less formation of morphine will lead to a poor analgesic effect. This could be the case with some SSRIs such as fluoxetine.

Oxycodone undergoes N-demethylation to noroxycodone and O-demethylation to oxymorphone. CYP3A4 and CYP3A5 displayed the highest activity for oxycodone N-demethylation. CYP2D6 had the highest activity for O-demethylation. A high interindividual variability in the activity of these enzymes because of genetic polymorphisms and/or drug-drug interactions is well established and can cause insufficient pain relief or adverse effects [11].

3.2. Dual or multimechanism opioids

Methadone is a synthetic opioid with potent analgesic effects. Although it is commonly associated with treatment of opioid addiction, its unique pharmacokinetics and pharmacodynamics make it a valuable option in the management of chronic pain.

Methadone has various mechanisms of action. As well as acting through binding to μ and δ opioid receptors centrally and in the periphery, it also acts inhibiting serotonin and noradrenalin reuptake and as a noncompetitive N-methyl-D-aspartate (NMDA) receptor antagonist. These multiple action mechanisms give it advantages over other opioids. NMDA antagonism is also believed to attenuate tolerance [12–16]. These combined mechanisms are the cause of its efficacy in chronic and neuropathic pain [17].

The available methadone hydrochloride on the market is a racemic mixture of two stereoisomers: (R)- and (S)-methadone. Both enantiomers are responsible for its analgesic effect: the (R)-enantiomer exerting most of its opioid effect and acting as a NMDA antagonist and the (S)-methadone having NMDA receptor antagonism and inhibiting serotonin and noradrenalin reuptake [18–20].

Taken orally and at steady state methadone is subjected to first-pass effect. It has a variable bioavailability (41–95%) and 60–90% is bound to plasma proteins, mainly to alpha-1acid glycoprotein (AGP) due to its basic properties. AGP is one of the major acute phase proteins in humans, rats, mice and other species so its serum concentration increases in response to systemic tissue injury, inflammation or infection [21]. As pain and inflammation are nearly always associated with each other, a higher protein binding could be found in patients with chronic pain in comparison with healthy volunteers [22].

Methadone is extensively metabolized in the liver by the enzymes of the P450 cytochrome system (CYP3A4, CYP2B6, CYP2D6, CYP2C19 and other enzymes to a lesser extent) and in the gastrointestinal tract by CYP3A4. CYP3A4 content is much higher in the intestine than in the liver [23]. Methadone is also a substrate of P-glycoprotein (P-gp) [24], efflux transporter, which is expressed in several eliminating tissues (intestine, liver and kidneys) [25]. Due to the induction of its own metabolism (CYP3A4 and/or P-glycoprotein induction), reported by some authors, elimination half-life is longer after the first dose (36.7 h) [26] than during maintenance treatment [27, 28].

According to previous studies carried out by our group in other drugs [29], methadone must induce both CYP3A4 and P-glycoprotein for explaining the nonlinearity in drug response when daily dose is changed as it is shown in **Figure 1** with patients whose blood concentrations were analyzed in our therapeutic drug service.

Hence, a nonlinear relationship between steady state methadone plasma concentrations and methadone daily dose could be explained by induction of both the enzyme and the transporter, reducing its bioavailability and increasing its clearance. The hypothesis of efflux transporter induction is reinforced by the fact that patients treated chronically with methadone, developed higher saliva/plasma drug concentration ratio [30], probably due to the transporter overexpression at the luminal membrane of the acini cells and those surrounding the salivary ducts [31].

http://dx.doi.org/10.5772/66444

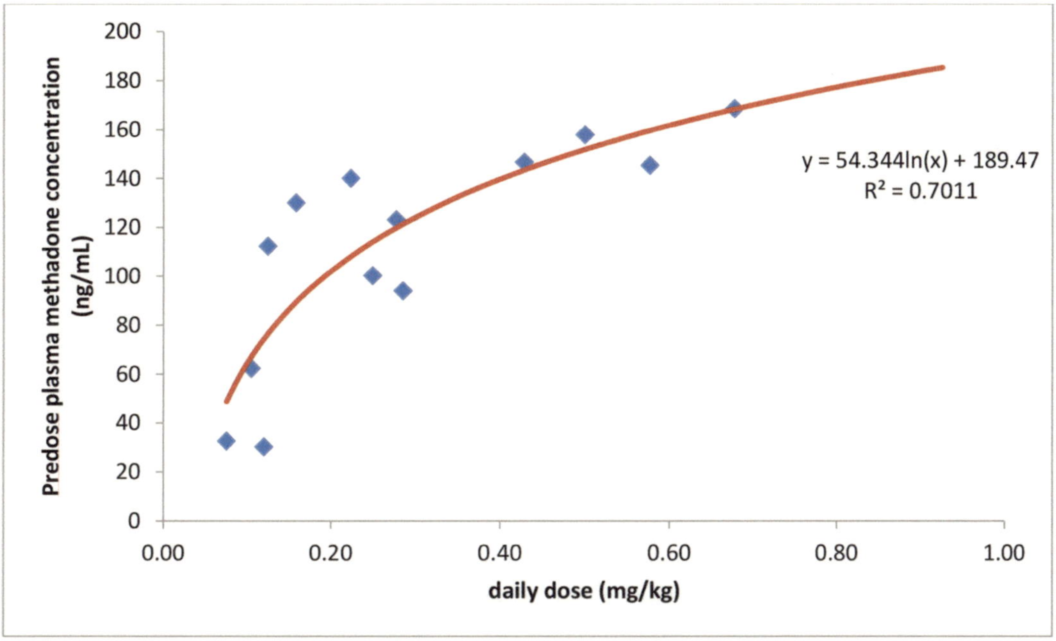

Figure 1. Predose plasma concentration of methadone (ng/mL) versus methadone daily dose (mg/kg).

Our research group has also identified methadone recirculation process via gastric secretion and intestinal reabsorption using saliva as biological fluid [32] as it can be observed in **Figure 2**.

A possible explanation for the appearance of these peaks is that, unlike NSAIDs, methadone is a basic drug and may be secreted into the stomach, to a greater extent once a meal was taken, and then reabsorbed from the intestine. Such secretions could be due to both the pH gradient between plasma (pH 7.4) and the gastric juice (pH 1.2), and the increased blood flow rate and gastric fraction of the cardiac output that takes place after food intake. The knowledge on methadone gastric secretion could have impact in the clinical setting in case of methadone intoxication. The administration of activated charcoal could be a solution as methadone reentries could be interrupted resulting in a more rapid drug elimination rate.

Tramadol has shown another mechanism of action other than acting as an agonist of μ receptors. Inhibition of noradrenalin (NA) and serotonin (5-HT) reuptake makes a significant contribution to the analgesic action of this drug by blocking nociceptive impulses at the spinal level. Tramadol is extensively metabolized in the liver and has one main major metabolite, O-desmethyltramadol. Both the parent drug and the metabolite drug contribute to the analgesic effect, but the metabolite has a significantly higher affinity for opioid receptors than tramadol [33]. CYP2D6 is responsible for the metabolite formation, and CYP2D6 gene is highly polymorphic so for poor metabolizers pain relief could be insufficient.

Serotonin syndrome is a potentially life-threatening syndrome that may occur with the use of tramadol or methadone, especially if other medications such as antidepressants or other

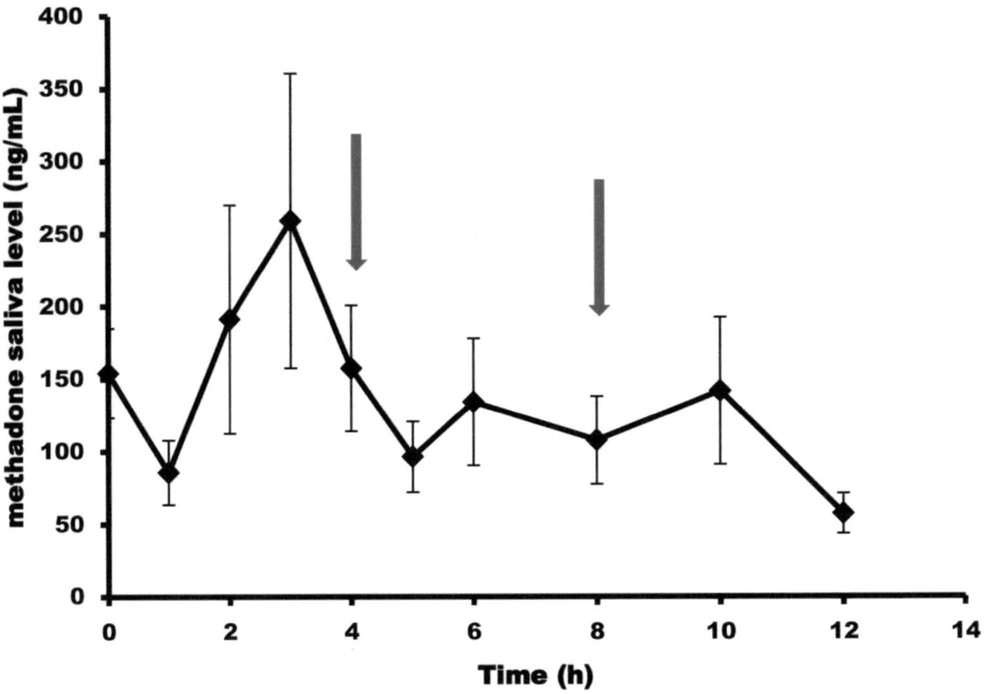

Figure 2. Mean saliva methadone concentration-time curve after administration of methadone dose with standard error in eight patients. The arrows represent meals intake.

drugs that impair the metabolism of these drugs (CYP2D6 and CYP3A4 inhibitors) are used concurrently. Symptoms include changes in mental status (e.g., agitation, hallucinations and coma), autonomic instability (e.g., tachycardia, labile blood pressure and hyperthermia), neuromuscular aberrations (e.g., hyperreflexia and incoordination) and/or gastrointestinal symptoms (e.g., nausea, vomiting and diarrhea).

During platelet activation, serotonin, along with other aggregating factors, becomes a stimulus for platelet aggregation. A transporter protein is necessary to transport serotonin into the platelet. Methadone, tramadol and SSRIs are antagonists of this transporter, and because platelets do not produce serotonin, they are dependent on plasma uptake of serotonin [34]. It is plausible that these drugs could increase bleeding risks as the blockade of the serotonin transporter could lead to a decreased concentration of serotonin within the platelet [35].

Inhibition of serotonin reuptake has been associated with the syndrome of inappropriate antidiuretic hormone secretion (SIADH) and hyponatremia [36]. SIADH is more likely in some populations, including people who are elderly or who take diuretics [37].

Lastly, both S- and R-form of methadone inhibit the cardiac potassium channel leading to prolonged action potentials that are expressed as long QT intervals resulting in potentially fatal polymorphic ventricular tachycardia: torsades de pointes (TdP). The risk of acquired QT prolongation and TdP is more pronounced in patients receiving more than one QT-prolonging drug simultaneously (e.g., escitalopram, citalopram, paroxetine, sertraline and venlafaxine) [38].

4. Antidepressants

4.1. Serotonin and noradrenalin reuptake inhibitors

TCAs exerting inhibition of 5-HT and NA reuptake, such as amitriptyline, appear to be effective analgesics. The pain relief from amitriptyline is generally moderate and is accompanied by side effects. TCAs block receptors of other neurotransmitters: histamine H1, muscarinic and nicotinic cholinergic and alpha-adrenergic. These actions explain certain side effects such as dry mouth, constipation, sedation, postural hypotension, etc [3]. For this reason, TCAs must be used with caution in patients with a history of cardiovascular disease, glaucoma, urinary retention and autonomic neuropathy, and with extreme caution in elderly patients.

Venlafaxine and duloxetine exhibit 5-HT and NA reuptake inhibition, but unlike amitriptyline and other TCAs, they lack significant affinity for muscarinic, histamine H1 and alpha-1 adrenergic receptors.

4.2. Selective serotonin reuptake inhibitors

The SSRIs are not so effective in treating pain. They can be considered as first-line agents when treatment of the depression is the priority, if TCAs are contraindicated or venlafaxine has failed. When using SSRIs, it is important to be aware of the metabolism in the liver by cytochrome P450 isoenzymes and potential interactions as most of them are enzymes inhibitors. Citalopram and escitalopram have the least impact on the cytochrome P450 isoenzymes [3, 39].

5. Anticonvulsants

Certain anticonvulsants exhibit analgesic action in neuropathic pain. This is on the basis of their ability to reduce neuronal excitability [40]. The most well-studied agents are gabapentin, pregabalin and carbamazepine; however, there is growing evidence that lamotrigine, topiramate and oxcarbazepine can act as analgesic too [40–42].

Gabapentin and pregabalin were originally developed as a structural analogue of gamma-aminobutyric acid (GABA), but do not actually bind to GABA or affect GABA reuptake or metabolism. They bind to the $\alpha 2$-δ subunit of voltage-dependent calcium channels and thus may modulate presynaptic release of excitatory neurotransmitters.

Carbamazepine remains the most successful first-line approach in treatment of trigeminal neuralgia [43, 44]. Its mechanism in stabilizing neuronal excitability is through sodium channel blockade.

Carbamazepine is extensively metabolized in the liver and the intestine by the isoenzyme CYP3A4 and is a substrate of multidrug resistance protein (MRP2) [45].

Like methadone, carbamazepine induces both CYP3A4 and P-glycoprotein explaining, in this way, the nonlinearity in drug response when daily dose is changed. This fact was confirmed by our studies [46].

6. Cannabis

Multiple lines of evidence support the important role of the endocannabinoid system in modulating pain and inflammation [47–54]. The potential value of the cannabinoids for medicinal purposes arose from the discovery of endogenous cannabinoid receptors: CB1 (mostly in the central nervous system) and CB2 (mostly in peripheral tissues) [55, 56]. The best-studied cannabinoids in *Cannabis* involved in having potential analgesic properties are tetrahydrocannabinol (THC) and cannabidiol (CBD).

CB1 is predominantly responsible for the psychoactive effects of THC, and the stimulation of this receptor plays a role in regulating pain, stress responses, energy regulation and lipogenesis, and immune function. CB2 is expressed on immune cells, so it is thought to serve an important role in immune function and inflammation. CBD, lacking psychoactivity compared to THC, agonist activity at CB2 receptors seems to account for its anti-inflammatory properties.

These cannabinoids are rapidly metabolized in the liver and intestine, undergoing extensive hepatic first-pass metabolism. Cannabinoids are distributed throughout the body; they are highly lipid-soluble and accumulate in fatty tissue. The release of cannabinoids from fatty tissue is responsible for their prolonged elimination half-lives [57, 58].

Precaution must be taken when CBD is used in conjunction with many other drugs due to its inhibition of several cytochrome P450 isoenzymes (CYP1A2, CYP2B6, CYP2C9, CYP2D6 and CYP3A4) and efflux transporters (P-glycoprotein). This is important in the management of chronic pain, since many conventionally used analgesics (opioids, SNRIs and SSRIs) are metabolized via these pathways (mainly CYP2D6 and CYP3A4) and/or are efflux transporters substrates [59, 60].

The growing number of preclinical studies and clinical trials with compounds that modulate the endocannabinoid system will probably result in novel therapeutic approaches in the treatment of pain for which current drugs do not fully address the patients' need.

7. Conclusions

The management of chronic pain requires an interdisciplinary approach. Only understanding pain perception and the knowledge of the multifactorial nature of pain could lead to individualizing analgesic therapy.

Author details

Marta Vázquez* and Pietro Fagiolino

*Address all correspondence to: mvazquez@fq.edu.uy

Pharmaceutical Sciences Department, Faculty of Chemistry, Universidad de la República, Montevideo, Uruguay

References

[1] Vos T, Flaxman AD, Naghavi M, et al. Years lived with disability (YLDs) for 1160 sequelae of 289 diseases and injuries 1990–2010: a systematic analysis for the Global Burden of Disease Study 2010. Lancet 2012;380:2163–96.

[2] Woolf CJ, Max MB. Mechanism based pain diagnosis: issues for analgesic drug development. Anesthesiology 2001;95:241–9.

[3] Lynch ME, Watson CPN. The pharmacotherapy of chronic pain: a review. Pain Res Manage 2006;11(1):11–38.

[4] Levesque LE, Brophy JM, Zhang B. The risk for myocardial infarction with cyclooxygenase-2 inhibitors: a population study in elderly adults. Ann Intern Med 2005;142:481–9.

[5] Galli G, Panzetta G. Do nonsteroidal antiinflammatory drugs and COX-2 selective inhibitors have different renal effects? J Nephrol 2002;15:480–8.

[6] Lorier M, Magallanes L, Ibarra M, Guevara N, Vázquez M, Fagiolino P. Stereoselective pharmacokinetics of ketoprofen after oral administration of modified-release formulations in Caucasian healthy subjects. Eur J Drug Metab Pharmacokinet 2015. doi:10.1007/s13318-015-0313-2.

[7] Jaeschke H. Acetaminophen: dose-dependent drug hepatotoxicity and acute liver failure in patients. Dig Dis 2015;33(4):464–71.

[8] Vázquez M, Fagiolino P, De Nucci G, Parrillo S, Piñeyro A. Post-prandial reabsorption of paracetamol. Eur J Drug Metab and Pharmacokinet 1993 (Special Issue: 177–83. Proceedings of the 5th. Eur. Cong. Biopharm. Pharmacokinet., Brussel (Belgium), 1993).

[9] Chen ZR, Somogyi AA, Bochner F. Polymorphic O-demethylation of codeine. Lancet 1988;2:914–5.

[10] Chen ZR, Somogyi AA, Reynolds G, Bochner F. Disposition and metabolism of codeine after single and chronic doses in one poor and seven extensive metabolizers. Br J Clin Pharmacol 1991;31:381–90.

[11] Lalovic B, Phillips B, Risler LL, Howald W, Shen DD. Quantitative contribution of CYP2D6 and CYP3A to oxycodone metabolism in human liver and intestinal microsomes. Drug Metab Dispos 2004;32(4):447–54.

[12] Ebert B, Thorkildsen C, Andersen S, Chritup LL, Hjeds H. Opioid analgesics as noncompetitive N-methyl-D-aspartate (NMDA) antagonists. Biochem Pharmacol 1998;56:553–9.

[13] Codd EE, Shank RP, Schupsky JJ, Raffa RB. Serotonin and norepinephrine uptake inhibiting activity of centrally acting analgesics: structural determinants and role in antinociception. J Pharmacol Exp Ther 1995;274:1263–70.

[14] Ripamonti C, Zecca E, Bruera E. An update on the clinical use of methadone for cancer pain. Pain 1997;70:109–15.

[15] Dickenson AH. NMDA receptor antagonists: interactions with opioids. Acta Anaesthesial Scand 1997;41:112–5.

[16] Mao J. NMDA and opioid receptors: their interactions in antinociception, tolerance and neuroplasticity. Brain Res Rev 1999;30:289–304.

[17] Gagnon B, Almahrezi A, Schreier G. Methadone in the treatment of neuropathic pain. Pain Res Manag 2003;8:149–54.

[18] Shimoyama N, Shimoyama M, Elliot KJ, Inturrisi CE. d-Methadone is antinociceptive in the rat formalin test. JPET 1997;283:648–65.

[19] Gorman AL, Elliot KJ, Inturrisi CE. The d-and l-isomers of methadone bind to the non-competitive site on the N-methyl-D-aspartate (NMDA) receptor in rat forebrain and spinal cord. Neurosci Lett 1993;223:5–8.

[20] Davis AM, Inturrisi CE.d-Methadone blocks morphine tolerance and N-methyl-D-aspartate-induced hyperalgesia. JPET 1999;289:1048–53.

[21] Fournier T, Medjoubi-N N, Porquet D. Alpha-1-acid glycoprotein. Biochim Biophys Acta 2000;1482(1–2):157–71.

[22] Belpaire FM, De Rick A, Dello C, Fraeyman N, Bogaert MG. Alpha 1-acid glycoprotein and serum binding of drugs in healthy and diseased dogs. J Vet Pharmacol Ther 1987;10(1):43–8.

[23] von Ritcher O, Burk O, Fromm MF, et al. Cytochrome P450 3A4 and P-glycoprotein expression in human small intestinal enterocytes and hepatocytes: a comparative analysis in paired tissue specimens. Clin Pharmacol Ther 2004;75:172–83.

[24] Crettol S, Digon P, Golay KP, Brawand M, Eap CB. In vitro P glycoprotein mediated transport of (R)-, (S)-, (R, S)-methadone, LAAM and their main metabolites. Pharmacology 2007;80:304–311.

[25] Couture L, Nash JA, Turgeon J. The ATP-binding cassette transporters and their implication in drug disposition: a special look at the heart. Pharmacol Rev 2006;58:244–58

[26] Vinson RK. Pharmacokinetics of a new immediate-release methadone tablet formulation with decreased in vitro solubility. Clin Drug Investig 2012;32:487–95.

[27] Lugo RA, Satterfield KL, Kern SE. Pharmacokinetics of methadone. J Pain Palliat Care Pharmacother 2005;19(4):13-24.

[28] Eap CB, Buclin T, Bauman P. Interindividual variability of the clinical pharmacokinetics of methadone: implication for the treatment of opioid dependence. Clin Pharmacokinet 2002;41:1153–93.

[29] Fagiolino P, Vázquez M, Eiraldi R, Maldonado C, Scaramelli A. Influence of Efflux transporters on drug metabolism. Theoretical approach for bioavailability and clearance prediction. Clin Pharmacokinet 2011;50(2):75–80.

[30] Bermejo AM, Lucas ACS, Tabernero MJ. Saliva/plasma ratio of methadone and EDDP. J Anal Toxicol 2000;24:70–1.

[31] Uematsu T, Yamaoka M, Doto R, Tanaka H, Matsuura T, Furusawa K. Expression of ATP-binding cassette transporter in human salivary ducts. Arch Oral Biol 2003;48(1):87–90.

[32] Vázquez M, Fagiolino P, Lorier M, Guevara N, Maldonado C, Ibarra M, Montes MJ, Retamoso I. Secondary-peak profile of methadone in saliva after administration of multiple doses in patients with chronic pain. Curr Top Pharmacol 2015;19:21–6.

[33] Gillen C, Haurand M, Kobelt DJ, Wnendt S. Affinity, potency and efficacy of tramadol and its metabolites at the cloned human mu-opioid receptor. Naunyn Schmiedebergs Arch Pharmacol 2000;362(2):116–21.

[34] de Abajo FJ. Effects of selective serotonin reuptake inhibitors on platelet function: mechanisms, clinical outcomes and implications for use in elderly patients. Drugs Aging 2011;28:345–67.

[35] Hougardy DM, Egberts TC, van der Graaf F, Brenninkmeijer VJ, Derijks LJ. Serotonin transporter polymorphism and bleeding time during SSRI therapy. Br J Clin Pharmacol 2008;65:761–6.

[36] Lane RM. SSRIs and hyponatraemia. Br J Clin Pract 1997;51:144–6.

[37] Rottmann CN. SSRIs and the syndrome of inappropriate antidiuretic hormone secretion. Am J Nurs 2007;107:51–58.

[38] Wiśniowska B, Tylutki Z, Wyszogrodzka G, Pola S. Drug-drug interactions and QT prolongation as a commonly assessed cardiac effect—comprehensive overview of clinical trials. BMC Pharmacol Toxicol 2016;17:12 doi:10.1186/s40360-016-0053-1

[39] Lynch ME. Antidepressants as analgesics. A review of random controlled trials examining analgesic effects of antidepressant agents. J Psychiatry Neurosci 2001;26:30–6.

[40] Chong MS, Libretto SE. The rationale and use of topiramate for treating neuropathic pain. Clin J Pain 2003;19:59–68.

[41] Finnerup NB, Sindrup SH, Bach FW, Johannesen IL, Jensen TS. Lamotrigine in spinal cord injury pain: a randomized controlled trial. Pain 2002;96:375–83.

[42] Guay DP. Oxcarbazepine, topiramate, zonisamide, and levetiracetam: potential use in neuropathic pain. Am J Geriatr Pharmacother 2003;1:18–37.

[43] Al-Quliti KW.Update on neuropathic pain treatment for trigeminal neuralgia. The pharmacological and surgical options. Neurosciences 2015;20(2):107–14.

[44] Watson CPN. Management issues of neuropathic trigeminal pain from a medical perspective. J Orofac Pain 2004;18:366–73.

[45] Geissmann T, May K, Modess C et al. Carbamazepine regulates intestinal P-glycoprotein and multidrug resistance protein MRP2 and influences disposition of tanilolol in humans. Clin Pharmacol Ther 2004;76:192–200.

[46] Maldonado C, Fagiolino P, Vázquez M, Eiraldi R, Alvariza S, Bentancour C, Alvarez P. Time-dependent and concentration efflux transporter. A preliminary assessment from salivary drug monitoring. Lat Am J Pharm 2011;30(5):908–12.

[47] Notcutt W, Price M, Miller R, et al. Initial experiences with medicinal extracts of cannabis for chronic pain: results from 34 "N of 1" studies. Anaesthesia 2004;59:440–52.

[48] Wade DT, Makela P, Robson P, et al. Do cannabis-based medicinal extracts have general or specific effects on symptoms in multiple sclerosis? A double-blind, randomized, placebo-controlled study on 160 patients. Mult Scler 2004;10:434–41.

[49] Svendsen KB, Jensen TS, Bach FW. Does the cannabinoid dronabinol reduce central pain in multiple sclerosis? Randomised double blind placebo controlled crossover trial. BMJ 2004;329:253.

[50] Zajicek JP, Sanders HP, Wright DE, et al. Cannabinoids in multiple sclerosis (CAMS) study: safety and efficacy data for 12 months follow up. J Neurol Neurosurg Psychiatry 2005;76:1664–9.

[51] Rog DJ, Nurmiko T, Friede T, et al. Randomized controlled trial of cannabis based medicine in central neuropathic pain due to multiple sclerosis. Neurology 2005;65:812–19.

[52] Holdcroft A, Maze M, Dore C, et al. A multicenter dose-escalation study of the analgesic and adverse effects of an oral cannabis extract (Cannador) for postoperative pain management. Anesthesiology 2006;104:1040–6.

[53] Desphande A. Efficacy and adverse effects of medical marijuana for chronic non cancer pain. Can Fam Physician 2015;61(8):e372–81.

[54] Petzke F, Enax-Krumova EK, Häuser W. Efficacy, tolerability and safety of cannabinoids for chronic neuropathic pain: a systematic review of randomized controlled studies. Schmerz 2016;30(1):62–88.

[55] Matsuda LA, Stephen JL, Micheal J, Young C, Bonner TI. Structure of a cannabinoid receptor and functional expression of the cloned cDNA. Nature 1990;346:561–4.

[56] Galiegue S, Mary S, Marchand J, et al. Expression of central and peripheral cannabinoid receptors in human immune tissues and leukocyte subpopulations. Eur J Biochem 1995;232:54–61.

[57] Cuhha JM, Carlini EA, Pereira AE. Chronic administration of cannabidiol to healthy volunteers and epileptic patients. Pharmacology 1980;21:175–8.

[58] Borgelt LM, Franson KL, Nussbaum AM, Wang GS. The pharmacologic and clinical effects of medical cannabis. Pharmacotherapy 2013;33:195–209.

http://dx.doi.org/10.5772/66444

[59] Yamaori S, Kushihara M, Yamamoto I, Watanabe K. Characterization of major phyto-cannabinoids, cannabidiol and cannabinol, as isoform-selective and potent inhibitors of human CYP1 enzymes. Biochem Pharmacol 2010;79:1691–8.

[60] Zhu HJ, Wang JS, Markowitz JS, Donovan JL et al. Characterization of P-glycoprotein inhibition by major cannabinoids from marijuana. JPET 2006;317(2):850–7.

Chapter 4

Patient-Controlled Analgesia (PCA) in Acute Pain: Pharmacological and Clinical Aspects

Marcos Tadeu Parron Fernandes,
Fernanda Bortolanza Hernandes,
Thaís Natália de Almeida, Vitor Pinheiro Sobottka,
Regina Célia Poli-Frederico and
Karen Barros Parron Fernandes

Additional information is available at the end of the chapter

http://dx.doi.org/10.5772/67299

Abstract

Moderate or severe pain are important sources of complications as well as morbidity and mortality in the postoperative period after surgical procedures. Patient-controlled analgesia (PCA) is an effective strategy for postoperative analgesia, since it may provide suitable analgesic dose just after system activation, with reduced periods of pain and an increase in patients' satisfaction. Although intravenous and epidural routes are the typical approaches used for PCA, regional patient-controlled analgesia has been shown to be an effective alternative providing a higher standard of analgesia with lower incidence of adverse effects. New devices and routes of PCA administration (transdermal, sublingual, inhalation, and oral routes) have shown to be promising alternatives in clinical studies. Nowadays, there is still no consensus regarding which is the best route or drug used since clinical efficacy/safety depends on the complex comprehension of the drugs pharmacokinetic profile through different routes of administration. Additionally, pharmacoeconomic studies are needed to evaluate the cost-effectiveness of these approaches.

Keywords: patient-controlled analgesia, opioids, acute pain, analgesic medication, morphine

1. Introduction

The International Association for Study of Pain defines pain as an unpleasant experience, with or without tissue damage, which can be related to individual memories, life expectations and emotions [1]. The painful experience involves interpretation of biological aspects of pain and its interaction with social and cultural characteristics [2].

In surgical procedures, moderate to severe pain can be observed in up to 40% of cases [3], representing an important source of complications as well as morbidity and mortality in the postoperative period [4]. Postoperative pain can limit mobility and respiratory function, increasing the incidence of atelectasis, pneumonia and thromboembolic events [5, 6].

Moreover, the lack of adequate pain control in acute situations can lead to chronic pain, with deleterious effects for the patient and health-related quality of life [7]. Despite these findings, between 50% to 75% of those submitted to major surgery do not receive enough analgesic medication, increasing the risk of complications and length of stay and costs for the health system [8].

Morphine was isolated by a German pharmacist Friedrich Wilhem Sertürner in 1806 and, after that, opioids have become widely used in clinical practice for pain control. Later in 1844, parenteral administration of morphine has started after the introduction of glass syringe [2].

In 1963, Roe demonstrated that administration of small doses of intravenous morphine allowed a better pain control compared to intramuscular injections [9]. Sechzer, in 1968, was the first to evaluate the quality of analgesia after administration of small doses of opioids *per* patient request, performing the first patient-controlled analgesia (PCA). Due to complex logistic to meet the requests of many patients, which would require numerous nursing staff, Sechzer and other doctors began to develop equipment prototypes for analgesic administration with reduced costs. The first PCA pump available for marketing was named "Cardiff Palliator" and it was developed in the Welsh National School of Medicine in 1973 [10, 11].

Since then, several drugs and routes of administration have been used in PCA, with differences in analgesic efficacy, tolerability profile, adverse effects, and procedure-related complications as well as patient satisfaction [12].

2. PCA: principles and pharmacological aspects

The principle of intravenous PCA was first described by Austin et al. in 1980, after he administrated small increasing doses of meperidine and measured the plasma levels, demonstrating the dose-related analgesic effect in patients [13].

Despite being associated with the idea of pump with intravenous opioids, there are several routes of administration, drugs, and equipment that can be used in this mode of analgesia. It is essential that, for the PCA recommendation, individual pain pattern and intensity be considered.

The patients must be previously and duly enlightened on the technical procedure and their consent should be obtained. As desirable characteristics of PCA, we can highlight the adequate pain relief according to individual requirements, the tolerance and safety profile of drugs administered, the high level of patients' satisfaction and minimal complications related to technological aspects [12].

In order to understand the effectiveness of PCA, we need to understand the concept of "minimal effective analgesic concentration (MEAC)." The MEAC is defined as the smallest concentration at which the pain is relieved [13].

Considering the existence of individuals' variability, the MEAC cannot be determined from the plasma levels of opioids. It is known that the plasma concentration is a function related to the dose, dosage intervals, gender and age of the patient. It can be calculated based on pharmacokinetic concepts such as volume of distribution and distribution and elimination rates. However, in clinical situations, the plasma levels are not able to predict the pattern of analgesic response [14]. Tamsen et al. showed that the MEAC has a direct correlation with preoperative concentrations of endogenous opioids and substance P in the cerebral spinal fluid. Obviously, the achievement of these measurements is restricted in clinical practice [15].

For the PCA effectiveness, the MEAC should be achieved by titration, which means that the drug is administered as a *bolus* of small doses until the establishment of an adequate analgesia pattern is obtained. Considering the acute postoperative pain, this can be done in the post-anesthetic recovery room, before patient discharge. From this reference dose, the equipment is regulated in order to maintain the plasma concentration of analgesic levels of MEAC or slightly above it, looking for adequate pain control with minimal adverse effects. The goal of this approach is to prevent the occurrence of sharp peaks and troughs in plasma concentrations in a standard that seeks the lowest level of oscillation of concentrations, ideally as close to a continuous infusion [16].

Regardless of the route or administered drug, the two main types of PCA are: the demand dosing (the fixed dose which is self-administered intermittently) and continuous infusion associated with demand dosing (the constant-rate fixed background infusion is supplemented by patient demand dosing), whereas the principles of a fixed infusion administration as well as principles of variation of the infusion rates managed by a period of time are considered [17].

Some basic principles and technical parameters are common to several modalities. They are initial loading dose, demand dose, interval lockout, and background infusion rate.

The initial dose usually is not administered by the patient, since the goal of first administration is to promote adequate pain control or prevent the early pain manifestation. This approach allows the establishment of the demand dose, also called PCA dose or *bolus* dose, which will be administered by the patient when he shoots the demand button.

The lockout interval is a set period in which the equipment does not perform a new infusion of demand. During the interval lockout, if the patient triggers the button, he/she will not receive the medication. Normally, the equipment has a sound signal connected to the drive, regardless of the infusion, so that the patient does not know whether his/her requests were effective. The lockout interval has the primary function of security by preventing the administration of an overdose of analgesic drugs. The background infusion rate is a given infusion rate in a continuous manner, independent of the patient's wish (also called continuous infusion). The

1-h and/or 4-h limits, depending on the equipment configuration, it has the function to limit the total cumulative dose in the period of 1 or 4 h in order to reduce the adverse effects and ensure the patient safety [11, 18].

Considering the advances in the development of drug delivery systems, the use of infusion pumps for patient-controlled analgesia (PCA) and analgesia epidural catheter with opioids are considered the most powerful strategies to control of postoperative pain. However, there are doubts about the advantages and limitations of these different forms of PCA.

The basal opioid administration doses may be administered concurrently with the administration of opioids by PCA techniques. However, the basal administration increases the risk of respiratory depression without providing necessarily an additional analgesia pattern [19].

PCA different modalities can minimize the occurrence of gaps in analgesic administration, supplying analgesic dosage immediately after the system activation, providing more uniform analgesia and eliminating painful waiting periods between the patient's request and drug administration.

3. PCA modalities

Electronic PCA pumps have several models in the market, including small portable devices nowadays. Since the first commercially available PCA pump ("Cardiff Palliator"), PCA devices have evolved enormously in technological sophistication, ease of use, flexibility and portability.

3.1. Intravenous PCA (IV-PCA)

Currently, IV-PCA is one of the most used techniques for acute pain control. Its use is suitable for virtually any patient undergoing surgery that are cursed with postoperative pain of moderate or severe intensity [18]. Many studies have demonstrated the efficacy, safety, and patient satisfaction with PCA intravenously. A meta-analysis involving 115 randomized clinical trials demonstrated that this technique provides greater efficacy when compared to intramuscular administration of analgesics [20]. Another study showed that, among patients who received IV-PCA, 36% experienced moderate to severe pain in the first 24 h after surgery when compared to 67% of important painful experience among patients who received intramuscular opioids [21]. Moreover, it was verified that the IV-PCA is associated with a higher rate of patient satisfaction [22].

Despite the possibility that IV-PCA may be combined to a basal opioids infusion, it was shown that the incidence of respiratory depression with IV-PCA was much smaller (0.19% versus 0.29%) when compared to the combination of this technique with systemic infusion of opioids (1.09–3% versus 8%) [23].

IV-PCA is associated with potential complications inherent in the technique, which are operator-dependent. Errors may occur in the drug administration, usually by programming failures on infusion pump [24] and they may result in inadequate pain control, heavy sedation, respiratory depression, and, eventually, death of the patient [25]. Currently, many infusion pumps feature smart devices that are equipped with an integrated software library on dosing regimens of different drugs, thus avoiding underdosing or overdosing. In these models, the smart bombs are programmed to stop operation or to alert clinicians when doses exceed the limits [26].

However, serious errors can still occur even with smart bombs. According to the Food and Drug Administration (FDA), 56,000 adverse events with these smart bombs during the period 2005–2009 have been reported [27].

Several complications may be observed from the IV-PCA, such as clogging or dislodgement of catheters, intervals between the administrations of opiates for maintenance of analgesic effect [28]. Still, this technique implies in risk for adverse effects related to opioids [29].

Furthermore, IV-PCA limits mobility and it reduces the comfort of the patient who is connected to the infusion pump, which can be minimized by using more modern compact equipment. Zafar et al. [30] reported that about 21% of patients who received IV-PCA complained of reduced mobility. It is worth noting, finally, the economic aspect, as a limitation of the technique, as well as the need of equipment (infusion pump) and the discarding of remaining solutions after the PCA use, causing unnecessary costs for health services [12, 30].

The major drugs used in this system are the opioid analgesics, such as morphine, hydromorphone, fentanyl, sufentanil and tramadol [31]. Meperidine is no longer considered a valid option for PCA as its toxic metabolite may be accumulated, especially in patients with abnormal kidney function [32]. Therefore, meperidine has not been recommended for acute pain [33].

3.1.1. Morphine

Morphine is the most common opioid used for IV-PCA and it is considered the gold standard for this procedure. Although many studies have demonstrated its clinical safety, adverse effects such as nausea, vomiting, itching, urinary retention, sedation and respiratory depression may occur. Its active metabolite morphine-6-glucuronide (M6G) have analgesic action but presents risk of adverse effects. As the M6G has renal elimination, the use of morphine should be done with caution in patients with impaired renal function and the elderly [34, 35]. The low therapeutic index of morphine in IV-PCA was shown in preclinical models, indicating that morphine cannot be the best option for all patients for pain relief in the postoperative period [31].

The usual morphine dose and the recommended parameters are: demand dose: 1–2 mg; lockout period: 6–10 min; continuous basal infusion dose: 0–2 mg/h [11].

3.1.2. Hydromorphone

Hydromorphone has been used in patients with impaired renal function or with a history of allergy to morphine. It is mainly metabolized by the liver and it is, approximately, five times more potent than morphine. Clinical effects of hydromorphone are dose-dependent and its adverse event profile is morphine-like [11, 36]. A systematic review of adverse events associated with the postoperatory use of six different opioids (buprenorphine, fentanyl, hydromorphone, meperidine, morphine, and sufentanil) showed that after meperidine (proscribed, 67.9%), the opioid with the highest incidence of central nervous system side effects was hydromorphone (42.7%). Furthermore, at higher doses, hydromorphone can cause excitation [37].

Due to the similarity between morphine and hydromorphone, errors have been reported in programming the IV-PCA pump. Considering that these agents have significant differences in their clinical potency, inadvertent hydromorphone administration can result in serious complications [38].

Doses and recommended parameters are: demand dose: 0.2–0.4 mg; lockout period: 6–10 min; continuous basal infusion dose: 0–0.4 mg/h [11].

3.1.3. *Fentanyl*

Fentanyl is 80–100 times more potent than morphine and it may cause less respiratory depression when compared with morphine. It has no active metabolites, and it has a wider therapeutic index than morphine in preclinical models [39].

In a retrospective cohort study of 8955 patients who received one of the three opioids for postoperative pain (morphine, fentanyl or meperidine), the incidence of respiratory depression was 0.6% in the group of patients who received fentanyl, compared to 2.8% among patients who received morphine [40]. Although apparently it may be associated with smaller risk of respiratory depression when compared to morphine, fentanyl can be associated with more device programming errors, since this drug is dosed in micrograms [40, 41].

Because of its high lipid solubility, fentanyl has a pharmacokinetic profile characterized by a rapid onset and short action. Therefore, some patients may need doses too frequently or require a basal infusion rate, which greatly increases the risk of respiratory depression. Due to its high volume of distribution, prolonged administration may result in a significant increase in drug half-life, with consequent raise in the incidence of adverse effects [42]. Given these pharmacokinetic characteristics, there are complaint reports of patients after fentanyl administration in IV-PCA [43].

Doses and recommended parameters: demand dose: 20–50 μg; lockout: 5–10 min; Basal continuous: 0–60 μg/h [11].

3.1.4. *Sufentanil*

Sufentanil is a fentanyl analog, being about 5–10 times more potent than Fentanyl itself. It represents the opioid with greater therapeutic index (25,000) used for postoperative pain in preclinical studies [39]. The high therapeutic index is clinically relevant for evoking a decreased risk of incidence of respiratory depression compared to morphine, fentanyl, and alfentanil [44]. In a randomized clinical trial with 30 volunteers, it was noted that sufentanil provided more effective analgesia and less respiratory depression when compared with fentanyl [44].

Sufentanil is highly lipophilic (twice more lipophilic than fentanyl) and it provides rapid onset of action and shorter effect duration when administered intravenously to PCA, justifying its rare use in this route. However, unlike fentanyl, its half-life of elimination does not increase with infusion time and it shows paradoxical increase in their concentration during the elimination phase [39]. A randomized clinical trial that compared plasma levels of sufentanil and fentanyl in 41 patients undergoing coronary artery bypass surgery, demonstrated the occurrence of peak plasma concentration (increase of 29–49%) from 4 to 15 h after administration *bolus* of fentanyl. On the other hand, only one patient had sufentanil treated with this paradoxical effect (43% increase). This peak in plasma concentration explains the occurrence of late respiratory depression in patients treated with fentanyl [45]. Therefore, considering their high therapeutic index and predictable pharmacokinetic profile, sufentanil represents a promising example of opioid that could be used to PCA cases requiring short duration of effect and availability intravenously.

The doses and the usual parameters are: demand dose: 4–6 μg; lockout: 5–10 min; continuous baseline: 0–8 μg/h [11].

3.1.5. Tramadol

Tramadol acts on opioid receptors with higher affinity for κ receptors than δ and μ receptors. It has an active metabolite, mono-O-desmethyl (M1), which has analgesic effect. In addition to the opioid agonist activity, tramadol analgesia is also promoted by inhibiting the central norepinephrine and serotonin reuptake. Tramadol potency compared to morphine is approximately 0.1. Several studies have shown that tramadol is a safe and an effective option for PCA, but with a higher incidence of nausea and vomiting [46, 47]. The recommended doses are: demand dose: 10–20 mg; lockout: 6–10 min; continuous baseline: 0–20 mg/h [11].

3.1.6. Oxycodone

Oxycodone is an opioid μ receptor agonist indicated for the treatment of moderate to severe pain. Despite being most frequently used orally, in recent years, its intravenous use has increased. Its potency is about 1/75 of fentanyl, and in some studies has shown great potency up to 1/60 [48, 49].

A randomized clinical trial with 82 patients compared IV-PCA with oxycodone and fentanyl. In this study, oxycodone demonstrated potency of 1/55 of fentanyl for the same levels of analgesia, being equally safe and the same incidence of adverse effects such as nausea, vomiting and sedation [45]. It is a drug with good efficacy and a promising role in the practice of PCA. Its use must be made on demand associated with basal infusion. The recommended doses are: demand bolus: 1 mg; lockout: 15 min; background infusion rate: 1 mg/h [50].

3.1.7. Other drugs

Other opioids have been less used in IV-PCA. The alfentanil, probably due to their pharmacokinetic characteristics, did not show good results and a demand dose was not established to present a satisfactory analgesia [51]. The remifentanil, because of their ultrashort half-life, does not have a favorable profile for PCA with some indication for analgesia for a short period such as during labor [52].

Other drugs have been used by some authors that are normally associated with morphine. Ketamine, which is an agonist of the NMDA receptor, and naloxone, which is an antagonist of opioid receptors, have shown conflicting results regarding the safety or quality of analgesia, and more studies are needed so that they can get their recommended use [18].

3.2. Epidural PCA

Epidural patient-controlled analgesia (EPCA) is the second most significant method used and studied within the PCA approach. Its use is mainly for control of acute postoperative pain, commonly in patients undergoing orthopedic, abdominal and thoracic surgery [12]. EPCA allows the use of opioids, local anesthetics, or a combination of both. Opioids epidural administered provide greater analgesic potency when compared to equivalent doses of opioid administered intravenously [53].

Although both opioids and local anesthetics represent feasible options, local anesthetics are the most appropriate strategies for patients sensitive to the opioids adverse effects, even though it is associated with a higher incidence of hypotension, motor block and urinary retention compared with the use of opioids [53]. Similarly to the PCA intravenous technique, EPCA allows patients to administer the medication in accordance with analgesic requirements. There is large evidence indicating that the EPCA represents a safe and effective method [46, 54]. A meta-analysis concluded that, regardless of the drug chosen, epidural provides a better analgesia pattern when compared to intravenous PCA technique [55].

In a population-based study of 2276 surgical patients, Kim et al. [56] discloses that ropivacaine with fentanyl was able to provide good quality analgesia for up to 48 h after the several surgical procedures, with limited side effects [56].

Unlike IV-PCA, the use of continuous infusion, coupled with the demand dose, have shown excellent results with minimal complications. Small doses of local anesthetics of long action combined with low doses of opioids (i.e., fentanyl or sufentanil) with continuous infusion rate associated with increments *bolus* may be combined [57, 58]. The following concentrations are recommended: bupivacaine: 0.05–0.125%; levobupivacaine: 0.05–0.125%; ropivacaine: 0.1–0.2%. Additionally, the following doses are recommended: demand dose: 2–4 ml; lockout: 10–20 min; continuous basal infusion: 4–10 ml/h [11].

Despite many advantages, EPCA also has limitations, especially considering the complexity of the procedure and technical staff training. In addition, there are reports of catheter migration which may lead to failure in the procedure in 17% of cases. It has been suggested that this technique has great effectiveness but it should be used with caution considering individual factors, in order to ensure patient safety [56].

3.3. Patient-controlled regional analgesia

There are several techniques that use catheters for the purpose of providing postoperative analgesia with little or no opioid use. In this model of patient-controlled regional analgesia, local anesthetics (ropivacaine, bupivacaine or levobupivacaine) are normally administered through a catheter located in perineural site, intraarticular region or surgical incision site. Eventually, a combination of local anesthetics and opioids can be administered by the infusion pump [12].

Several studies have addressed the effectiveness of this method for postoperative analgesia [59]. Vintar et al. [60] noted that about 80% of patients who received bupivacaine and ropivacaine at the incision site were satisfied with the outcome of the procedure and said they would use this treatment again.

Studies emphasizing the intraarticular administration of opioids and/or local anesthetics are rare. Vintar et al. [60], in a controlled clinical trial, describes that the group which received the combination of ropivacaine/morphine/ketorolac required less use of rescue analgesics in relation to other groups.

It is estimated that, during orthopedic surgery, drug administration by intraarticular can provide 12–15 h of analgesia [61]. In this context, the most efficient strategy would be the infusion of local anesthetics via epidural. Additionally, the brachial plexus, lumbar plexus and femoral nerve and sciatic nerve are examples of sites for drugs infusion. In a clinical trial, the PCRA ropivacaine 0.2% in the brachial plexus region was effective in shoulder orthopedic surgery regarding pain intensity, opioids' use as rescue medication, and less sleep disorders [61].

In a multicenter study involving orthopedic surgeries, the perineural ropivacaine administration by continuous infusion or PCRA was compared to intravenous morphine. Patients receiving morphine showed higher levels of postoperative pain and required higher consumption of analgesic as rescue medication, significantly increasing the side effects such as nausea, vomiting, dizziness and sleep disturbances [62].

3.4. Other modalities of patient-controlled analgesia

3.4.1. Transdermal

The iontophoretic fentanyl system (IONSYS; Ortho-McNeil, Raritan, NJ, USA) is a preprogrammed noninvasive method of PCA, which does not require venous access for drug administration. By adhesively secured to the outside of the arm or chest of the patient, fentanyl is transferred iontophoretically through intact skin. The system allows the transdermal administration of the drug for 10 min and a 10 min lockout interval between administrations [39].

However, the fentanyl dose administered over time is not constant. Whereas the target dose for the desired effect of fentanyl is 40 µg, it is estimated that the average dose is 16 µg after the initial application. Therefore, it would take a long period of time until the optimal dose is reached. Many patients do not receive adequate analgesia for up to 10 h after the start of the application [39].

Although clinical studies have suggested that the use of transdermal fentanyl could show similar efficacy to morphine in PCA intravenously in relation to the overall control of pain [12], there was a need for additional analgesia in 40% of patients involved in the first 3 h of treatment. Moreover, there were local side effects such as skin redness in about 60% of cases. This system was not marketed in the U.S. and it was withdrawn from the European market by the manufacturer due to a manufacturing error in some units [38].

3.4.2. *Sublingual*

A new sublingual administration system using sufentanil (AcelRx Pharmaceuticals, Redwood City, CA, USA) is designed as a microtablet coupled to a preprogrammed portable device with locking features and radio frequency identification to enable the characterization of a single user. Although intravenous sufentanil present a short half-life context-dependent due to its rapid redistribution, pharmacokinetic studies in healthy subjects showed that after sublingual administration, sufentanil has adequate profile for the postoperative analgesia [39].

Sufentanil NanoTabs® shows high bioavailability and plasma half-life and it is safer than the administration of the drug intravenously to avoid the need for frequent administrations of the lipophilic opioids commonly used for this procedure. Several clinical trials have demonstrated its efficacy in pain relief in different types of orthopedic and abdominal surgery, having been described few side effects to this method [38].

3.4.3. *Inhalation*

Several products using the inhalation of PCA to opioid administration are described in the literature. Thipphawong et al. [63] tested a morphine inhalation system (System AERx Pain Management; Aradigma Corporation, Hayward, CA, USA), which had desirable characteristics of a drug for PCA (possibility of multiple dosing with lock time between them and observed similar efficacy to morphine IV-PCA).

Similarly, fentanyl (AeroLEF, YM Biosciences, Mississauga, ON, Canada) also had proven to control postoperative pain following orthopedic surgery. However, further studies are needed to confirm the effectiveness of opioids in this route, especially clinical trials phase III and IV.

3.4.4. *Intranasal*

The intranasal opioid administration is possible, since the nasal mucosa has an extensive vascularization, providing rapid drug absorption and distribution [12].

The presentation of intranasal morphine (Rylomine®, Javelin Pharmaceuticals Inc., Cambridge, MA, USA) was effective for the control of postoperative pain in orthopedic surgery [64]. However, the single dose after a nasal administration does not have the desirable safety features of PCA models, such as the possibility of multiple dosages and lock scheduled time between applications. Other opioids have been tested for intranasal administration but similar to morphine, these devices also did not have the desirable features of a PCA device. In this context, Toussaint et al. [65] noted that intranasal fentanyl administration showed similar efficacy compared to IV-PCA fentanyl. Intranasal sufentanil was also successfully used both in adults and pediatric patients [64].

However, this route may have local adverse effects: nasal irritation, nasal congestion, upper respiratory tract infections, sinusitis, rhinitis, pharyngitis, or epistaxis, which may be a limitation of its clinical use [66].

http://dx.doi.org/10.5772/67299

3.4.5. Oral

Oral PCA device (Avancen, Mount Pleasant, SC, USA) is a drug unit coupled to a bracelet programmed to keep out of the drug for a predetermined time interval. After this lockout period, a green light indicates the possibility of new management. The equipment is compact and allows the patient to make the registration of pain on a scale of 0–10, providing feedback to the health team.

In a study of this device with hydromorphone administration, oxycodone and morphine, it was reported better control of pain in 95% of patients who used these devices when compared to the control group. Furthermore, it highlighted the ease of programming of this device by the health team [38].

Although this oral device for PCA is a good alternative, there are few studies regarding its safety. It is noteworthy of some shortcomings: lack of clinical efficacy in cases of moderate to severe pain, management failure in patients in whom oral administration is not available and uncertain absorption in the immediate postoperative period.

4. Conclusion

Patient-controlled analgesia (PCA) is a great option for acute pain control. Several advantages of this technique can be highlighted, such as higher analgesic standard with patient's satisfaction, and also minor side effects. However, there is still no consensus regarding which is the best route or drug used since clinical efficacy/safety depends on the complex comprehension of the pharmacokinetic drugs profile through different routes of administration. Additionally, pharmacoeconomic studies are needed to evaluate the cost-effectiveness of these approaches.

Author details

Marcos Tadeu Parron Fernandes[1,2], Fernanda Bortolanza Hernandes[3], Thaís Natália de Almeida[3], Vitor Pinheiro Sobottka[2], Regina Célia Poli-Frederico[4] and Karen Barros Parron Fernandes[4, 5]*

*Address all correspondence to: karenparron@gmail.com

1 Department of Anesthesiology, Irmandade da Santa Casa de Londrina Hospital (ISCAL), Londrina-PR, Brazil

2 Associate Professor, Department of Anesthesiology and Surgery, School of Medicine, Pontifical Catholic University of Parana (PUCPR), Londrina-PR, Brazil

3 School of Medicine, Pontifical Catholic University of Parana (PUCPR), Londrina-PR, Brazil

4 Associate Professor, Doctoral Program of Rehabilitation Sciences, University of Northern Parana (UNOPAR), Londrina-PR, Brazil

5 Institute of Education, Research and Innovation, Irmandade da Santa Casa de Londrina (ISCAL), Londrina-PR, Brazil

References

[1] Loeser JD, Treede RD. The Kyoto protocol of IASP Basic Pain Terminology. Pain 2008;137:473–77.

[2] Kopf A, Patel NB, editors. Guide for Pain Management in Low-Resources Settings. 1st ed. United States: International Association for the Study of Pain – IASP Press; 2010.

[3] Power I. Recent advances in postoperative pain therapy. Br J Anaesth 2005;95(1):43–51.

[4] Mueller XM, Tinguely F, Tevaearai HT, et al. Pain location, distribution and intensity after cardiac surgery. Chest 2000;118(2):391–6.

[5] Johnson D, Kelm C, Thomson D, et al. The effect of physical therapy on respiratory complications following cardiac valve surgery. Chest 1996;109(3):638–44.

[6] Ulke ZS, Senturk M. Non-analgesic effects of thoracic epidural anesthesia. Agri 2007;19(2):6–12.

[7] Boddy AP, Metha S, Rhodes M. The effect of intraperitoneal local anesthesia in laparoscopic cholecystectomy: a systematic review and meta-analysis. Anesth Analg 2006;103:682–88.

[8] Giacomazzi CM, Lagni VB, Monteiro MB. A dor pós-operatória como contribuinte do prejuízo na função pulmonar em pacientes submetidos a cirurgia cardíaca. Braz J Cardiovasc Surg 2006;21(4):386–92.

[9] Roe BB. Are postoperative narcotics necessary?. Arch Surg 1963;87:912–15.

[10] Evans JM, Rosen M, MacCarth J, Hogg MI. Apparatus for patient-controlled administration of intravenous narcotics during labour. Lancet 1976;I:17–8.

[11] Grass JA. Patient-controlled analgesia. Anesth Analg 2005;101:S44–61.

[12] Viscusi ER. Patient-controlled drug delivery for acute postoperative pain management: a review of current and emerging technologies. Reg Anesth Pain Med 2008;33(2):146–58.

[13] Austin KL, Stapleton JV, Mather LE. Relationship between blood meperidine concentrations and analgesic response: a preliminary report. Anesthesiology 1980;53:460–6.

[14] Dahlstrom B, Tamsen A, Paalzow L, Hartvig P. Patient-controlled analgesic therapy, Part IV: pharmacokinetics and analgesic plasma concentrations of morphine. Clin Pharmacokinet 1982;7:266–79.

[15] Tamsen A, Sakaruda T, Wahlstrom A, et al. Postoperative demand for analgesics in relation to individual levels of endorphines and substance P in cerebral spinal fluid. Pain 1982;13:171–82.

[16] Ferrante FM, Covino BG. Patient-controlled analgesia: a historical perspective. In: Ferrante FM, Ostheimer GW, Covino BG, editors. Patient-controlled Analgesia. Boston: Blackwell Scientific Publications; 1990, pp. 3–9.

[17] Ferrante FM. Patient-controlled analgesia: a conceptual framework for analgesic administration. In: Ferrante FM, Vadeboncouer TR, editors. Postoperative Pain Management. 1st ed. New York: Churchill Livingston; 1993, pp. 255–277.

[18] Mann C, Ouro-Bangna F, Eledjam JJ. Patient-controlled analgesia. Curr Drug Targets 2005;6:815–9.

[19] Hagle ME, Lehr VT, Brubakken K, Shippee A. Respiratory depression in adult patients with intravenous patient-controlled analgesia. Ortho Nurs 2004;23:18–27.

[20] Ballantyne JC, Carr DB, Chalmers TC, et al. Postoperative patient-controlled analgesia: meta-analyses of initial randomized controlled trials. J Clin Anesth 1993;5:182–93.

[21] Dolin SJ, Cashman JN, Bland JM. Effectiveness of acute postoperative pain management: I. Evidence from published data. Br J Anaesth 2002;89:409–23.

[22] Lebovits AH, Zenetos P, O'Neill DK, Cox D, Dubois MY, Jansen LA, Turndorf H. Satisfaction with epidural and intravenous patient-controlled analgesia. Pain Med. 2001;2:280–6.

[23] Schug SA, Torrie JJ. Safety assessment of postoperative pain management by an acute pain service. Pain 1993;55:387–91.

[24] Vicente KJ, Kada-Bekhaled K, Hillel G, Cassano A, Orser BA. Programming errors contribute to death from patient-controlled analgesia: case report and estimate of probability. Can J Anaesth 2003;50:328–32.

[25] Hankin CS, Schein J, Clark JA, Panchal S. Adverse events involving intravenous patient-controlled analgesia. Am J Health Syst Pharm 2007;64:1492–9.

[26] Rothschild JM, Keohane CA, Cook EF, et al. A controlled trial of smart infusion pumps to improve medication safety in critically ill patients. Crit Care Med 2005;33:533–40.

[27] Center for Devices and Radiological Health, US Food and Drug Administration. Infusion Pump Improvement Initiative. April 2010.

[28] Panchal SJ, Damaraju CV, Nelson WW, et al. System-related events and analgesic gaps during postoperative pain management with the fentanyl iontophoretic transdermal system and morphine intravenous patient-controlled analgesia. Anesth Analg 2007;105:1437–41.

[29] Miaskowski C. Patient-controlled modalities for acute postoperative pain management. J Perianesth Nurs 2005;20(4):255–67.

[30] Zafar SU, Hamid M, Hoda MQ. Patient controlled intravenous analgesia (PCIA) in postoperative surgical patients: an audit. J Pak Med Assoc 2004;54(7):353–6.

[31] Hutchison RW, Chon EH, Tucker WF, et al. A comparison of fentanyl, morphine and hydromorphone patient-controlled intravenous delivery for acute postoperative analgesia: a multicenter study of opioid-induced adverse reactions. Hosp Pharm 2006;41:659–63.

[32] Simopoulos TT, Smith HS, Peeters-Asdourian C, et al. Use of meperidine in patient-controlled analgesia and the development of a normeperidine toxic reaction. Arch Surg 2002;137:84–8.

[33] American Society of Pain. Principles of Analgesic Use in the Treatment of Acute Pain and Cancer Pain. 6th Edition: Glenvile, IL: American Society of Pain; 2008.

[34] Momeni M, Crucitti M, Kock MD. Patient-controlled analgesia in the management of postoperative pain. Drugs 2006;66:2321–37.

[35] Ratka A, Wittwer E, Baker L, et al. Pharmacokinetics of morphine, morphine-3-glucoronide, and morphine-6-glucoronide in health older men and women. Am J Pain Manage 2004;14:45–55.

[36] Hong D, Flood P, Diaz G. The side-effects of morphine and hydromorphone patient-controlled analgesia. Anesth Analg 2008;107:1384–9.

[37] Wheeler M, Oderda GM, Ashburn MA, et al. Adverse events associated with postoperative opioid analgesia: a systematic review. J Pain 2002;3:159–80.

[38] Palmer PP, Royal MA, Miller RD. Novel delivery systems for postoperative analgesia. Best Pract Res Clin Anaesthesiol 2014;18:81–90.

[39] Palmer PP, Miller RD. Current and developing methods of patient-controlled analgesia. Anesthesiol Clin 2010;28(4):587–99.

[40] Cepeda MS, Farrat JT, Baugarten M, et al. Side-effects of opioids during short term administration: effect of age, gender and race. Clin Pharmacol Ther 2003;74:102–12.

[41] Scott LJ. Fentanyl iontophoretic transdermal system: a review in acute postoperatory pain. Clin Drug Investig 2016;36:321–30.

[42] Egan TD, Lemmens HJ, Fiset P, et al. The pharmacokinetics of the new short-acting opioid remifentanil (GI87084B) in healthy adult male volunteers. Anesthesiology 1993;79:881–92.

[43] Prakash S, Fatima T, Pawar M. Patient-controlled analgesia with fentanyl for burn dressing changes. Anesth Analg 2004;99:552–5.

[44] Bailey PL, Streisand JB, East KA, et al. Differences in magnitude and duration of opioid-induced depression and analgesia with fentanyl and sufentanil. Anesth Analg 1990;70:8–15.

[45] Stoeckel H, Schuttler J, Magnussen H, et al. Plasma fentanyl concentrations and the occurrence of respiratory depression in volunteers. Br J Anaesth 1982;54:1087–95.

[46] Silvasti M, Pitaknen M. Patient-controlled epidural analgesia versus continuous epidural analgesia after total knee arthroplasty. Acta Anaesthesiol Scand 2001;45:471–6.

[47] Erolcay H, Yuceyar L. Intravenous patient-controlled analgesia after thoracotomy: a comparison of morphine with tramadol. Eur J Anaesthesiol 2003;20:141–6.

[48] Sjovall S, Kokki M, Kokki H. Laparoscopy surgery: a narrative review of pharmacotherapy in pain management. Drugs 2015;75(16):1867–89.

[49] Park JH, Lee C, Shin Y, An JH, Ban JS, Lee JH. Comparison of oxycodone and fentanyl for postoperative patient-controlled analgesia after laparoscopic gynecological surgery. Korean J Anesthesiol 2015;68:153–8.

[50] Jung KW, Kang HW, Park CH, Choi BH, et al. Comparison of the analgesic effect of patient-controlled oxycodone and fentanyl for pain management in patients undergoing colorectal surgery. Clin Exp Pharmacol Physiol 2016;43(8):745–52.

[51] Owen H, Brose WG, Plummer JL, Mather LE. Variables of patient-controlled analgesia. Test of an infusion-demand system using alfentanil. Anesthesia 1990;452–5.

[52] Thurlow JA, Laxton CH, Dick A, et al. Remifentanil by patient-controlled analgesia compared with intramuscular meperidine for pain relief in labor. Br J Anaesth 2002;88:374–8.

[53] Sinatra RS, Torres J, Bustos AM. Pain management after major orthopaedic surgery: current strategies and new concepts. J Am Acad Orthop Surg 2002;10:117–29.

[54] Saito M, Okutomi T, Kanai Y, Mochizuki J, Tani A, Aamano K, Hoka S. Patient-controlled epidural analgesia during labor using ropivacaine and fentanyl provides better maternal satisfaction with less local anesthetic requirement. J Anesth 2005;19:208–12.

[55] Wu CL, Cohen SR, Richman JM, et al. Efficacy of postoperative patient-controlled and continuous infusion epidural analgesia versus intravenous patient-controlled analgesia with opioids: a meta-analysis. Anesthesiology 2005;103:1079–88.

[56] Kim SH, Yoon KB, Yoon DM, et al. Patient-controlled epidural analgesia with ropivacaine and fentanyl: experience with 2,276 surgical patients. Korean J Pain 2005;26(1):39–45.

[57] Leon-Casasola OA, Parker BM, Lema MJ, Groth RI, Orsini-Fuentes J. Epidural analgesia versus intravenous patient-controlled analgesia. Differences in the postoperative course of cancer patients. Reg Anesth 1994;19(5):307–15.

[58] Liu SS, Allen HW, Olsson GL. Patient-controlled epidural analgesia with bupivacaine and fentanyl on hospital wards: prospective experience with 1,030 surgical patients. Anesthesiology 1998;88(3):688–95.

[59] Fredman B, Shapiro A, Zohar E, et al. The analgesic efficacy of patient-controlled ropivacaine instillation after Cesarean delivery. Anesth Analg 2000;91:1436–40.

[60] Vintar N, Pozlep G, Rawal N, Godec M, Rakovec S. Incisional self-administration of bupivacaine or propivacaine provides effective analgesia after inguinal hernia repair. Can J Anaesth 2002;49:481–86.

[61] Ilfeld BM, Morey TE, Wright TW, Chidgey LK, Enneking FK. Continuous interscalene brachial plexus block for postoperative pain control at home: a randomized, double-blinded, placebo-controlled study. Anesth Analg 2003;96:1089–95.

[62] Capdevila X, Dadure C, Bringuier S, Bernard N, Biboulet P, Gaertner E, Macaire P. Effect of patient-controlled perineural analgesia on rehabilitation and pain after ambulatory orthopedic surgery: a multicenter randomized trial. Anesthesiology 2006;105:566–73.

[63] Thipphawong JB, Babul N, Morishige RJ, Findlay HK, Reber KR, Millward GJ, Otulana BA. Analgesic efficacy of inhaled morphine in patients after bunionectomy surgery. Anesthesiology 2003;99(3):693–700.

[64] Stoker DG, Reber KR, Waltzman LS, et al. Analgesic efficacy and safety of morphine-chitosan nasal solution in patients with moderate to severe pain following orthopedic surgery. Pain Med 2008;9:3–12.

[65] Toussaint S, Maidl J, Schwagmeier R, Striebel HW. Patient-controlled intranasal analgesia: effective alternative to intravenous PCA for postoperative pain relief. Can J Anaesth 2000;47(4):299–302.

[66] Dale O, Hjortkjaer R, Kharasch ED. Nasal administration of opioids for pain management in adults. Acta Anaesthesiol Scand 2002;46:759–70.

Chapter 5

A Review of Intravenous Lidocaine Infusion Therapy for Paediatric Acute and Chronic Pain Management

Gillian R. Lauder

Additional information is available at the end of the chapter

http://dx.doi.org/10.5772/66771

To raise new questions, new possibilities, to regard old problems from a new angle, requires creative imagination and marks real advance in science.

Albert Einstein [1]

Abstract

Pediatric acute and chronic pain experiences involve the interaction of physiological, psychological, behavioural, developmental, pharmacological and situational factors. In the acute perioperative pain setting preventative multimodal analgesia is required to provide comfort and minimise the potential for "wind-up" and central sensitisation. When pain is recurrent, ongoing or chronic some children embark on a downward spiral of decreased physical, psychological and social functioning. The multidisciplinary team management approach is a well-established standard of care for children with complex chronic pain. Intravenous lidocaine has peripheral and central mediated analgesic, anti-inflammatory and anti-hyperalgesic properties. Intravenous lidocaine infusion therapy (IVLT) has been shown to be effective in the management of acute and chronic pain in adults. This chapter will present the rational for IVLT in pediatric pain management with emphasis on preventative multimodal therapy in acute pain and the multidisciplinary treatment approach in chronic pain. Large multi-centre randomised controlled trials are required to provide the evidence-base to confirm that IVLT is indeed an effective and safe treatment option in acute preventative multimodal analgesia and as an adjunct in the multidisciplinary care of chronic pain in the pediatric population.

Keywords: lidocaine, acute pain management, chronic pain management, paediatric

1. Introduction

1.1. Paediatric pain

Pain is described as an unpleasant sensory and emotional sensation associated with actual or potential tissue damage [2]. Pain is a normal physiological response to injury that protects an injured area at the time of healing. The experience of pain is the consequence of neuro-inflammatory activity and its interaction with complex peripheral and central nervous information-processing networks. It is not a simple hardwired impulse to sense message. The complex sequence of electrochemical events that take place from the site of injury to perception of pain is known as nociception. External noxious energy from the site of injury is converted into electrophysiological activity (transduction). This coded information is relayed via multiple parallel ascending pathways through the spinal cord to the brainstem, thalamus and sensory cortex (transmission). Incoming nociceptive traffic can be modified at any point in this transmission pathway by descending inhibitory pathways (modulation) [3]. The periaqueductal grey region, within the midbrain, and the periventricular grey matter connect anatomically with the rostroventral medulla and send descending excitatory projections to the dorsal horn of the spinal cord. Finally, connections between the thalamus and other higher cortical centres integrate the autonomic, affective and emotional responses to give a cumulative perception of pain [4]. It is important to note that pain pathways show remarkable neuroplasticity, changing phenotype in response to sustained inputs [5].

The paediatric experience of pain is influenced by many factors including the degree of tissue damage, age, sex, pharmacogenetic profile, previous pain experiences, cognitive factors, emotional issues, behavioural aspects, family background, environment, peer groups and culture. Due to the diverse interplay of these factors, there is substantial inter-individual variability in pain perception for different child/youths who have undergone the same surgical insult. In addition inter-individual variability in response to medications due to pharmacogenetic, sex, cultural, cognitive and emotional factors means that the analgesic response to doses of analgesia medication is also not predictable. Hence, the nature of pain as a sensation and its overall significance to a child/youth is unique. The resulting uncertainty in an individual child's pain perception and response to medications dictate that pain therapy is targeted according to ongoing individual assessment and response. Safe clinical practice requires appropriate understanding of pain pathophysiology, different pain models, pain assessment in different aged children and the age-related changes in the pharmacokinetics and pharmacodynamics of analgesics in infants and children. In an effort to comprehend why IVLT is effective, it is essential to understand some the mechanisms integral to pain physiology and pathophysiology.

1.2. Pain physiology and pathophysiology

Nociceptors are the free nerve endings of primary afferent pain nerve fibres responsible for the detection of noxious (unpleasant) stimuli, transforming the stimuli into electrical signals that are conducted to the central nervous system. Nocioceptors are distributed throughout the body and can be stimulated by mechanical, thermal or chemical stimuli.

Tissue injury induces an inflammatory reaction with an increase in acute phase proteins and the release of vasoactive mediators from mast cells and platelets. This inflammatory reaction includes activation of the kinin, complement and cytokine systems with release of inflammatory markers such as endothelin, prostaglandin E2, leukotrienes, substance P, bradykinin, cytokines, serotonin and adrenaline. These inflammatory markers induce peripheral nocioceptor sensitization and increased neuronal excitability [6–8]. These changes are partly caused by a change in levels of growth factors such as nerve growth factor, brain-derived neurotrophic factor, neuotrophin-3 and glial-cell derived neurotrophic factor [5].

Activation of nocioceptors creates energy that is converted into electrophysiological activity and transduced. Action potentials are created by activity of voltage-gated sodium and potassium channels which then propagate through axons to synapse in the dorsal horn [9]. The spinal-dorsal horn receives this nocioceptive information principally from primary afferent A-delta and C fibres. A-delta fibres are medium diameter myelinated axons that transmit acute afferent, localized sharp pain sensation. C fibres are small diameter un-myelinated afferents and convey delayed poorly localized pain. In the dorsal horn depolarization opens voltage-gated calcium channels (VGCC) which release substance P and glutamate that activate second-order neurons.

Following injury, the inflammatory mediators released also activate G-protein-coupled receptors expressed on sensory neurons. These are of fundamental importance for intra- and inter-cellular communication pathways [10] and play an important role in pain modulation and inflammation [11, 12]. It is relevant to note that cell membranes of injured peripheral nerves can exhibit an increased density in sodium channels and produce ectopic impulse generation and persistent spontaneous discharge in these nerves, their dorsal root ganglia, as well as neighbouring un-injured neurons [13–20]. As these spontaneous discharges have been shown to develop in both myelinated and un-myelinated nerve fibres, it is evident that ectopic activity can arise in both nociceptors and low-threshold mechanoreceptors [21]. Voltage-gated sodium channels (VGSC) with distinct gating and pharmacological properties have been reported to be upregulated in adult neurons by injury or disease [22]. An increased expression of sodium channels in dorsal root ganglia and around the injury site of injured axons contributes to spontaneous firing of nerve fibres after injury [23]. Changes in expression of sodium channels also occur in chronic neuropathic and inflammatory pain states [20, 24–28]. Changes in the properties and expression of voltage-gated calcium channels are also observed in neuropathic pain [29].

The non-selective cation channels, which make up the transient receptor potential (TRP) family of ion channels, are also key components in nocioception [30–32] and neurogenic inflammation [33, 34]. The transient receptor potential vanilloid 1 (TRPV1) and ankyrin 1 (TRPA1) channels are members of this TRP family. TRPV1 and TRPA1 are expressed on some sensory nerves and dorsal root ganglia [35]. They inter-link considerably with each other in terms of function, except, only TRPV1 is activated by vanilloids, like capsaicin (the piquant component of chili peppers). About 97% of TRPA1-expressing sensory neurons express TRPV1, while 30% of TRPV1-expressing neurons express TRPA1 [36]. TRPA1 is a molecular sensor of potentially toxic chemicals [37, 38] and is also activated by low temperatures [38, 39], mechanical stimuli [40, 41], and elevation of intra-cellular Ca^{2+} [42]. TRPA1 is, therefore, involved in the generation of pain signals associated with exposure to noxious chemicals, cold and mechanical stimuli [31].

In animal models of inflammatory and neuropathic pain, TRPA1 is up-regulated in sensory neurons [43, 44] and TRPA1 antagonists have been found to exhibit analgesic properties [45–47].

The terminals of C and A-delta fibres are concentrated in the superficial dorsal horn, C and Ad fibres terminate in lamina I (marginal zone) and lamina II (substantia gelatinosa) with some Ad fibres also terminating in lamina V. These fibres activate second-order neurons as well as modulatory inter-neurons (located in laminae V and VI). Primary afferent terminals release a number of excitatory neurotransmitters including glutamate and substance P.

Primary afferent nociceptive inputs synapse in the dorsal horn utilizing alpha-amino-3-hydroxy-5-methyl-4-iso-xazolepropionate (AMPA), neurokinin-1, and calcitonin gene-related peptide. Glutamate has a fundamental role in the activation of both AMPA and N-methyl-D-aspartate (NMDA) receptors in the dorsal horn, which generate excitatory post-synaptic potentials. Substance P belongs to the neurokinin group of small peptides, its effects are mediated by its binding to the NK1 receptor. The substance P-NK1 (SP-NK1) receptor system is present in only a minority of neurons (5–7%) and only in certain areas of the central nervous system. Release of substance P is induced by injurious stimuli, and the extent of its release is proportional to the strength and frequency of stimulation.

Glycine also serves an important role in central neurotransmission. It is an inhibitory neurotransmitter, and a co-agonist with glutamate at the NMDA receptor. These actions depend on extracellular glycine levels, which are regulated by glycine transporters. Ablation or silencing of spinal glycinergic neurons induces hyperalgesia and spontaneous pain behaviours, while their activation evokes analgesia against acute and chronic pain in rodents [48]. During high neuronal activity, glycine released from inhibitory inter-neurons escapes from the synaptic cleft, reaches nearby NMDA receptors and stimulates the NMDA receptor.

It is important to realize that different pain states (i.e. neuropathic/cancer/inflammatory) do create a unique but different set of neurochemical changes within sensory neurons, dorsal root ganglia and the spinal cord [5, 49].

Information from second-order neurons is relayed via the spinal cord to the brainstem and thalamus. Connections between the thalamus and higher cortical centres integrate the affective and autonomic responses to pain perception. In addition, descending axons from the brainstem synapse and release serotonin, noradrenaline and enkephalins in dorsal horn to also modify nociceptive transmission.

Primary afferent A-beta fibres are large-diameter myelinated nerves, which transmit mechanical information such as light touch. A-beta fibres do not usually activate nociceptive neurons and therefore do not transmit pain. The terminals of A-beta fibres are concentrated in the deeper dorsal horn and mainly target excitatory and inhibitory inter-neurons. However, the dorsal horn neuronal interconnections are modified and modulated under pathological conditions, such as peripheral nerve injury or peripheral tissue inflammation from injury or surgery [50–52]. Peripheral injuries may trigger on-going increases in the excitability of neurons (sensitization). This occurs at the level of the primary afferent nociceptive peripheral neuron (peripheral sensitization) and at the dorsal horn of the spinal cord (central sensitization).

Reduction in the threshold for activation of nociceptive neurons is manifest as allodynia (a non-painful stimulus perceived as painful) and hyperalgesia (a mild painful stimulus perceived as severe or long-lasting pain). Allodynia or touch-evoked pain is A-beta mediated [53].

Complex interactions occur in the dorsal horn between afferent neurons, inter-neurons and descending modulatory pathways (see below). These interactions determine activity of the secondary afferent neurons. Glycine and gamma-aminobutyric acid (GABA) are important neurotransmitters acting at inhibitory inter-neurons.

Neuropathic pain may involve anomalous excitability in the dorsal horn, resulting from multiple functional alterations including; loss of function of inhibitory inter-neurons, reduced effectiveness of the inhibitory neurotransmitters, sprouting of wide dynamic neurons and activation of microglia, the immune cells of the CNS [54–56]. Microglia activate, respond and transform to reactive states through hypertrophy and proliferation [57, 58]. These activated microglia induce/enhance production and release of pro-inflammatory cytokines and brain-derived neurotrophic factor [59], which modulate the activity of dorsal-horn neurons [60].

"Wind up" is physiological activation in the spinal cord after an intense or persistent barrage of afferent nociceptive impulses [57, 61]. Central sensitization refers to enhanced excitability of dorsal-horn neurons and is characterized by increased spontaneous activity, enlarged receptive field areas, and an increase in responses evoked by large and small calibre primary afferent fibres. IASP taxonomy defines central sensitization as increased responsiveness of nociceptive neurons in the central nervous system to their normal or sub-threshold afferent input [2]. Secondary hyperalgesia (hyperalgesia in undamaged tissue adjacent to the area of actual tissue damage) is due to an increased receptive field and reduced threshold of wide dynamic neurons in the dorsal horn.

Central sensitization and wind-up intensify pain perception, and both depend on activation of N-methyl-D-aspartate (NMDA) receptors. Pain memories imprinted within the central nervous system by NMDA-receptor activation produce hyperalgesia and allodynia. NMDA glutaminergic synapses do not participate significantly in primary nociceptive transmission, but instead in spinal sensitization. NMDA blockade in the spinal cord does not prevent primary afferent transmission of nociceptive information to the thalamus. Therefore, any attempt to reduce pain needs to target nociception, as well as wind up and central sensitization.

The increased barrage of pain impulses secondary to peripheral and central sensitization confers change within the nervous system known as neuroplasticity. That is, the nervous system undergoes maladaptive changes in response to incoming pain signals by reorganizing its structure, function and connections. Patients with ongoing or chronic pain demonstrate such structural brain changes as well as abnormal functioning of the inhibitory pain-modulatory system [62]. In addition, in chronic-pain conditions, the primary brain areas accessed through classical acute pain pathways decrease in their activation incidence and pre-frontal cortex activity increases [63]. A simplified depiction of acute and chronic pain pathways is depicted in **Figures 1** and **2**.

For more detailed information, please review "The Basic Science of Pain" by Philip Peng (https://itunes.apple.com/ca/book/the-basic-science-of-pain/id1174147456?mt=11).

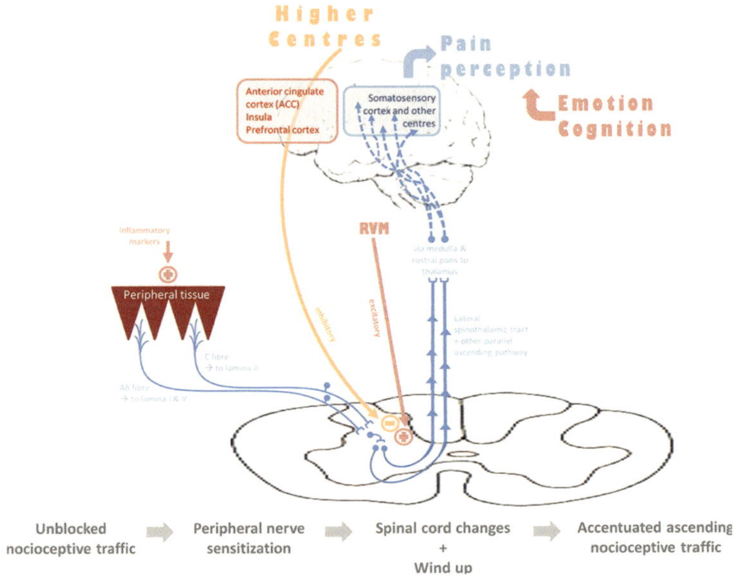

Figure 1. Simplified acute pain pathways.

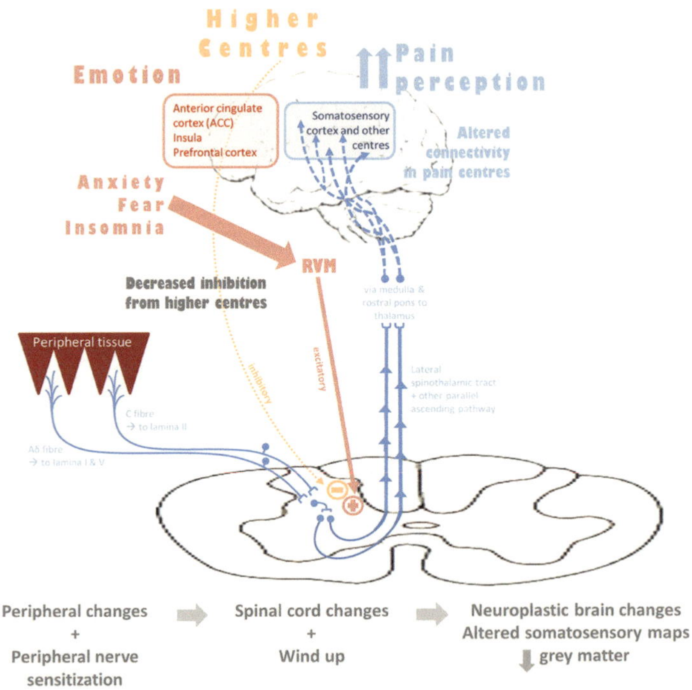

Figure 2. Simplified chronic pain pathophysiology.

http://dx.doi.org/10.5772/66771

1.3. Impacts of poorly managed acute pain

When acute pain is not well-managed, deleterious effects on physiology, functional recovery and psychology can develop. Changes include increased morbidity such as nausea, emesis, poor oral fluid intake, sleep disturbance and behavioural changes. Ongoing discomfort and distress have a negative impact on child and family satisfaction and may be associated with poor recovery, anxiety, fear and reduced quality of life measures [64–71].

Physical and psychological responses to pain not only affect children's health directly but may also predispose them to develop chronic post-surgical pain (CPSP). Chronic pain affects approximately 20% of the adult population of which 22.5% develop their condition after surgery [72]. CPSP occurs following 10–50% of adult operations in which 2–10% of these adult patients will experience severe chronic pain [73]. The incidence of CPSP in the adult population is found to depend on a number of perioperative factors, which include genetic predisposition, younger age, degree of pre-operative anxiety, degree of catastrophization, depression, pre-operative pain status, the surgical pain model, surgical technique, length of surgery and the quality of acute post-operative pain management [73–76]. CPSP will often be neuropathic, resulting from nerve damage during surgery. CPSP studies in children are limited with a preliminary incidence of CPSP reported as 13–25% [77–80]. Prospective studies after spine surgery have also demonstrated prevalence rates of CPSP between 11 and 22% with risk factor for development of CPSP including high levels baseline pain intensity, anxiety and older age [81–83]. Recently, Rabbitts et al. found two distinct pain trajectories following major surgery in children; most children follow a positive early recovery pathway, whereas 22% follow a late recovery trajectory. One of the factors of the late recovery group was the presence of baseline parental catastrophizing (not child/youth catastrophizing) [84]. Nikolajsen and Brix also identified factors for risk of CPSP in children as older age, pre-op pain, acute postoperative pain and psychological factors, especially anxiety [85]. Some of these children/youth will go on to develop chronic pain in adulthood [86]. All these complications of poorly managed acute pain ultimately increase healthcare utilization and have an economic cost for both families and the health-care service. It is, therefore, essential to minimize post-surgical pain to prevent pain-related complications. This may be achievable with the adoption of preventative multimodal analgesia to minimize nociceptive traffic and reduce wind up and central sensitisation.

1.4. Preventative multimodal analgesia

Preventative analgesia is defined as analgesia that is provided by an intervention given in the perioperative period, which may be before or after incision and surgery, that reduces analgesic requirements for post-operative pain for a period longer than the duration of action for the analgesic intervention. Consideration needs to be given, not only to efficacy of analgesia regimens, but also that the duration pain management so that it spans the whole painful experience from incision to healing [87, 88]. Preventative analgesia differs from pre-emptive analgesia, where an analgesic intervention is administered pre-operatively with the aim to provide improved analgesia post-operatively compared with the identical analgesic intervention administered after incision or in the post-operative period [89].

Multimodal analgesia utilises combinations of analgesics that act by different modes to enable a reduction in analgesic requirements of each type of medication and therefore reduce side-effect profiles. The components of multimodal analgesia are shown in **Table 1**. A multimodal approach provides significant benefits, which include reduction in; pain intensity, opioid dose requirements, and opioid-related adverse events [68, 90–93]. In the acute perioperative pain setting, preventative multimodal analgesia is required not only to provide comfort but also to minimise the potential for "wind-up" and central sensitisation. Therefore, directly impacting, the mechanisms may induce the development of CPSP or chronic pain [94].

Acetaminophen
NSAID's including COX-2 inhibitors
Local anaesthetic agents
Opioids
Anxiolytics
Adjuvant medications: ketamine, clonidine, dexmedetomidine, pregabalin/gabapentin
Non-pharmacological techniques:
Education
Hypnosis
Cognitive behavioural therapy; relaxation/imagery/controlled breathing
TENS
Acupuncture
Massage
Distraction techniques (games/videos/virtual reality/computer games)

Table 1. Multimodal analgesia comprises a combination of the following modalities.

Although multimodal analgesia has been shown to be effective in reducing pain in children [95, 96], it should be remembered that many drugs used worldwide for paediatric pain management do not have approved labelling for use in children [97]. Drug dosing recommendations based on clinical evidence and experience, not based on evidence may well put children/youth at risk for medication-related adverse events [98].

A limited number of well-conducted, prospective randomized controlled trials have demonstrated improved clinical outcomes with respect to analgesia and opioid-related side effects with multimodal (vs. single) therapy [92, 93, 99]. However, there is an urgent need for research evaluating, which preventive multimodal analgesic regimens are most effective for different paediatric acute pain settings or surgical models of pain, the most appropriate timing of administration and which of these decrease or prevent long-term pain after surgery. In the meantime, paediatric acute pain teams need to develop surgery specific multimodal analgesia guidelines [100], assess effectiveness and respond quickly when the regime proves inadequate for an individual child/youth.

Good quality acute pain management enhances functional recovery, improves long-term functional outcomes [101] and improves patient and family satisfaction [93, 102].

Non-pharmacological techniques are an extremely useful component of multimodal therapy [103–105]; unfortunately, they are under-utilised in hospitalised children [106]. The mainstay of acute pain management for children and youths resides in the use of opioid analgesia, but opioid use is associated with a significant side effect profile (see **Table 2**). Adverse effects (except allergy) are dose-related and may be relieved by minimizing the opioid dose, conversion to a different opioid and/or using non-opioid adjuvants. IVLT is a useful adjuvant for specific acute pain procedures.

Sedation
Respiratory depression
Nausea and vomiting
Pruritus
Meiosis
Urinary retention
Ileus/constipation
Myoclonic jerks
Dysphoria/hallucinations
Opioid-induced hyperalgesia [107]
Long term opioids in mice cause dose-dependent enhanced sarcoma-induced bone loss, fracture and bone pain [108]
Decreased regional grey matter volume [109]
Inhibit cellular and humoral immune function in humans [110]
Tolerance: physiologic adaptation that results in a decreased medication effect at its current dose or when needing a higher dose to maintain the desired analgesic effect [65]
Dependence: physiologic effect of opioid use resulting in withdrawal symptoms following abrupt discontinuation of opioids or after administration of opioid antagonist [65]
Long term potential for addiction (unlikely in pediatric, short-term, acute postoperative opioid therapy)
Long term endocrine effects [111]
Potential for diversion and abuse of prescription opioids in community [112]

Table 2. Adverse effects of opioids.

2. Intravenous lidocaine therapy

2.1. Lidocaine pharmacology

Local anaesthetics are primarily used for local infiltration, nerve blocks and regional anaesthesia. Analgesia results from blockade of voltage-gated Na^+ channels that prevent action potential initiation and propagation. Local anaesthetics impede sodium ion access to the axon interior, probably by physically occluding the trans-membrane sodium channels. This is a reversible process, which does not damage the nerve. Depolarization cannot take place when the sodium channel is blocked, so the axon remains polarized. A local anaesthetic regional or nerve block is, therefore, a reversible, non-depolarization block. In contrast, systemically administered local anaesthetics produce analgesia at plasma levels well below that required to block an action potential. Systemic administration of local anaesthetic is most recognized with lidocaine due to its widespread use for anti-arrhythmic treatment [113–115].

Lidocaine is an amide local anaesthetic and a Class Ib cardiac anti-dysrhythmic agent [116]. Therapeutic plasma levels and duration of IVLT for acute pain management are not well defined, although the optimal therapeutic range for acute pain treatment appears to be between 1 and 5 μg/ml [6, 24, 117–120]. Only preservative free formulations should be given intravenously. Bolus administration of 2 mg/kg and a continuous infusion of 2–5 mg/kg/h have shown to reach plasma levels of 1–4 μg/ml [121]. After a bolus injection or continuous administration for up to 12 h, the half-life of lidocaine is about 100 minutes and shows linear pharmacokinetics [122].

Lidocaine metabolism occurs rapidly in the liver by cytochrome P450 isoforms CYP1A2 and 3A4, as outlined in **Figure 3**. Lidocaine undergoes oxidative N-dealkylation, to a number of metabolites that include monoethylglycinexylidide (MEGX) and glycinexylidide (GX), and N-ethylglycine (NEG), all of which have a glycine-like moiety. Less than 10% of lidocaine is excreted unchanged by the kidneys. MEGX is an active metabolite and has 80% potency of lidocaine at VGSC's. GX is also active but NEG is inactive. Following intravenous administration, MEGX concentrations in serum range from 11 to 36% of the lidocaine concentration. All lidocaine metabolites are excreted by the kidneys. The half-life of lidocaine elimination from the plasma following IV administration is 81–149 min (mean 107 ± 22 SD, n = 15). The systemic clearance is 0.33–0.90 l/min (mean 0.64 ± 0.18 SD, n = 15). Children older than 6–7 months of age distribute and eliminate intravenous lidocaine in the same manner as adults [123].

In infants less than 6–7 months of age liver metabolism is immature so metabolism of drugs is delayed, and plasma protein levels are lower [124]. There are low levels of plasma alpha-1-acid glycoprotein, which increases the free fraction of circulating lidocaine and therefore increases the risk of toxicity [125]. IVLT in high doses (6–8mg/kg/h without a bolus dose) has used to treat neonatal seizures but the risk-benefit indication is considerably different than for pain management [126]. For these reasons, IVLT for pain management cannot be recommended in infants until more evidence of efficacy and safety in this population are available.

2.2. Safety of IVLT for pain management

A major advantage with IVLT is that appropriate use in adults is not associated with a significant side-effect profile [7, 127, 128]. In adults, a 100 mg bolus followed by an infusion at 1 mg/min, which approximates to 1mg/kg/h, produces a plasma level of just over 1 μg/ml in normal individuals with no co-morbidities [129]. IVLT doses used to manage pain are usually in the range of 1–2 mg/kg/h. Plasma levels at this rate of infusion are generally less than 3–5 μg/ml, but awake patients may complain of light-headedness, perioral numbness, dizziness and or sedation. Toxic plasma lidocaine levels are considered to be in the >6 μg/ml range [130]. Early signs of local anaesthetic systemic toxicity (LAST) will present as perioral numbness, metallic taste, tinnitus, visual and auditory disturbances, paresthesias, nausea, dizziness and drowsiness [7, 131–133]. Due to the short half-life of lidocaine, the symptoms of LAST are easily reversible by lowering or discontinuing the infusion. To provide some perspective, lidocaine effects at higher plasma levels are more serious; at 8 μg/ml, patients experience visual or auditory disturbances, dissociation, muscle twitching, and decreased blood pressure. At 12 μg/ml, convulsions can occur; at 16 μg/ml, coma may develop, and at levels above 20 μg/ml respiratory arrest and cardiovascular collapse ensue [132]. Physicians administering IVLT must be aware of algorithms of care to prevent, recognise and treat LAST when it occurs [134].

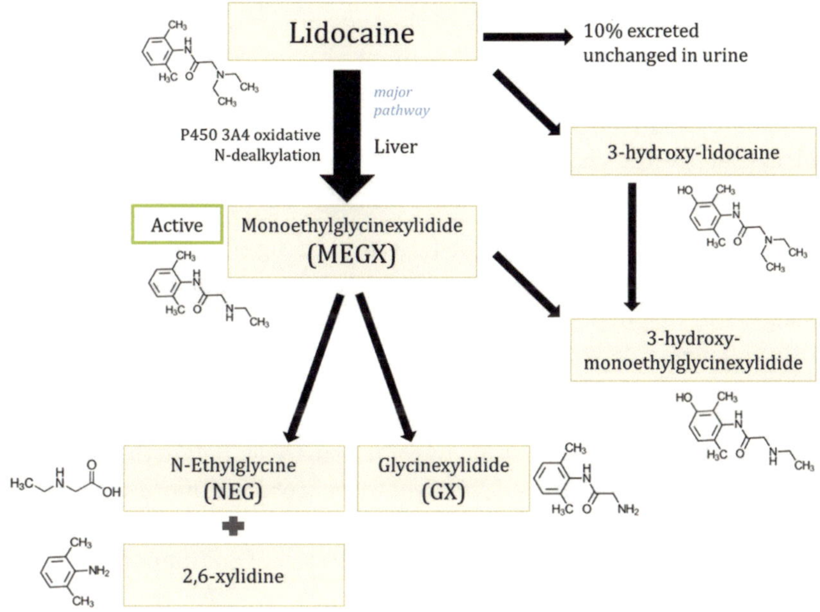

Figure 3. Lidocaine metabolism.

Contraindications to IVLT include allergy to amide local anaesthetics, significant cardiac disease, heart block, seizures, liver disease and/or significant renal impairment.

2.3. The rationale for IVLT in the management of pain

Studies in animal preparations clearly indicate that systemically administered lidocaine can silence ectopic discharges without blocking nerve conduction [135, 136]. Systemic administration of local anaesthetics provides clinical analgesia in a broad range of neuropathic pain states [23, 117, 137–140]. IVLT induces global analgesia and dampens the neuro-inflammatory response in pain [126, 141–144]. Lidocaine exerts its different effects on the neuro-inflammatory response by inhibiting ion channels and receptors. The exact lidocaine plasma level and duration of infusion required to produce this effect are unknown; however, it occurs at levels below those required for action potential initiation and propagation for neural blockade. It is also not known if plasma lidocaine concentration correlates with analgesic effect in a dose dependent manner as different channels and receptors are modulated at different plasma lidocaine concentrations [145].

Intravenous lidocaine has peripherally and centrally mediated analgesic, anti-inflammatory and anti-hyperalgesic properties. Its analgesic properties reflect the variable dose, time dependent, multimodal aspect of its action on voltage-gated channels receptors and neurotransmitters that affect nociceptive transmission pathways [24, 45, 146–148]. In vitro, low dose lidocaine inhibits voltage-gated sodium channels (VGSC), some potassium channels, the glycinergic system, and G-protein coupled receptors. Higher dose lidocaine blocks voltage-gated calcium channels, other potassium channels, and NMDA receptors [145, 149, 150]. Lidocaine dosages needed for voltage-gated sodium channel blockade range from 60 to 200 μM, whereas voltage-gated calcium channel blockade occurs at higher doses in the 1–10 mM range [6, 151–153]. A number of different sodium channel isoforms exist with distinct tissue distribution and possibly distinct physiological functions. Some of these isoforms have been shown to be up-regulated in inflammatory and neuropathic pain states [28, 154–156]. Lidocaine blocks all sodium channel isoforms but differences in isoform sensitivity to lidocaine could be an explanation for efficacy in various different pain models.

Animal studies demonstrate that systemic lidocaine changes conduction in neurons of the dorsal horn, dorsal root ganglion and hyper-excitable neuromas without affecting normal nerve conduction [23, 135, 157]. Cell membranes of injured peripheral nerves express sodium channels with unusual density and produce persistent spontaneous discharges that maintain a central hyper-excitable state [20]. Ectopic discharges can be initiated along the injured nerve, in the dorsal root ganglion, and in peripheral neuromata [157–161]. Lidocaine inhibits these aberrant electrical discharges at concentrations well below those necessary to produce conduction blockade in nerves. Dorsal-horn neurons are more sensitive to lidocaine compared with peripheral neurons [135]. The high susceptibility of hyper-excitable neurons to lidocaine may be attributed to the changed expression of sodium channels during nerve injury [28].

Analgesic effects are thought to be mediated by the inhibition of Na channels, NMDA, and G-protein-coupled receptors that lead to the suppression of spontaneous impulses generated from injured nerve fibres and the proximal dorsal root ganglion [23, 117, 159, 162].

While the main mechanism of the therapeutic action of lidocaine is considered to be blockade of voltage-gated channels, lidocaine may also have a desensitizing effect on TRP channels. This may reflect the prolonged analgesic effects sometimes seen that outlast the expected presence of lidocaine in the tissue [163].

Anti-inflammatory effects are attributable to attenuation of neurogenic inflammation and subsequent blockade of neural transmission at the site of tissue injury. Lidocaine inhibits the migration of granulocytes and release of lysosomal enzymes which leads to decreased release of pro- and anti-inflammatory cytokines [146, 162, 164–167]. Animal studies demonstrate that these anti-inflammatory effects of lidocaine are mediated by inhibition of VGSC, G-protein-coupled receptors and ATP-sensitive potassium channels.

The anti-hyperalgesic effect of lidocaine is presumed to result from the suppression of peripheral and central sensitization through a combination of nociceptor blockade, dampening of the neuro-inflammatory response to pain, NMDA receptor inhibition and modulation of the glycinergic system [25, 168–173]. Low dose lidocaine (10 μM) enhances and high dose (1 mM) inhibits glycinergic signalling [174]. The lidocaine metabolite, N-ethylglycine (NEG) is a substrate of the glycine reuptake transporter so it competes with endogenous and synaptically released glycine for reuptake leading to increased extracellular and synaptic glycine levels [172]. This would explain why NEG has been shown to induce analgesia in rodent models of neuropathic and inflammatory pain but has minor effects on Na^+ channels [172]. The lidocaine metabolite MEGX has been shown to inhibit the glycine transporter which will also increase glycine levels [172].

2.4. A central effect of systemic lidocaine

On-going input from peripheral nociceptors which is blocked by local anaesthetics is used to explain dependence of pain syndromes on peripheral inputs [175]. However, IVLT also has a central effect reducing components of pain caused by central nervous system injuries [176]. Systemically administered lidocaine has been shown to suppress capsaicin-induced hyperalgesia by a central mode of action, whilst concurrently reducing acute chemically induced pain by a peripheral mode of action [114]. Descending facilitatory pain transmission from the rostroventromedial medulla may also be suppressed by lidocaine [177, 178].

2.5. Role of IVLT in acute perioperative pain

Lidocaine infusions were described to be effective in the relief of acute post-surgical pain as early as 1961 [179]. Since then many other studies have confirmed the analgesic effects of lidocaine in patients with acute pain, such as Stayer's report on the safe and successful use of continuous pleural lidocaine after thoracotomy in children [180]. In 2012, Sun et al. published a meta-analysis of randomized controlled trials examining systemic lidocaine for post-operative analgesia and recovery after abdominal surgery [181]. It showed a decrease in post-operative pain intensity, opioid consumption, time to first bowel movement, and hospital length of stay. The most widely used lidocaine infusion regimen was a bolus of 1.5 mg/kg lidocaine followed by an infusion of 1.5–2 mg/kg/h.

The current evidence for using IV lidocaine for perioperative pain is based on four systematic reviews and one Cochrane review [128, 182–185]. In the most recent Cochrane review Kranke et al., reviewed only perioperative studies where the IVLT had been started intra-operatively prior to incision and continued at least until the end of surgery. Forty studies met the inclusion criteria. Primary outcomes measures required were pain score (0–10 cm, 0–100 mm visual analogue scale, (VAS), numeric rating scale (NRS), post-operative ileus, and functional gastrointestinal recovery (either time to defaecation, time to first flatus, or time to first bowel movement/sounds). Secondary outcomes sought included length of hospital stay, functional post-operative neuropsychological status scales, surgical complications (such as post-operative infections, thromboembolism, wound breakdown), patient satisfaction (satisfaction survey), cessation of the intervention, intra-operative opioid requirements, opioid requirements during the postoperative period and any adverse events (e.g. post-operative nausea and vomiting (PONV), death, dysrhythmias or signs of lidocaine toxicity).

Intravenous lidocaine administration was initiated with a bolus dose in 64% of the included trials. The subsequent infusion ranged from 1 to 3 mg/kg/h but most commonly was 1.5 mg/kg/h. In five studies, no bolus dose was given prior to the start on the intravenous infusion of lidocaine [186–190].

The lidocaine infusion was terminated either at skin closure or the end of the surgical procedure [45, 186, 188, 190–206]; 1 h after surgery/skin closure [207–212]; 1 h after arrival in the post anaesthesia care unit (PACU) [213]; 4 h post-operatively [214]; up to 8 h post-operatively (or at PACU discharge whichever occurred earlier) [187]; after a total of 12 h [215]; 24 h post-operatively [216–223]; 48 h post-operatively [215, 224–226]; or on the day of return of bowel function or, at the latest, on the fifth post-operative day [189]. One study did not report the cessation time for the lidocaine infusion [227].

In this review, intravenous lidocaine was used in a variety of surgical procedures such as abdominal surgeries, tonsillectomy, orthopaedic, cardiac, and ambulatory surgeries. It was found to be useful only in abdominal surgery, where anaesthetic and opioid requirements were significantly reduced in the perioperative period. Several studies reported a decrease in pain intensity (pain at rest, cough, and movement), opioid requirements, and opioid-related side-effects, such as PONV. A decrease in the duration of post-operative ileus was also seen and is attributed to a combination of opioid-sparing effect, anti-inflammatory actions, decreased sympathetic tone and the direct effect of lidocaine on intestinal smooth muscle. These benefits did not translate to expedited discharge from PACU nor have a positive effect on ambulatory surgeries.

2.6. Role of lidocaine in paediatric acute perioperative pain

None of the studies included in the most recent Cochrane review for IVLT in acute pain management were paediatric. There is currently only one randomized controlled trial of IVLT in a paediatric acute pain population [228]. This study demonstrated decreased hospital stay, decreased rescue analgesia requirements, decreased cortisol levels and earlier return of bowel function with IVLT (1.5mg/kg bolus followed by 1.5mg/kg/h infusion) compared to placebo followed abdominal surgery. Until further evidence of paediatric analgesic efficacy and safety are available doses have to be translated from adult practice. It is not clear what dose regime and plasma concentration provide the best analgesic efficacy for particular surgical models of pain. Pain management remains an off-label indication for the use of IVLT, and the paediatric continuous infusion dosing quoted in the drug information documentation (0.5–3 mg/kg/h) refers to its use as an anti-arrhythmic agent.

The author uses IVLT as an adjunct in preventative multimodal analgesia for major paediatric (non-infant) surgical procedures where a regional or neuraxial analgesia technique has to be avoided or is contra-indicated. Typical procedures include scoliosis surgery, laparoscopic abdominal surgery and external frame fixator procedures. Lidocaine infusion regimes are typically 1 mg/kg bolus dose followed by an infusion with 2 mg/kg/h started prior to incision and continued until just after surgical closure. With extensive surgical times, the IVLT is decreased to 1.5 mg/kg/h after 8 h. It is essential to understand that there is little data to confirm the appropriate dosing and safe lidocaine levels in the paediatric population. However, clinical evaluation would suggest that the use of intravenous lidocaine therapy, in this manner, has beneficial effects on paediatric post-operative pain, opioid requirements and child/youth sense of wellbeing, especially in the first 24 h. In an attempt to determine appropriate research questions and outcome measures we have retrospectively reviewed 24 paediatric scoliosis cases. Twelve children undergoing idiopathic scoliosis correction (posterior instrumentation and fusion only) between January 2012 and March 2014, where intra-operative IV lidocaine infusion was administered were compared against twelve matched controls. The lidocaine group received a total dose of 14.17 ± 2.39 mg/kg, given over 6.45 ± 0.74 h. Both groups were comparable with respect to age, gender, body mass index (BMI), number of levels instrumented and surgical duration. Morphine consumption within the first 48 h post-operatively was significantly lower in the IVLT group [229]. Despite the small sample size and the retrospective nature of this case matched chart review the significant opioid-sparing effect in the post-operative period with the use of intra-operative IV lidocaine infusion merits further study. Prospective, randomized controlled trials are recommended.

2.7. Role of lidocaine in preventative analgesia

In many studies, the analgesic effect has persisted after the lidocaine infusion was discontinued, which suggests prevention of peripheral and/or central hypersensitivity [209, 211]. Perioperative lidocaine has been found to have a preventive effect on post-operative pain for up to 72 h after abdominal surgery [211]. A randomized, double-blind, placebo-controlled study of 36 adult patients undergoing breast cancer surgery showed that perioperative intravenous lidocaine (bolus of IV lidocaine 1.5 mg/kg followed by a continuous infusion of lidocaine 1.5 mg/kg/h) was associated with decreased incidence and severity of chronic pain after breast surgery. Two (11.8%) patients in the lidocaine group and 9 (47.4%) patients in the control group reported CPSP at 3 months follow-up ($P = 0.031$) [209]. Secondary hyperalgesia (area of hyperalgesia over length of surgical incision) was significantly less in the lidocaine group compared with control group (0.2 ± 0.8 vs. 3.2 ± 4.5 cm; $P = 0.002$). The authors concluded that IV perioperative lidocaine decreases the incidence and severity of CPSP after breast cancer surgery siting prevention of the induction of central hyperalgesia is a potential mechanism [209].

2.8. Multi-disciplinary team management of children with chronic pain

Chronic pain is pain that persists for more than 3 months and often years beyond the expected time to heal from injury, surgery or onset of a painful condition. It occurs in one in five adults and is a significant cause of suffering and disability worldwide. Although mainly a disease of adults, it does occur in children and youths with slightly more than one child/youth in every twenty reporting a chronic pain issue. A Canadian study of 495 schoolchildren aged 9–13, reported that more than half reported having experienced at least one recurrent pain (headache, stomach pain or 'growing pains'). 46% of this population reported a 'long-lasting' pain, however, the authors classified 6% as having chronic pain [230]. A Statistics Canada health report identifies chronic pain among 2.4% of males and 5.9% of females aged 12–17 years [231].

Typical types of chronic pain seen in children and youths include headaches, complex regional pain syndrome (CRPS), recurrent abdominal pain, limb and other musculoskeletal pains. Girls are three times more likely to report chronic pain than boys [232, 233]. Abdominal pain is significantly more likely to be reported by girls and limb pain (or growing pains/muscle aches) is significantly more likely to be reported by boys [230, 233, 234]. Although prevalence of chronic pain in school children varies from 9 to 32% [235, 236] and is on an increase [234], the reported prevalence exceeds the prevalence of school aged children seeking medical care for pain [237]. Cross-sectional and/or retrospective studies may not reflect the true picture and call for more longitudinal research to establish the actual prevalence and impacts of ongoing pain in children and youths has been advocated [238].

Some children with severe chronic pain embark on a downhill spiral of decreased physical, psychological and social functioning [239]. This includes loss of mobility with inability to participate in physical or sporting activities, poor sleep, difficulty concentrating on school work, school absenteeism, social isolation and family stress [240]. As chronic pain persists, the child can experience increased pain intensity, distress, sadness, anxiety, depression resulting in very poor quality of life [241]. The impact of chronic pain on the family matches the adverse impact experienced by families caring for children at home with severe cerebral palsy or birth defects [242–244]. Direct and indirect costs such as loss of earnings, adaptations to housing, over-the-counter medications and care assistance managing a child with chronic pain are considerable [245–248].

When entangled in the disordered lifestyle associated with chronic pain the child/youth and their family require coordinated integrated care to affect a recovery. The multi-disciplinary team management approach, based on pharmacology, physiotherapy and psychology (the 3P approach), is now well established to be the standard of care for children with chronic pain. This method involves looking beyond a child's pathology in isolation and engages multiple specialists to optimize the child/youth's psychological and emotional wellbeing, physical function and pharmacological therapy [247, 249–251]. This process requires adoption of a self-management approach and reduced reliance on medical investigation and intervention. Children and youth with significant pain-related disability have been shown to derive significant improvements in functional ability after participating in an intensive pain rehabilitation program employing daily physical, occupational and psychological therapies [247, 248, 252, 253].

Multi-disciplinary treatment goals are targeted to each individual child/youth after careful consideration of the medical history, pain history, examination and relevant investigations. How each therapeutic modality of care is balanced is dependent on the individual child and takes into consideration the type and duration of pain, as well as the impact of pain on particular biopsychosocial aspects of the child's life. Early recognition and appropriate '3P' management is the key to success. Within the context of the coordinated multi-disciplinary approach, IVLT can serve as a useful adjunct to concurrent physical, and psychological interventions to manage chronic pain in children and youths [133, 254, 255]. IVLT needs to be explained and utilized in a way that does not negate the multi-disciplinary teams attempts to promote self-management and de-medicalization.

Determining or predicting suitability for successful pharmacological treatment requires attention to a number of factors. It is essential to consider any available evidence (often lacking especially in the paediatric population), drug responsiveness (matching the predicted mechanism of action of the drug with the pathophysiology of the pain condition), side effect profile, goals of therapy and the possible impact of the pharmacological intervention to the holistic plan of self-management and return to function for the individual child/youth. One of the goals of therapy is a shift away from a change in the pain rating and pain responsiveness to restoration of physical and social functioning. For some children pharmacological therapy is not required to achieve this goal. Timing of pharmacological intervention is also important. For some children ensuring that self-management strategies and attempts at return to function are initiated prior to pharmacological intervention may decrease a reliance on medications to initiate or promote change. Not all children and youths will have a predictable or positive response to the types of medications used in chronic pain. Some will require a trial of more than one type of pharmacological agent. To minimize side-effect profiles only the lowest effective dose should be used. Different pharmacological agents may have to be used in a tiered proportional manner, balancing risk versus benefits but with the over-riding aim to improve quality of life. As the simplest most appropriate pharmacological strategy should be trialled first it is important to briefly discuss topical lidocaine.

2.9. The use of topical lidocaine therapy in paediatric chronic pain

For the purpose of this review topical lidocaine refers to q12h 5% lidocaine patch or compounded 5% lidocaine applied under an occlusive dressing (12 h on, 12 h off) administered daily. Topical lidocaine should only be applied to intact skin over a localised painful area. It is assumed that topical lidocaine works by blocking sodium channels on C, A-delta [256] and A-beta nerve fibres [257]. Allodynia is a prominent component of neuropathic pain, which is A-beta mediated and driven by central sensitization [80]. Topical lidocaine reduces nociceptor discharge at the level of the skin, to enable a light mechanical stimulus to induce a sense of touch, not pain. The analgesic effects of topical lidocaine probably do not require anaesthesia to the skin [258]. When lidocaine patches are used according to the recommended dosing instructions, only 3 ± 2% of the dose applied is expected to be absorbed. Repeated application of three lidocaine patches, used for 3 days simultaneously (12 h on, 12 h off), indicates that the lidocaine concentration does not incrementally increase with ongoing daily use. Pain relief from topical lidocaine occurs despite the extremely low systemic lidocaine plasma levels achieved. These plasma levels range from 0.13 to 0.23 μg/ml [259, 260], which is approximately one-tenth of the effective level obtained with IVLT. Despite this, neuropathic pain patients achieve pain relief from topical lidocaine [259, 261–267]. Lidocaine patches also produce analgesia in patients with painful diabetic neuropathy [268], Complex regional pain syndrome (CRPS) [269] and non-neuropathic conditions such as osteoarthritis and low-back pain [261, 270–273]. Systemic side effects are extremely rare and topical lidocaine is therefore recommended as a first-line therapy for all children and youths with localized peripheral neuropathic pain or CRPS and definitely before consideration of IVLT.

2.10. Selection criteria for the use of IVLT in paediatric chronic pain

Lidocaine's short serum half-life of 120 min dictates that the analgesic effect disappears a few hours after treatment so this should completely preclude its use for chronic pain issues. However, prolonged relief has been reported in animal models [274] and in some non-randomized [255, 275] and randomized trials [175, 276, 277]. The Canadian Pain Society states that "intravenous lidocaine infusions are generally safe and can provide significant pain relief for 2–3 weeks at a time" [278]. The 2012 neuropathic pain interventional guidelines by Mailis and Taenzer issue a Grade B recommendation for IV lidocaine at 5–7.5 mg/kg, with relief expected to last in the range of hours to 4 weeks [279]. Clinical studies show analgesic effects of intravenously administered sodium channel blockers especially in pain conditions where hyperalgesia is prominent [114, 139, 143, 144, 276, 277, 280–282]. Chronic pain conditions, in which reports of IVLT have been beneficial include peripheral nerve injury [283], neuropathic pain [7, 16, 274, 276, 279, 284–286], CRPS [255, 287], headaches [133, 288, 289], cancer therapy, spinal cord injury [176] and fibromyalgia [290].

There is a distinct lack of evidence to support the use of IVLT for paediatric chronic pain management. Criteria and dosing guidelines are institutionally formulated based on clinical experience, but equate with dose regimes previously reported to manage chronic pain in adolescents and young adults [133], see **Table 3**.

1.	Child/youth is fully integrated into multi-disciplinary care
2.	Their pain syndrome is considered to be lidocaine-responsive
3.	The pain is not amenable to the use of topical lidocaine
4.	Patients have no contra-indication to the use of systemic lidocaine such as major cardiac dysfunction, liver dysfunction, renal impairment, seizure activity, or allergy to amide local anaesthetics
5.	Child/youth capable of verbally communicating analgesic response and symptoms of potential local anaesthetic toxicity.
6.	A high-acuity environment capable of providing continuous ECG monitoring, oxygen saturation, and frequent blood pressure measurements, plus access to healthcare personnel skilled in resuscitation and airway management.

Table 3. BCCH institutional selection criteria for initial IVLT in children/youth.

2.11. IV lidocaine infusion protocol at BC children's hospital

Initial infusion:

- Location: post-anaesthetic care unit
- Monitors: as dictated by CPSBC guideline

- Loading dose: 1 mg/kg bolus
- Infusion: 5 mg/kg delivered over 1 h
- Total dose: 6 mg/kg (loading dose + infusion)

IVLT should only be administered within a high-acuity environment such as a paediatric intensive care unit, high-acuity unit, step-down unit, or post-anaesthetic care unit.

The College of Physicians and Surgeons of British Columbia published out of hospital Pain Infusion Clinic guidelines in 2014. The guidelines are intended only for the treatment of adults, and to the best of our knowledge, no such guidelines exist for the paediatric population. Of note, they require two appropriately trained nurses or one anaesthesiologist plus one nurse to be present in the room at all times during a lidocaine infusion, as well as one-to-one nursing for the first hour of the infusion. If the patient remains stable and not overly sedated, then the nursing ratio can be dropped to one nurse per two patients. An anaesthesiologist must be present on site until the patient is suitable for discharge. Required equipment includes an ECG monitor, suction, oxygen source and delivery systems, intravenous supplies, emergency medications, a light source, and emergency power and lighting. Lidocaine infusions are to be administered by a programmable device with a locked control panel and delivered via a dedicated intravenous line. Loading doses are to be given only by an anaesthesiologist. Patient and vital sign monitoring should be performed every 5 min for the first 15 min, every 15 min for the next 45 min, and then every hour until the infusion is complete, then 30 min after discontinuation of the infusion [291].

2.12. Selection criteria for repeat IVLT in paediatric chronic pain

There is also a distinct lack of evidence to support the use of repeated IVLT for chronic pain management. The following criteria and dosing guidelines are also institutionally formulated based on clinical experience, see **Table 4**.

1.	Child/youth is fully integrated into multi-disciplinary care
2.	The pain syndrome is lidocaine-responsive based on previous lidocaine infusion.
3.	The pain is not amenable to the use of topical lidocaine
4.	The child/youth demonstrates some improvement in functional activity following on from previous lidocaine infusion
5.	Child/youth has no contra-indication to the use of systemic lidocaine such as major cardiac dysfunction, liver dysfunction, seizure activity, or allergy to amide local anaesthetics.
6.	Child/youth capable of verbally communicating analgesic response and symptoms of potential local anaesthetic toxicity.
7.	A high-acuity environment capable of providing continuous ECG monitoring, oxygen saturation, and frequent blood pressure measurements, plus access to healthcare personnel skilled in resuscitation and airway management.

Table 4. BCCH selection criteria for repeat systemic lidocaine therapy in child/youth.

Second infusion:

- Location and monitors as for initial infusion
- Loading dose: 1 mg/kg bolus
- Infusion increased to 7 mg/kg over 90 min
- Total dose: 8 mg/kg (loading dose + infusion)
- Time between infusions: usually a month

Third infusion:

- Location and monitors as above
- Loading dose: 1 mg/kg bolus
- Infusion increased to 9 mg/kg over 90–120 min
- Total dose: 10 mg/kg (loading dose + infusion)
- Time between infusions: usually a month

2.13. Continuous subcutaneous lidocaine therapy

If IVLT is effective or partially effective, the patient can be started on a 5-day continuous subcutaneous (SC) infusion if pain is hampering for restoration of function/physical activity (**Table 5**). SC infusions use an elastomer pump which delivers a set volume of lidocaine per hour (depending on the pump used), usually 5 ml/h, which approximately equates with 2 mg/kg/h using 2% lidocaine for a patient who is 50 kg. The infusion only runs whilst the patient is awake so that they can self-report any symptoms, which may suggest lidocaine toxicity.

1.	Child/youth is fully integrated into multi-disciplinary care
2.	Their pain syndrome is lidocaine-responsive.
3.	The pain is not amenable to the use of topical lidocaine
4.	Child/youth has no contra-indication to the use of systemic lidocaine.
5.	Child/youth capable of verbally communicating analgesic response and symptoms of early local anaesthetic toxicity.
6.	The child has previously experienced a lidocaine infusion in a high acuity environment without complication.
7.	The child/youth demonstrates some improvement in functional activity following on from previous lidocaine infusion/s.
8.	The child/youth and their principal carer demonstrate the ability to follow safety instructions.
9.	Appropriate homecare support, immediate telephone contact with healthcare team and follow-up are in place.

Table 5. BCCH selection criteria for subcutaneous lidocaine therapy in child/youth.

http://dx.doi.org/10.5772/66771

2.14. BCCH experience of lidocaine infusions for chronic pain

Of 336 new children/youth seen as out-patients by one pain physician in our institution over a 6.5 year time frame, only 45 (13%) were considered appropriate for trial of IVLT; 36/45 (80%) of these patients were females. The diagnoses, IVLT treatments and outcomes for these 45 children/youth are shown in **Tables 6** and 7.

	n (%), N = 45
Diagnosis	
Complex regional pain syndrome (CRPS)	24 (53%)
Neuropathic pain	7 (16%)
Headaches	4 (9%)
Diffuse muscular/whole body pain	4 (9%)
Other	6 (13%)
IVLT sessions	
1 IVLT session only	19 (42%)
2 IVLT sessions	19 (42%)
3 IVLT sessions	6 (13%)
4 IVLT sessions	1 (2%)

Table 6. Diagnoses and number of IVLT treatments received as part of 3P treatment package.

Improved outcome reported	Success ratio*
Physical functioning	32/43 (74%)
Pain	32/45 (71%)
Mood related to pain	22/31 (71%)
School	16/26 (62%)
Sleep	17/29 (59%)
Social functioning	8/21 (38%)

*Number of patients reporting improvement / number reporting issue prior to treatment.

Table 7. Improved outcomes reported by patients following 3P treatment including intravenous lidocaine therapy (IVLT).

It is clear that not all children and youth with chronic pain are candidates for IVLT. Focus should be on pain conditions with a neuropathic or central element. However, when appropriately selected, and integrated in multi-disciplinary care, IVLT can be part of the reason that children and youth experience less pain facilitating healthier sleep, improved physical activities, and return to school. It is also clear that not all children/youth considered appropriate for IVLT respond positively. This needs to be clearly outlined with a plan of management prior to embarking on an IVLT therapy.

2.15. The mechanism and effects of IVLT in chronic pain

The specific effects of IVLT rely on the pharmacological action of lidocaine. However, other elements of care are also critically important especially the psychosocial dynamics of the diagnosis and treatment process. Three mechanisms contribute to improvement in a patient's pain or functioning; the specific or intended effects of treatment, natural history of the disease and non-specific effects of treatment [292].

One non-specific treatment effect likely to improve treatment outcomes is high pre-treatment expectations of recovery [293–299]. Factors shown to modulate pre-treatment expectations include dispositional optimism [300–302], sex [297, 303], age [303], education level [297, 303], clinician-patient interactions [304] and degree of psychological distress [297]. Expectations can be enhanced by verbal suggestions, conditioning and imagery [299]. Influences likely to improve treatment outcomes include high expectations, no pre-existing mood disorder, low levels of anxiety, acceptance of the chronic pain diagnosis, a desire to get better, a need to return to a previous level of functioning, motivation and good clinician-to-child relationship and trust in the healthcare team.

Children and youth with chronic pain will require a lot of effort on the part of the clinicians to establish trust as they have met with many previous different healthcare workers; they may have been given mixed messages regarding the aetiology of pain, and potentially exposed to a negative encounter (not feeling believed that they have pain, lack of empathy, poor communication, lack of appropriate help).

To gain a child or youth's trust and that of their parents requires good communication [304–306]. This demands devotion of enough time to listen and extract a precise pain history, use of appropriate language and terminology, developmentally appropriate explanation of concepts [307] as well as understanding family culture, beliefs, hopes and fears. Trust necessitates that; potentially embarrassing questions are asked separately and in confidence and that the healthcare team convey empathy and expertise/credibility in chronic pain management. Introducing appropriate humour into the dialogue also helps to establish good rapport. It is also important to explain to a child/youth with ongoing pain that the healthcare team will attempt to minimise any pain on examination. During the initial assessment good education, establishing an agreed workable goal-directed and achievable management plan positively alters patient outlook as well as responses to treatment [298, 308]. Communicating positive expectations of treatment also contributes to decreased pain and improved functioning [309–311].

Psycho-social effects such as sadness, frustration, anxiety, anger, catastrophization or depression are the detrimental factors that are associated with continuation or worsening of pain. If these psychological factors remain unrecognized and untreated, they become barriers to the onward progress of any chronic pain management plan.

Without the evidence of a randomised double-blind placebo controlled trial, it is not easy to discern the over-riding beneficial therapeutic modality in the chronic pain case series presented. It could be argued that IVLT responsiveness, in tandem with good rapport and trust in the healthcare team, represents a placebo response. Such a response is defined as 'the psychobiological response seen after administration of a non-therapeutic modality'. Placebo treatments have known effects on endogenous pharmacology, as well as the cognitive and conditioning systems in humans [312–319]. The placebo response rate is higher in children compared with adults [320, 321]. Patient expectations and the doctor-patient relationship contribute to placebo analgesia responses and are unique to the individual [322]. The respiratory centres, serotonin secretion, hormone secretion, immune responses and heart function are also involved in the biological response to placebo analgesic treatments [319]. There is evidence that endogenous endorphins play a role as some placebo analgesic responses are reversed with naloxone [318, 323]. When considering non-analgesia placebo responses, dopamine also plays a major role [324]. Placebo response, or not, IVLT is a short intervention with minimal side effect profile, it is a worthwhile component of therapy that helps effect a turnaround to recovery in a child or youth who may have had pain and disability for many months prior to the intervention.

In an effort to increase the effectiveness of multi-disciplinary pain programs, more research is needed to further investigate pharmacological advances, psychological therapies and physiotherapy techniques that work for different ages, different types of pain and at different times in the chronic pain journey. It is clear that we also need to research and adopt clinical strategies aimed at optimising placebo and non-specific treatment effects in the paediatric population.

3. Conclusion

Intravenous lidocaine has peripherally and centrally mediated analgesic, anti-inflammatory and anti-hyperalgesic properties [176] with minimal side-effect profile if used at appropriate dosing in properly selected children/youths. It is ideally placed to be a useful adjunct in perioperative pain management to improve comfort, reduce opioid requirements and reduce the attendant opioid side effect profile.

The analgesic properties reflect the variable dose, time dependant, multimodal aspect of its action on voltage-gated Na channels and other receptors that affect nociceptive transmission pathways [23, 24, 45, 117, 146–148, 159, 162]. The anti-inflammatory effects of lidocaine are attributable to attenuation of neurogenic inflammation and subsequent blockade of neural transmission at the site of tissue injury [146, 162, 164, 165, 167].

The anti-hyperalgesic effect of lidocaine, through suppression of peripheral and central sensitization also diminishes the neuro-inflammatory response to pain [25, 168–171, 173, 325]. A basic understanding of pain physiology and pathophysiology is essential to understand how these three beneficial components of IVLT are effecting this response.

Evidence from adult work and clinical experience with paediatric patients indicates that IVLT is a modality, which needs to be considered for major surgical procedures where a regional technique is not indicated. This has promise to improve post-operative pain, reduce opioid requirements and prevent central sensitisation. More work needs to be done to demonstrate effective dose response and plasma levels of lidocaine that are associated with analgesic efficacy for different surgical pain models and whether continuation of the infusion into the post-operative phase will further reduce acute or chronic postsurgical pain.

Chronic pain of childhood is an extremely complex condition that can have devastating effects on physical, psychological and social functioning. The inter-disciplinary team management approach, based on pharmacology, physiotherapy and psychology, is the standard of care for children with severe or ongoing chronic pain. IVLT is a modality that may be considered when the history and examination findings confirm a central, neuropathic or CRPS aspect of the presenting pain. The current lack of evidence-base to support this recommendation does necessitate full disclosure of risks and benefits for informed consent and shared decision making to occur. IVLT must be explained in the right context as a small part of the multi-disciplinary care package, which focuses on de-medicalization and self-management. A singular focus on reducing pain intensity without considering improvement in physical activity, social functioning and overall quality of life is distinctly misguided. Treatment expectations need to be clear that IVLT is used to improve comfort to enable physiotherapy/physical functioning to go ahead and needs to be performed in tandem with all the other multi-disciplinary aspects of care.

Pain clinicians need to engage in large multi-site randomised controlled trials to provide the evidence-base to determine that IVLT is indeed an effective and safe treatment option in acute preventative multimodal analgesia and as an adjunct in the multi-disciplinary care of chronic pain in the paediatric population.

Acknowledgements

Nick West for his help with preparation of this chapter. Dr. T. Oberlander and Dr. C. Montgomery for their helpful reviewer comments.

Author details

Gillian R. Lauder

Address all correspondence to: glauder@cw.bc.ca

Department of Anesthesia, BC Children's Hospital, Vancouver, BC, Canada

References

[1] Einsten A, Infield L. The Evolution of Physics. New York: Simon & Schuster; 1938. 95 p.

[2] IASP Taxonomy [Internet]. The International Association for the Study of Pain. 2014 [cited 2016 Sep 16]. Available from: http://www.iasp-pain.org/Education/Content.aspx?ItemNumber=1698

[3] Ren K, Dubner R. Descending modulation in persistent pain: an update. Pain. 2002 Nov;100(1–2):1–6.

[4] Jensen KB, Regenbogen C, Ohse MC, Frasnelli J, Freiherr J, Lundström JN. Brain activations during pain: a neuroimaging meta-analysis of patients with pain and healthy controls. Pain. 2016 Jun;157(6):1279–86.

[5] Hunt SP, Mantyh PW. The molecular dynamics of pain control. Nat Rev Neurosci. 2001 Feb;2(2):83–91.

[6] Hollmann MW, Fischer LG, Byford AM, Durieux ME. Local anesthetic inhibition of m1 muscarinic acetylcholine signaling. Anesthesiology. 2000 Aug;93(2):497–509.

[7] Mao J, Chen LL. Systemic lidocaine for neuropathic pain relief. Pain. 2000;87(1):7–17.

[8] Ji RR, Xu ZZ, Strichartz G, Serhan CN. Emerging roles of resolving in the resolution of inflammation and pain. Trends Neurosci. 2011 Nov;34(11):599–609.

[9] Waxman SG, Zamponi GW. Regulating excitability of peripheral afferents: emerging ion channel targets. Nat Neurosci. 2014 Feb;17(2):153–63.

[10] Hollmann MW, McIntire WE, Garrison JC, Durieux ME. Inhibition of mammalian Gq protein function by local anesthetics. Anesthesiology. 2002 Dec;97(6):1451–7.

[11] Tappe-Theodor A, Constantin CE, Tegeder I, Lechner SG, Langeslag M, Lepcynzsky P, et al. Gα(q/11) signaling tonically modulates nociceptor function and contributes to activity-dependent sensitization. Pain. 2012 Jan;153(1):184–96.

[12] Malin SA, Molliver DC. Gi- and Gq-coupled ADP (P2Y) receptors act in opposition to modulate nociceptive signaling and inflammatory pain behavior. Mol Pain. 2010;6:21.

[13] Black JA, Liu S, Tanaka M, Cummins TR, Waxman SG. Changes in the expression of tetrodotoxin-sensitive sodium channels within dorsal root ganglia neurons in inflammatory pain. Pain. 2004 Apr;108(3):237–47.

[14] Matzner O, Devor M. Hyperexcitability at sites of nerve injury depends on voltage-sensitive Na+ channels. J Neurophysiol. 1994 Jul;72(1):349–59.

[15] Wall PD, Devor M. Sensory afferent impulses originate from dorsal root ganglia as well as from the periphery in normal and nerve injured rats. Pain. 1983 Dec;17(4):321–39.

[16] Tremont-Lukats IW, Challapalli V, McNicol ED, Lau J, Carr DB. Systemic administration of local anesthetics to relieve neuropathic pain: a systematic review and meta-analysis. Anesth Analg. 2005;101(6):1738–49.

[17] Dong XW, Goregoaker S, Engler H, Zhou X, Mark L, Crona J, et al. Small interfering RNA-mediated selective knockdown of Na(V)1.8 tetrodotoxin-resistant sodium channel reverses mechanical allodynia in neuropathic rats. Neuroscience. 2007 May 11;146(2):812–21.

[18] Nieto FR, Entrena JM, Cendán CM, Pozo E Del, Vela JM, Baeyens JM. Tetrodotoxin inhibits the development and expression of neuropathic pain induced by paclitaxel in mice. Pain. 2008 Jul 31;137(3):520–31.

[19] Baron R. Peripheral neuropathic pain: from mechanisms to symptoms. Clin J Pain. 2000 Jun;16(2 Suppl):S12–20.

[20] Cepeda MS, Lau J, Carr DB. Defining the therapeutic role of local anesthetic sympathetic blockade in complex regional pain syndrome: a narrative and systematic review. Clin J Pain. 2002;18(4):216–33.

[21] Devor M, Seltzer Z. Pathophysiology of damaged nerves in relation to chronic pain. In: Wall P, Melzack R, editors. Textbook of Pain. 4th ed. London, UK: Churchill Livingstone; 1999. pp. 129–64.

[22] Dib-Hajj SD, Cummins TR, Black JA, Waxman SG. Sodium channels in normal and pathological pain. Annu Rev Neurosci. 2010;33:325–47.

[23] Devor M, Wall PD, Catalan N. Systemic lidocaine silences ectopic neuroma and DRG discharge without blocking nerve conduction. Pain. 1992 Feb;48(2):261–8.

[24] Amir R, Argoff CE, Bennett GJ, Cummins TR, Durieux ME, Gerner P, et al. The role of sodium channels in chronic inflammatory and neuropathic pain. J Pain. 2006 May;7(5 Suppl 3):S1–29.

[25] Vranken JH. Elucidation of pathophysiology and treatment of neuropathic pain. Cent Nerv Syst Agents Med Chem. 2012 Dec;12(4):304–14.

[26] Dib-Hajj SD, Black JA, Waxman SG. Voltage-gated sodium channels: therapeutic targets for pain. Pain Med. 2009 Oct;10(7):1260–9.

[27] Liu M, Wood JN. The roles of sodium channels in nociception: implications for mechanisms of neuropathic pain. Pain Med. 2011 Jul;12(Suppl 3):S93–9.

[28] Levinson SR, Luo S, Henry MA. The role of sodium channels in chronic pain. Muscle Nerve. 2012 Aug;46(2):155–65.

[29] Perret D, Luo ZD. Targeting voltage-gated calcium channels for neuropathic pain management. Neurotherapeutics. 2009 Oct;6(4):679–92.

[30] Montell C. The history of TRP channels, a commentary and reflection. Pflügers Arch Eur J Physiol. 2011 May 2;461(5):499–506.

[31] Nilius B, Owsianik G. The transient receptor potential family of ion channels. Genome Biol. 2011;12(3):218.

[32] Damann N, Voets T, Nilius B. TRPs in our senses. Curr Biol. 2008 Sep 23;18(18):R880–9.

[33] Geppetti P, Nassini R, Materazzi S, Benemei S. The concept of neurogenic inflammation. BJU Int. 2008 Mar;101(Suppl 3):2–6.

[34] Fernandes ES, Russell FA, Spina D, McDougall JJ, Graepel R, Gentry C, et al. A distinct role for transient receptor potential ankyrin 1, in addition to transient receptor potential vanilloid 1, in tumor necrosis factor α-induced inflammatory hyperalgesia and Freund's complete adjuvant-induced monarthritis. Arthritis Rheum. 2011 Mar;63(3):819–29.

[35] Anand U, Otto WR, Facer P, Zebda N, Selmer I, Gunthorpe MJ, et al. TRPA1 receptor localisation in the human peripheral nervous system and functional studies in cultured human and rat sensory neurons. Neurosci Lett. 2008 Jun;438(2):221–7.

[36] Fernandes E, Fernandes M, Keeble J. The functions of TRPA1 and TRPV1: moving away from sensory nerves. Br J Pharmacol. 2012 May;166(2):510–21.

[37] Jordt S-E, Bautista DM, Chuang H, McKemy DD, Zygmunt PM, Högestätt ED, et al. Mustard oils and cannabinoids excite sensory nerve fibres through the TRP channel ANKTM1. Nature. 2004 Jan 15;427(6971):260–5.

[38] Story GM, Peier AM, Reeve AJ, Eid SR, Mosbacher J, Hricik TR, et al. ANKTM1, a TRP-like channel expressed in nociceptive neurons, is activated by cold temperatures. Cell. 2003 Mar 21;112(6):819–29.

[39] Bandell M, Story GM, Hwang SW, Viswanath V, Eid SR, Petrus MJ, et al. Noxious cold ion channel TRPA1 is activated by pungent compounds and Bradykinin. Neuron. 2004 Mar;41(6):849–57.

[40] Brierley SM, Castro J, Harrington AM, Hughes PA, Page AJ, Rychkov GY, et al. TRPA1 contributes to specific mechanically activated currents and sensory neuron mechanical hypersensitivity. J Physiol. 2011 Jul 15;589(14):3575–93.

[41] Corey DP, García-Añoveros J, Holt JR, Kwan KY, Lin SY, Vollrath MA, et al. TRPA1 is a candidate for the mechanosensitive transduction channel of vertebrate hair cells. Nature. 2004 Dec 9;432(7018):723–30.

[42] Doerner JF, Gisselmann G, Hatt H, Wetzel CH. Transient receptor potential channel A1 Is directly gated by calcium ions. J Biol Chem. 2007 May 4;282(18):13180–9.

[43] Obata K, Katsura H, Mizushima T, Yamanaka H, Kobayashi K, Dai Y, et al. TRPA1 induced in sensory neurons contributes to cold hyperalgesia after inflammation and nerve injury. J Clin Invest. 2005 Sep 1;115(9):2393–401.

[44] Frederick J, Buck ME, Matson DJ, Cortright DN. Increased TRPA1, TRPM8, and TRPV2 expression in dorsal root ganglia by nerve injury. Biochem Biophys Res Commun. 2007 Jul 13;358(4):1058–64.

[45] Kuo CP, Jao SW, Chen KM, Wong CS, Yeh CC, Sheen MJ, et al. Comparison of the effects of thoracic epidural analgesia and i.v. infusion with lidocaine on cytokine response, postoperative pain and bowel function in patients undergoing colonic surgery. Br J Anaesth. 2006;97(5):640–6.

[46] Chen J, Joshi SK, DiDomenico S, Perner RJ, Mikusa JP, Gauvin DM, et al. Selective blockade of TRPA1 channel attenuates pathological pain without altering noxious cold sensation or body temperature regulation. Pain. 2011 May;152(5):1165–72.

[47] Petrus M, Peier AM, Bandell M, Hwang S, Huynh T, Olney N, et al. A role of TRPA1 in mechanical hyperalgesia is revealed by pharmacological inhibition. Mol Pain. 2007;3(1):40.

[48] Foster E, Wildner H, Tudeau L, Haueter S, Ralvenius WT, Jegen M, et al. Targeted ablation, silencing, and activation establish glycinergic dorsal horn neurons as key components of a spinal gate for pain and itch. Neuron. 2015 Mar;85(6):1289–304.

[49] Honore P, Rogers SD, Schwei MJ, Salak-Johnson JL, Luger NM, Sabino MC, et al. Murine models of inflammatory, neuropathic and cancer pain each generates a unique set of neurochemical changes in the spinal cord and sensory neurons. Neuroscience. 2000;98(3):585–98.

[50] Todd AJ. Neuronal circuitry for pain processing in the dorsal horn. Nat Rev Neurosci. 2010 Dec;11(12):823–36.

[51] Braz J, Solorzano C, Wang X, Basbaum AI. Transmitting pain and itch messages: a contemporary view of the spinal cord circuits that generate gate control. Neuron. 2014 May 7;82(3):522–36.

[52] Prescott SA, Ma Q, De Koninck Y. Normal and abnormal coding of somatosensory stimuli causing pain. Nat Neurosci. 2014 Feb;17(2):183–91.

[53] Campbell JN, Raja SN, Meyer RA, Mackinnon SE. Myelinated afferents signal the hyperalgesia associated with nerve injury. Pain. 1988 Jan;32(1):89–94.

[54] Petrenko AB, Yamakura T, Baba H, Shimoji K. The role of N-methyl-D-aspartate (NMDA) receptors in pain: a review. Anesth Analg. 2003 Oct;1108–16.

[55] Tsuda M, Masuda T, Tozaki-Saitoh H, Inoue K. Microglial Regulation of neuropathic pain. J Pharmacol Sci. 2013;121(2):89–94.

[56] Tsuda M. Microglia in the spinal cord and neuropathic pain. J Diabetes Investig. 2016 Jan;7(1):17–26.

[57] Costigan M, Scholz J, Woolf CJ. Neuropathic Pain: a maladaptive response of the nervous system to damage. Annu Rev Neurosci. 2009 Jun;32(1):1–32.

[58] Inoue K, Tsuda M. Microglia and neuropathic pain. Glia. 2009 Nov 1;57(14):1469–79.

[59] Trang T, Beggs S, Wan X, Salter MW. P2X4-receptor-mediated synthesis and release of brain-derived neurotrophic factor in microglia is dependent on calcium and p38-mitogen-activated protein kinase activation. J Neurosci. 2009 Mar 18;29(11):3518–28.

[60] McMahon SB, Malcangio M. Current challenges in glia-pain biology. Neuron. 2009 Oct;64(1):46–54.

[61] Woolf CJ, Salter MW. Neuronal plasticity: increasing the gain in pain. Science. 2000 Jun 9;288(5472):1765–9.

[62] Seifert F, Maihöfner C. Functional and structural imaging of pain-induced neuroplasticity. Curr Opin Anaesthesiol. 2011 Oct;24(5):515–23.

[63] Apkarian AV, Bushnell MC, Treede RD, Zubieta JK. Human brain mechanisms of pain perception and regulation in health and disease. Eur J Pain. 2005 Aug;9(4):463–84.

[64] Sutters KA, Miaskowski C. Inadequate pain management and associated morbidity in children at home after tonsillectomy. J Pediatr Nurs. 1997 Jun;12(3):178–85.

[65] McCaffrey M, Pasero C. Pain: Clinical Manual. St. Louis, MO: Mosby; 1999.

[66] Kokki H. Current management of pediatric postoperative pain. Expert Rev Neurother. 2004 Mar;4(2):295–306.

[67] Strassels S, McNicol E, Wagner A, Rogers W, Gouveia W, Carr D. Persistent postoperative pain, health-related quality of life, and functioning 1 month after hospital discharge. Acute Pain. 2004;6(3):95–104.

[68] Sinatra R. Causes and consequences of inadequate management of acute pain. Pain Med. 2010 Dec;11(12):1859–71.

[69] Ruscheweyh R, Deppe M, Lohmann H, Stehling C, Flöel A, Ringelstein BE, et al. Pain is associated with regional grey matter reduction in the general population. Pain. 2011 Apr;152(4):904–11.

[70] Power NM, Howard RF, Wade AM, Franck LS. Pain and behaviour changes in children following surgery. Arch Dis Child. 2012 Oct;97(10):879–84.

[71] Rabbitts JA, Palermo TM, Zhou C, Mangione-Smith R. Pain and health-related quality of life after pediatric inpatient surgery. J Pain. 2015 Dec;16(12):1334–41.

[72] Crombie IK, Davies HT, Macrae WA. Cut and thrust: antecedent surgery and trauma among patients attending a chronic pain clinic. Pain. 1998 May;76(1–2):167–71.

[73] Kehlet H, Jensen TS, Woolf CJ. Persistent postsurgical pain: risk factors and prevention. Lancet (London, England). 2006 May 13;367(9522):1618–25.

[74] Macrae WA. Chronic post-surgical pain: 10 years on. Br J Anaesth. 2008 Jul;101(1):77–86.

[75] Poleshuck EL, Katz J, Andrus CH, Hogan LA, Jung BF, Kulick DI, et al. Risk factors for chronic pain following breast cancer surgery: a prospective study. J Pain. 2006 Sep;7(9):626–34.

[76] Poobalan AS, Bruce J, Smith WCS, King PM, Krukowski ZH, Chambers WA. A review of chronic pain after inguinal herniorrhaphy. Clin J Pain. 2003;19(1):48–54.

[77] Aasvang EK, Kehlet H. Chronic pain after childhood groin hernia repair. J Pediatr Surg. 2007 Aug;42(8):1403–8.

[78] Fortier MA, Chou J, Maurer EL, Kain ZN. Acute to chronic postoperative pain in children: preliminary findings. J Pediatr Surg. 2011 Sep;46(9):1700–5.

[79] Kristensen AD, Pedersen TAL, Hjortdal VE, Jensen TS, Nikolajsen L. Chronic pain in adults after thoracotomy in childhood or youth. Br J Anaesth. 2010 Jan;104(1):75–9.

[80] Pagé MG, Stinson J, Campbell F, Isaac L, Katz J. Identification of pain-related psychological risk factors for the development and maintenance of pediatric chronic postsurgical pain. J Pain Res. 2013;6:167–80.

[81] Connelly M, Fulmer RD, Prohaska J, Anson L, Dryer L, Thomas V, et al. Predictors of postoperative pain trajectories in adolescent idiopathic scoliosis. Spine (Phila Pa 1976). 2014 Feb 1;39(3):E174–81.

[82] Landman Z, Oswald T, Sanders J, Diab M, Spinal Deformity Study Group. Prevalence and predictors of pain in surgical treatment of adolescent idiopathic scoliosis. Spine (Phila Pa 1976). 2011 May 1;36(10):825–9.

[83] Sieberg CB, Simons LE, Edelstein MR, DeAngelis MR, Pielech M, Sethna N, et al. Pain prevalence and trajectories following pediatric spinal fusion surgery. J Pain. 2013 Dec;14(12):1694–702.

[84] Rabbitts JA, Zhou C, Groenewald CB, Durkin L, Palermo TM. Trajectories of postsurgical pain in children: risk factors and impact of late pain recovery on long-term health outcomes after major surgery. Pain. 2015 Nov;156(11):2383–9.

[85] Nikolajsen L, Brix LD. Chronic pain after surgery in children. Curr Opin Anaesthesiol. 2014 Oct;27(5):507–12.

[86] Finley G, Franck L, Grunau R, von Baeyer C. Why children's pain matters. Pain Clin Updat. 2005;13(4):1–6.

[87] Katz J, Clarke H, Seltzer Z. Review article: Preventive analgesia: quo vadimus? Anesth Analg. 2011 Nov;113(5):1242–53.

[88] Vadivelu N, Mitra S, Schermer E, Kodumudi V, Kaye AD, Urman RD. Preventive analgesia for postoperative pain control: a broader concept. Local Reg Anesth. 2014;7:17–22.

[89] McQuay HJ. Pre-emptive analgesia. Br J Anaesth. 1992 Jul;69(1):1–3.

[90] Kehlet H, Dahl JB. The value of "multimodal" or "balanced analgesia" in postoperative pain treatment. Anesth Analg. 1993 Nov;77(5):1048–56.

[91] Lavand'homme P, De Kock M, Waterloos H. Intraoperative epidural analgesia combined with ketamine provides effective preventive analgesia in patients undergoing major digestive surgery. Anesthesiology. 2005 Oct;103(4):813–20.

[92] Gilron I, Orr E, Tu D, Mercer CD, Bond D. A randomized, double-blind, controlled trial of perioperative administration of gabapentin, meloxicam and their combination for spontaneous and movement-evoked pain after ambulatory laparoscopic cholecystectomy. Anesth Analg. 2009 Feb;108(2):623–30.

[93] White PF, Sacan O, Tufanogullari B, Eng M, Nuangchamnong N, Ogunnaike B. Effect of short-term postoperative celecoxib administration on patient outcome after outpatient laparoscopic surgery. Can J Anaesth = J Can d'anesthésie. 2007 May;54(5):342–8.

[94] Andreae MH, Andreae DA. Regional anaesthesia to prevent chronic pain after surgery: a Cochrane systematic review and meta-analysis. Br J Anaesth. 2013 Nov 1;111(5):711–20.

[95] White PF. Multimodal analgesia: its role in preventing postoperative pain. Curr Opin Investig Drugs. 2008 Jan;9(1):76–82.

[96] Moizo E, Berti M, Marchetti C, Deni F, Albertin A, Muzzolon F, et al. Acute Pain Service and multimodal therapy for postsurgical pain control: evaluation of protocol efficacy. Minerva Anestesiol. 2004 Nov;70(11):779–87.

[97] Lenk C. Off-label drug use in paediatrics: a world-wide problem. Curr Drug Targets. 2012 Jun;13(7):878–84.

[98] Horen B, Montastruc J-L, Lapeyre-Mestre M. Adverse drug reactions and off-label drug use in paediatric outpatients. Br J Clin Pharmacol [Internet]. 2002 Dec;54(6):665–70. Available from: http://www.pubmedcentral.nih.gov/articlerender.fcgi?artid=PMC1874497

[99] Kehlet H, Dahl JB. Assessment of postoperative pain--need for action! Pain. 2011 Aug;152(8):1699–700.

[100] Brouwers MC, Kho ME, Browman GP, Burgers JS, Cluzeau F, Feder G, et al. AGREE II: advancing guideline development, reporting and evaluation in health care. CMAJ. 2010 Dec 14;182(18):E839–42.

[101] Morrison RS, Magaziner J, McLaughlin MA, Orosz G, Silberzweig SB, Koval KJ, et al. The impact of post-operative pain on outcomes following hip fracture. Pain. 2003 Jun;103(3):303–11.

[102] Kankkunen P, Vehviläinen-Julkunen K, Pietilä AM, Kokki H, Halonen P. Parents' perceptions and use of analgesics at home after children's day surgery. Paediatr Anaesth. 2003 Feb;13(2):132–40.

[103] Liossi C, White P, Hatira P. Randomized clinical trial of local anesthetic versus a combination of local anesthetic with self-hypnosis in the management of pediatric procedure-related pain. Health Psychol [Internet]. 2006 May;25(3):307–15. Available from: http://www.ncbi.nlm.nih.gov/pubmed/16719602

[104] Tsao JCI, Zeltzer LK. Complementary and alternative medicine approaches for pediatric pain: a review of the state-of-the-science. Evid Based Complement Alternat Med. 2005 Jun;2(2):149–59.

[105] Pillai Riddell RR, Racine NM, Gennis HG, Turcotte K, Uman LS, Horton RE, et al. Non-pharmacological management of infant and young child procedural pain. Cochrane database Syst Rev. 2015;12:CD006275.

[106] Stevens BJ, Abbott LK, Yamada J, Harrison D, Stinson J, Taddio A, et al. Epidemiology and management of painful procedures in children in Canadian hospitals. CMAJ. 2011 Apr 19;183(7):E403–10.

[107] Silverman SM. Opioid induced hyperalgesia: clinical implications for the pain practitioner. Pain Physician. 2009;12(3):679–84.

[108] King T, Vardanyan A, Majuta L, Melemedjian O, Nagle R, Cress AE, et al. Morphine treatment accelerates sarcoma-induced bone pain, bone loss, and spontaneous fracture in a murine model of bone cancer. Pain. 2007 Nov;132(1–2):154–68.

[109] Younger JW, Chu LF, D'Arcy NT, Trott KE, Jastrzab LE, Mackey SC. Prescription opioid analgesics rapidly change the human brain. Pain. 2011 Aug;152(8):1803–10.

[110] Sacerdote P, Bianchi M, Gaspani L, Manfredi B, Maucione A, Terno G, et al. The effects of tramadol and morphine on immune responses and pain after surgery in cancer patients. Anesth Analg. 2000 Jun;90(6):1411–4.

[111] Seyfried O, Hester J. Opioids and endocrine dysfunction. Br J Pain. 2012 Feb;6(1):17–24.

[112] Dowden SJ. Considerations of non-medical use of prescription opioids (NMUPO) in pediatric pain management. Pediatr Pain Lett 2014.

[113] Koppert W, Zeck S, Sittl R, Likar R, Knoll R, Schmelz M. Low-dose lidocaine suppresses experimentally induced hyperalgesia in humans. Anesthesiology. 1998 Dec;89(6):1345–53.

[114] Koppert W, Ostermeier N, Sittl R, Weidner C, Schmelz M. Low-dose lidocaine reduces secondary hyperalgesia by a central mode of action. Pain. 2000 Mar;85(1–2):217–24.

[115] Pinter A, Dorian P. Intravenous antiarrhythmic agents. Curr Opin Cardiol. 2001 Jan;16(1):17–22.

[116] Mazoit JX, Dalens BJ. Pharmacokinetics of local anaesthetics in infants and children. Clin Pharmacokinet. 2004;43(1):17–32.

[117] Tanelian DL, MacIver MB. Analgesic concentrations of lidocaine suppress tonic A-delta and C fiber discharges produced by acute injury. Anesthesiology. 1991 May;74(5):934–6.

[118] Wallace MS, Laitin S, Licht D, Yaksh TL. Concentration-effect relations for intravenous lidocaine infusions in human volunteers: effects on acute sensory thresholds and capsaicin-evoked hyperpathia. Anesthesiology. 1997 Jun;86(6):1262–72.

[119] Collinsworth KA, Kalman SM, Harrison DC. The clinical pharmacology of lidocaine as an antiarrhythymic drug. Circulation. 1974 Dec;50(6):1217–30.

[120] Wallace MS, Ridgeway BM, Leung AY, Gerayli A, Yaksh TL. Concentration-effect relationship of intravenous lidocaine on the allodynia of complex regional pain syndrome types I and II. Anesthesiology. 2000 Jan;92(1):75–83.

[121] Tsai PS, Buerkle H, Huang LT, Lee TC, Yang LC, Lee JH. Lidocaine concentrations in plasma and cerebrospinal fluid after systemic bolus administration in humans. Anesth Analg. 1998 Sep;87(3):601–4.

[122] LeLorier J, Grenon D, Latour Y, Caillé G, Dumont G, Brosseau A, et al. Pharmacokinetics of lidocaine after prolonged intravenous infusions in uncomplicated myocardial infarction. Ann Intern Med. 1977 Dec;87(6):700–6.

[123] Finholt DA, Stirt JA, DiFazio CA, Moscicki JC. Lidocaine pharmacokinetics in children during general anesthesia. Anesth Analg. 1986 Mar;65(3):279–82.

[124] Skinner A V. Neonatal pharmacology. Anaesth Intensive Care Med. 2011 Mar;12(3): 79–84.

[125] van den Broek MPH, Huitema ADR, van Hasselt JGC, Groenendaal F, Toet MC, Egberts TCG, et al. Lidocaine (Lignocaine) dosing regimen based upon a population pharmacokinetic model for preterm and term neonates with seizures. Clin Pharmacokinet. 2011 Jul;50(7):461–9.

[126] Lundqvist M, Ågren J, Hellström-Westas L, Flink R, Wickström R. Efficacy and safety of lidocaine for treatment of neonatal seizures. Acta Paediatrica. 2013 Sep;102(9):863–7.

[127] Challapalli V, Tremont-Lukats IW, McNicol ED, Lau J, Carr DB. Systemic administration of local anesthetic agents to relieve neuropathic pain. Cochrane database Syst Rev. 2005;(4):CD003345.

[128] Kranke P, Jokinen J, Pace NL, Schnabel A, Hollmann MW, Hahnenkamp K, et al. Continuous intravenous perioperative lidocaine infusion for postoperative pain and recovery. Cochrane database Syst Rev. 2015;7:CD009642.

[129] Rowland M, Thomson PD, Guichard A, Melmon KL. Disposition kinetics of lidocaine in normal subjects. Ann N Y Acad Sci. 1971 Jul 6;179:383–98.

[130] Ciechanowicz S, Patil V. Lipid emulsion for local anesthetic systemic toxicity. Anesthesiol Res Pract. 2012;2012:1–11.

[131] Kosharskyy B, Almonte W, Shaparin N, Pappagallo M, Smith H. Intravenous infusions in chronic pain management. Pain Physician. 2013;16:231–249.

[132] Ferrini R, Paice JA. How to initiate and monitor infusional lidocaine for severe and/or neuropathic pain. J Support Oncol. 2004;2(1):90–4.

[133] Mooney JJ, Pagel PS, Kundu A. Safety, Tolerability, and short-term efficacy of intravenous lidocaine infusions for the treatment of chronic pain in adolescents and young adults: a preliminary report. Pain Med. 2014;1–6.

[134] Neal JM, Deck JJ, Kopacz DJ, Lewis MA. Hospital discharge after ambulatory knee arthroscopy: a comparison of epidural 2-chloroprocaine versus lidocaine. Reg Anesth Pain Med. 2001;26(1):35–40.

[135] Sotgiu ML, Biella G, Castagna A, Lacerenza M, Marchettini P. Different time-courses of i.v. lidocaine effect on ganglionic and spinal units in neuropathic rats. Neuroreport. 1994 Apr 14;5(8):873–6.

[136] Omana-Zapata I, Khabbaz MA, Hunter JC, Bley KR. QX-314 inhibits ectopic nerve activity associated with neuropathic pain. Brain Res. 1997 Oct 17;771(2):228–37.

[137] Abram SE, Yaksh TL. Systemic lidocaine blocks nerve injury-induced hyperalgesia and nociceptor-driven spinal sensitization in the rat. Anesthesiology. 1994 Feb;80(2):383–91; discussion 25A.

[138] Yaksh TL. Spinal systems and pain processing: development of novel analgesic drugs with mechanistically defined models. Trends Pharmacol Sci. 1999 Aug;20(8):329–37.

[139] Ferrante FM, Paggioli J, Cherukuri S, Arthur GR. The analgesic response to intravenous lidocaine in the treatment of neuropathic pain. Anesth Analg. 1996 Jan;82(1):91–7.

[140] Kalso E, Tramèr MR, McQuay HJ, Moore RA. Systemic local-anaesthetic-type drugs in chronic pain: a systematic review. Eur J Pain. 1998 Mar;2(1):3–14.

[141] Hollmann MW, Durieux ME. Local anesthetics and the inflammatory response: a new therapeutic indication? Anesthesiology. 2000 Sep;93(3):858–75.

[142] Kastrup J, Angelo H, Petersen P, Dejgård A, Hilsted J. Treatment of chronic painful diabetic neuropathy with intravenous lidocaine infusion. Br Med J (Clin Res Ed). 1986 Jan 18;292(6514):173.

[143] Lindström P, Lindblom U. The analgesic effect of tocainide in trigeminal neuralgia. Pain. 1987 Jan;28(1):45–50.

[144] Rowbotham MC, Reisner-Keller LA, Fields HL. Both intravenous lidocaine and morphine reduce the pain of postherpetic neuralgia. Neurology. 1991 Jul;41(7):1024–8.

[145] van der Wal SEI, van den Heuvel SAS, Radema SA, van Berkum BFM, Vaneker M, Steegers MAH, et al. The in vitro mechanisms and in vivo efficacy of intravenous lidocaine on the neuroinflammatory response in acute and chronic pain. Eur J Pain. 2016 May;20(5):655–74.

[146] Lahav M, Levite M, Bassani L, Lang A, Fidder H, Tal R, et al. Lidocaine inhibits secretion of IL-8 and IL-1beta and stimulates secretion of IL-1 receptor antagonist by epithelial cells. Clin Exp Immunol. 2002;127(2):226–33.

[147] Olschewski A, Olschewski H, Bräu ME, Hempelmann G, Vogel W, Safronov B V. Effect of bupivacaine on ATP-dependent potassium channels in rat cardiomyocytes. Br J Anaesth. 1999 Mar;82(3):435–8.

[148] Wolff M, Schnöbel-Ehehalt R, Mühling J, Weigand MA, Olschewski A. Mechanisms of lidocaine's action on subtypes of spinal dorsal horn neurons subject to the diverse roles of Na(+) and K(+) channels in action potential generation. Anesth Analg. 2014 Aug;119(2):463–70.

[149] Akaike N, Ito H, Nishi K, Oyama Y. Further analysis of inhibitory effects of propranolol and local anaesthetics on the calcium current in Helix neurones. Br J Pharmacol. 1982 May;76(1):37–43.

[150] Oyama Y, Sadoshima J, Tokutomi N, Akaike N. Some properties of inhibitory action of lidocaine on the Ca^{2+} current of single isolated frog sensory neurons. Brain Res. 1988 Mar 1;442(2):223–8.

[151] Sugiyama K, Muteki T. Local anesthetics depress the calcium current of rat sensory neurons in culture. Anesthesiology. 1994 Jun;80(6):1369–78.

[152] Hirota K, Browne T, Appadu BL, Lambert DG. Do local anaesthetics interact with dihydropyridine binding sites on neuronal L-type Ca^{2+} channels? Br J Anaesth. 1997 Feb;78(2):185–8.

http://dx.doi.org/10.5772/66771

[153] Hollmann MW, Ritter CH, Henle P, de Klaver M, Kamatchi GL, Durieux ME. Inhibition of m3 muscarinic acetylcholine receptors by local anaesthetics. Br J Pharmacol. 2001 May;133(1):207–16.

[154] Gould HJ, England JD, Liu ZP, Levinson SR. Rapid sodium channel augmentation in response to inflammation induced by complete Freund's adjuvant. Brain Res. 1998 Aug 17;802(1–2):69–74.

[155] Coward K, Plumpton C, Facer P, Birch R, Carlstedt T, Tate S, et al. Immunolocalization of SNS/PN3 and NaN/SNS2 sodium channels in human pain states. Pain. 2000 Mar;85(1–2):41–50.

[156] Coward K, Jowett A, Plumpton C, Powell A, Birch R, Tate S, et al. Sodium channel beta1 and beta2 subunits parallel SNS/PN3 alpha-subunit changes in injured human sensory neurons. Neuroreport. 2001 Mar 5;12(3):483–8.

[157] Abdi S, Lee DH, Chung JM. The anti-allodynic effects of amitriptyline, gabapentin, and lidocaine in a rat model of neuropathic pain. Anesth Analg. 1998 Dec;87(6):1360–6.

[158] Wall PD, Gutnick M. Properties of afferent nerve impulses originating from a neuroma. Nature. 1974 Apr 26;248(5451):740–3.

[159] Chabal C, Russell LC, Burchiel KJ. The effect of intravenous lidocaine, tocainide, and mexiletine on spontaneously active fibers originating in rat sciatic neuromas. Pain. 1989 Sep;38(3):333–8.

[160] Kajander KC, Wakisaka S, Bennett GJ. Spontaneous discharge originates in the dorsal root ganglion at the onset of a painful peripheral neuropathy in the rat. Neurosci Lett. 1992 Apr 27;138(2):225–8.

[161] Stebbing MJ, Bornstein JC. Electrophysiological analysis of the convergence of peripheral inputs onto neurons of the coeliac ganglion in the guinea pig. J Auton Nerv Syst. 1994;46(1–2):93–105.

[162] Woolf CJ, Wiesenfeld-Hallin Z. The systemic administration of local anaesthetics produces a selective depression of C-afferent fibre evoked activity in the spinal cord. Pain. 1985 Dec;23(4):361–74.

[163] Docherty RJ, Ginsberg L, Jadoon S, Orrell RW, Bhattacharjee A. TRPA1 insensitivity of human sural nerve axons after exposure to lidocaine. Pain. 2013;154(9):1569–77.

[164] Huang YH, Tsai PS, Kai YF, Yang CH, Huang CJ. Lidocaine inhibition of inducible nitric oxide synthase and cationic amino acid transporter-2 transcription in activated murine macrophages may involve voltage-sensitive Na+ channel. Anesth Analg. 2006 Jun;102(6):1739–44.

[165] Lee PY, Tsai PS, Huang YH, Huang CJ. Inhibition of toll-like receptor-4, nuclear factor-κb and mitogen-activated protein kinase by lignocaine may involve voltage-sensitive sodium channels. Clin Exp Pharmacol Physiol. 2008 Sep;35(9):1052–8.

[166] de Klaver MJM, Buckingham M-G, Rich GF. Lidocaine attenuates cytokine-induced cell injury in endothelial and vascular smooth muscle cells. Anesth Analg. 2003 Aug;97(2):465–70, table of contents.

[167] Sotgiu ML, Lacerenza M, Marchettini P. Selective inhibition by systemic lidocaine of noxious evoked activity in rat dorsal horn neurons. Neuroreport. 1991 Aug;2(8):425–8.

[168] Muth-Selbach U, Hermanns H, Stegmann JU, Kollosche K, Freynhagen R, Bauer I, et al. Antinociceptive effects of systemic lidocaine: involvement of the spinal glycinergic system. Eur J Pharmacol. 2009 Jun 24;613(1–3):68–73.

[169] Gronwald C, Vegh V, Hollmann MW, Hahnenkamp A, Garaj V, Hahnenkamp K. The inhibitory potency of local anesthetics on NMDA receptor signalling depends on their structural features. Eur J Pharmacol. 2012 Jan 5;674(1):13–9.

[170] Sugimoto M, Uchida I, Mashimo T. Local anaesthetics have different mechanisms and sites of action at the recombinant N-methyl-D-aspartate (NMDA) receptors. Br J Pharmacol. 2003 Mar;138(5):876–82.

[171] Parsons CG. NMDA receptors as targets for drug action in neuropathic pain. Eur J Pharmacol. 2001 Oct 19;429(1–3):71–8.

[172] Werdehausen R, Kremer D, Brandenburger T, Schlösser L, Jadasz J, Küry P, et al. Lidocaine metabolites inhibit glycine transporter 1: a novel mechanism for the analgesic action of systemic lidocaine? Erratum Anesthesiology. 2012 Jan;116(6):1404.

[173] Werdehausen R, Mittnacht S, Bee LA, Minett MS, Armbruster A, Bauer I, et al. The lidocaine metabolite N-ethylglycine has antinociceptive effects in experimental inflammatory and neuropathic pain. Pain. 2015 Sep;156(9):1647–59.

[174] Hara K, Sata T. The effects of the local anesthetics lidocaine and procaine on glycine and γ-aminobutyric acid receptors expressed in xenopus oocytes. Anesth Analg. 2007 Jun;104(6):1434–9.

[175] Richards N, McMahon SB. Targeting novel peripheral mediators for the treatment of chronic pain. Br J Anaesth. 2013 Jul;111(1):46–51.

[176] Attal N, Gaudé V, Brasseur L, Dupuy M, Guirimand F, Parker F, et al. Intravenous lidocaine in central pain: a double-blind, placebo-controlled, psychophysical study. Neurology. 2000 Feb 8;54(3):564–74.

[177] Ossipov MH, Lai J, Malan TP, Porreca F. Spinal and supraspinal mechanisms of neuropathic pain. Ann N Y Acad Sci. 2000;909:12–24.

[178] Chen Q, King T, Vanderah TW, Ossipov MH, Malan TP, Lai J, et al. Differential blockade of nerve injury-induced thermal and tactile hypersensitivity by systemically administered brain-penetrating and peripherally restricted local anesthetics. J Pain. 2004 Jun;5(5):281–9.

[179] Bartlett EE, Hutserani O. Xylocaine for the relief of postoperative pain. Anesth Analg. 1961;40:296–304.

[180] Stayer SA, Pasquariello CA, Schwartz RE, Balsara RK, Lear BR. The safety of continuous pleural lignocaine after thoracotomy in children and adolescents. Paediatr Anaesth. 1995;5(5):307–10.

http://dx.doi.org/10.5772/66771

[181] Sun Y, Li T, Wang N, Yun Y, Gan TJ. Perioperative systemic lidocaine for postoperative analgesia and recovery after abdominal surgery. Dis Colon Rectum. 2012;55(11):1183–94.

[182] Macintyre P, Schug S, Scott D, Visser E, Walker S. APM:SE Working Group of the Australian and New Zealand College of Anaesthetists and Faculty of Pain Medicine. In: Acute Pain Management: Scientific Evidence. 3rd ed. Melbourne: ANZCA & FPM; 2010.

[183] McCarthy GC, Megalla S a, Habib AS. Impact of intravenous lidocaine infusion on postoperative analgesia and recovery from surgery: a systematic review of randomized controlled trials. Drugs. 2010 Jun 18;70(9):1149–63.

[184] Vigneault L, Turgeon AF, Côté D, Lauzier F, Zarychanski R, Moore L, et al. Perioperative intravenous lidocaine infusion for postoperative pain control: a meta-analysis of randomized controlled trials. Can J Anaesth. 2011 Jan;58(1):22–37.

[185] Weibel S, Jokinen J, Pace NL, Schnabel A, Hollmann MW, Hahnenkamp K, et al. Efficacy and safety of intravenous lidocaine for postoperative analgesia and recovery after surgery: a systematic review with trial sequential analysis. Br J Anaesth. 2016 Jun;116(6):770–83.

[186] Cui W, Li Y, Li S, Wang R, Li J. Systemic administration of lidocaine reduces morphine requirements and postoperative pain of patients undergoing thoracic surgery after propofol-remifentanil-based anaesthesia. Eur J Anaesthesiol. 2010 Jan;27(1):41–6.

[187] Farag E, Ghobrial M, Sessler DI, Dalton JE, Liu J, Lee JH, et al. Effect of perioperative intravenous lidocaine administration on pain, opioid consumption, and quality of life after complex spine surgery. Anesthesiology. 2013;119(4):932–40.

[188] Soltani H, Nasr M, Siadat Z. Effects of Lidocaine on Reducing the Need for Anesthetic Drugs during Ophthalmologic Surgeries. J Isfahan Med Sch. 2013;31(224):41–9.

[189] Swenson BR, Gottschalk A, Wells LT, Rowlingson JC, Thompson PW, Barclay M, et al. Intravenous lidocaine is as effective as epidural bupivacaine in reducing ileus duration, hospital stay, and pain after open colon resection: a randomized clinical trial. Reg Anesth Pain Med. 2010;35(4):370–6.

[190] Wu CT, Borel CO, Lee MS, Yu JC, Liou HS, Yi HD, et al. The interaction effect of perioperative cotreatment with dextromethorphan and intravenous lidocaine on pain relief and recovery of bowel function after laparoscopic cholecystectomy. Anesth Analg. 2005 Feb;100(2):448–53.

[191] Bryson GL, Charapov I, Krolczyk G, Taljaard M, Reid D. Intravenous lidocaine does not reduce length of hospital stay following abdominal hysterectomy. Can J Anaesth = J Can d'anesthésie. 2010 Aug;57(8):759–66.

[192] Choi SJ, Kim MH, Jeong HY, Lee JJ. Effect of intraoperative lidocaine on anesthetic consumption, and bowel function, pain intensity, analgesic consumption and hospital stay after breast surgery. Korean J Anesthesiol [Internet]. 2012 May;62(5):429–34. Available from: http://www.ncbi.nlm.nih.gov/pubmed/22679539

[193] De Oliveira GS, Fitzgerald P, Streicher LF, Marcus RJ, McCarthy RJ. Systemic lidocaine to improve postoperative quality of recovery after ambulatory laparoscopic surgery. Anesth Analg. 2012 Aug;115(2):262–7.

[194] De Oliveira GS, Duncan K, Fitzgerald P, Nader A, Gould RW, McCarthy RJ. Systemic lidocaine to improve quality of recovery after laparoscopic bariatric surgery: a randomized double-blinded placebo-controlled trial. Obes Surg. 2014 Feb;24(2):212–8.

[195] Kang H, Kim BG. Intravenous lidocaine for effective pain relief after inguinal herniorrhaphy: a prospective, randomized, double-blind, placebo-controlled study. J Int Med Res. 2011;39(2):435–45.

[196] Kim TH, Kang H, Hong JH, Park JS, Baek CW, Kim JY, et al. Intraperitoneal and intravenous lidocaine for effective pain relief after laparoscopic appendectomy: a prospective, randomized, double-blind, placebo-controlled study. Surg Endosc. 2011 Oct;25(10):3183–90.

[197] Kim TH, Kang H, Choi YS, Park JM, Chi KC, Shin HY, et al. Pre- and intraoperative lidocaine injection for preemptive analgesics in laparoscopic gastrectomy: a prospective, randomized, double-blind, placebo-controlled study. J Laparoendosc Adv Surg Tech A. 2013 Aug;23(8):663–8.

[198] Lauwick S, Kim DJ, Michelagnoli G, Mistraletti G, Feldman L, Fried G, et al. Intraoperative infusion of lidocaine reduces postoperative fentanyl requirements in patients undergoing laparoscopic cholecystectomy. Can J Anaesth = J Can d'anesthésie. 2008 Nov;55(11):754–60.

[199] Lauwick S, Kim DJ, Mistraletti G, Carli F. Functional walking capacity as an outcome measure of laparoscopic prostatectomy: the effect of lidocaine infusion. Br J Anaesth. 2009 Aug;103(2):213–9.

[200] Lee EH, Lee HM, Chung CH, Chin JH, Choi DK, Chung HJ, et al. Impact of intravenous lidocaine on myocardial injury after off-pump coronary artery surgery. Br J Anaesth. 2011 Apr;106(4):487–93.

[201] Omar A. Can systemic lidocaine be used in controlled hypotension? A double-blinded randomized controlled study in patients undergoing functional endoscopic sinus surgery. Egypt J Anaesth. 2013;29:295–300.

[202] Saadawy IM, Kaki AM, Abd El Latif AA, Abd-Elmaksoud AM, Tolba OM. Lidocaine vs. magnesium: effect on analgesia after a laparoscopic cholecystectomy. Acta Anaesthesiol Scand. 2010 May;54(5):549–56.

[203] Slovack M, Taylor B, Bryce R, D Ong. Does intravenous lidocaine infusion during video-assisted thoracoscopic surgery reduce postoperative analgesia? A randomized controlled study. Unpubl data Can J. Anesth. 2015; 62: 676–677.

[204] Wang D, Wu X, Li J, Xiao F, Liu X, Meng M. The effect of lidocaine on early postoperative cognitive dysfunction after coronary artery bypass surgery. Anesth Analg. 2002 Nov;95(5):1134–41, table of contents.

[205] Yang SY, Kang H, Choi GJ, Shin HY, Baek CW, Jung YH, et al. Efficacy of intraperitoneal and intravenous lidocaine on pain relief after laparoscopic cholecystectomy. J Int Med Res. 2014 Apr;42(2):307–19.

[206] Yardeni IZ, Beilin B, Mayburd E, Levinson Y, Bessler H. The effect of perioperative intravenous lidocaine on postoperative pain and immune function. Anesth Analg. 2009 Nov;109(5):1464–9.

[207] Baral BK, Bhattarai BK, Rahman TR, Singh SN, Regmi R. Perioperative intravenous lidocaine infusion on postoperative pain relief in patients undergoing upper abdominal surgery. Nepal Med Coll J. 2010 Dec;12(4):215–20.

[208] El-Tahan MR, Warda OM, Diab DG, Ramzy EA, Matter MK. A randomized study of the effects of perioperative i.v. lidocaine on hemodynamic and hormonal responses for cesarean section. J Anesth. 2009;23(2):215–21.

[209] Grigoras A, Lee P, Sattar F, Shorten G. Perioperative intravenous lidocaine decreases the incidence of persistent pain after breast surgery. Clin J Pain. 2012 Sep;28(7):567–72.

[210] Groudine SB, Fisher HA, Kaufman RP, Patel MK, Wilkins LJ, Mehta SA, et al. Intravenous lidocaine speeds the return of bowel function, decreases postoperative pain, and shortens hospital stay in patients undergoing radical retropubic prostatectomy. Anesth Analg. 1998 Feb;86(2):235–9.

[211] Koppert W, Weigand M, Neumann F, Sittl R, Schuettler J, Schmelz M, et al. Perioperative intravenous lidocaine has preventive effects on postoperative pain and morphine consumption after major abdominal surgery. Anesth Analg. 2004;98(4):1050–1055, table of contents.

[212] Martin F, Cherif K, Gentili ME, Enel D, Abe E, Alvarez JC, et al. Lack of impact of intravenous lidocaine on analgesia, functional recovery, and nociceptive pain threshold after total hip arthroplasty. Anesthesiology. 2008 Jul;109(1):118–23.

[213] McKay A, Gottschalk A, Ploppa A, Durieux ME, Groves DS. Systemic lidocaine decreased the perioperative opioid analgesic requirements but failed to reduce discharge time after ambulatory surgery. Anesth Analg. 2009 Dec;109(6):1805–8.

[214] Herroeder S, Pecher S, Schönherr ME, Kaulitz G, Hahnenkamp K, Friess H, et al. Systemic lidocaine shortens length of hospital stay after colorectal surgery: a double-blinded, randomized, placebo-controlled trial. Ann Surg. 2007 Aug;246(2):192–200.

[215] Mitchell SJ, Merry AF, Frampton C, Davies E, Grieve D, Mills BP, et al. Cerebral protection by lidocaine during cardiac operations: a follow-up study. Ann Thorac Surg. 2009 Mar;87(3):820–5.

[216] Cassuto J, Wallin G, Högström S, Faxén A, Rimbäck G. Inhibition of postoperative pain by continuous low-dose intravenous infusion of lidocaine. Anesth Analg. 1985 Oct;64(10):971–4.

[217] Grady M V, Mascha E, Sessler DI, Kurz A. The effect of perioperative intravenous lidocaine and ketamine on recovery after abdominal hysterectomy. Anesth Analg. 2012 Nov;115(5):1078–84.

[218] Kaba A, Laurent SR, Detroz BJ, Sessler DI, Durieux ME, Lamy ML, et al. Intravenous lidocaine infusion facilitates acute rehabilitation after laparoscopic colectomy. Anesthesiology. 2007 Jan;106(1):11-8-6.

[219] Rimbäck G, Cassuto J, Tollesson PO. Treatment of postoperative paralytic ileus by intravenous lidocaine infusion. Anesth Analg. 1990 Apr;70(4):414–9.

[220] Striebel HW, Klettke U. [Is intravenous lidocaine infusion suitable for postoperative pain management?]. Schmerz. 1992 Dec;6(4):245–50.

[221] Tikuišis R, Miliauskas P, Samalavičius NE, Žurauskas A, Samalavičius R, Zabulis V. Intravenous lidocaine for post-operative pain relief after hand-assisted laparoscopic colon surgery: a randomized, placebo-controlled clinical trial. Tech Coloproctol. 2014 Apr;18(4):373–80.

[222] Wallin G, Cassuto J, Högström S, Lindén I, Faxén A, Rimbäck G, et al. Effects of lidocaine infusion on the sympathetic response to abdominal surgery. Anesth Analg. 1987 Oct;66(10):1008–13.

[223] Wuethrich PY, Romero J, Burkhard FC, Curatolo M. No benefit from perioperative intravenous lidocaine in laparoscopic renal surgery: a randomised, placebo-controlled study. Eur J Anaesthesiol. 2012 Nov;29(11):537–43.

[224] Insler SR, O'Connor M, Samonte AF, Bazaral MG. Lidocaine and the inhibition of postoperative pain in coronary artery bypass patients. J Cardiothorac Vasc Anesth. 1995 Oct;9(5):541–6.

[225] Mathew JP, Mackensen GB, Phillips-Bute B, Grocott HP, Glower DD, Laskowitz DT, et al. Randomized, double-blinded, placebo controlled study of neuroprotection with lidocaine in cardiac surgery. Stroke. 2009 Mar;40(3):880–7.

[226] Wongyingsinn M, Baldini G, Charlebois P, Liberman S, Stein B, Carli F. Intravenous lidocaine versus thoracic epidural analgesia: a randomized controlled trial in patients undergoing laparoscopic colorectal surgery using an enhanced recovery program. Reg Anesth Pain Med [Internet]. 2011;36(3):241–8. Available from: http://www.ncbi.nlm.nih.gov/pubmed/21519309

[227] Kasten GW, Owens E. Evaluation of lidocaine as an adjunct to fentanyl anesthesia for coronary artery bypass graft surgery. Anesth Analg. 1986 May;65(5):511–5.

[228] El-Deeb A, El-Morsy GZ, Ghanem AA, Elsharkawy AA, Elmetwally AS. The effects of intravenous lidocaine infusion on hospital stay after major abdominal pediatric surgery. A randomized double-blinded study. Egypt J Anaesth. 2013 Jul;29(3):225–30.

[229] Umedaly A, Lowlaavar N, West N, Miyanji F, Lauder GR. Evaluation of Intra-operative Intravenouse Lidocaine Administration During Idiopathic Scoliosis Correction in

Children; A Retrospective Case-Matched Analysis. In: International Symposium on Pediatric Pain. Seattle, WA; 2015.

[230] van Dijk A, McGrath PA, Pickett W, VanDenKerkhof EG. Pain prevalence in nine- to 13-year-old schoolchildren. Pain Res Manag. 2006;11(4):234–40.

[231] Ramage-Morin PL, Gilmour H. Chronic pain at ages 12 to 44. Heal reports. 2010 Dec;21(4):53–61.

[232] Martin AL, McGrath PA, Brown SC, Katz J. Children with chronic pain: impact of sex and age on long-term outcomes. Pain. 2007 Mar;128(1–2):13–9.

[233] Perquin CW, Hazebroek-Kampschreur AA, Hunfeld JA, Bohnen AM, van Suijlekom-Smit LW, Passchier J, et al. Pain in children and adolescents: a common experience. Pain. 2000 Jul;87(1):51–8.

[234] Coffelt TA, Bauer BD, Carroll AE. Inpatient characteristics of the child admitted with chronic pain. Pediatrics. 2013 Aug;132(2):e422–9.

[235] Mikkelsson M, Salminen JJ, Kautiainen H. Non-specific musculoskeletal pain in pre-adolescents. Prevalence and 1-year persistence. Pain. 1997 Oct;73(1):29–35.

[236] Brun Sundblad GM, Saartok T, Engström L-MT. Prevalence and co-occurrence of self-rated pain and perceived health in school-children: age and gender differences. Eur J Pain. 2007 Feb;11(2):171–80.

[237] Watson KD, Papageorgiou AC, Jones GT, Taylor S, Symmons DPM, Silman AJ, et al. Low back pain in schoolchildren: occurrence and characteristics. Pain. 2002 May;97(1–2):87–92.

[238] Jones GT. Pain in children—a call for more longitudinal research. Pain. 2011 Oct;152(10):2202–3.

[239] Forgeron PA, King S, Stinson JN, McGrath PJ, MacDonald AJ, Chambers CT. Social functioning and peer relationships in children and adolescents with chronic pain: a systematic review. Pain Res Manag. 2010;15(1):27–41.

[240] Logan DE, Simons LE, Stein MJ, Chastain L. School impairment in adolescents with chronic pain. J Pain. 2008 May;9(5):407–16.

[241] Gold JI, Mahrer NE, Yee J, Palermo TM. Pain, fatigue, and health-related quality of life in children and adolescents with chronic pain. Clin J Pain. 2009 Jun;25(5):407–12.

[242] Vetter TR. A clinical profile of a cohort of patients referred to an anesthesiology-based pediatric chronic pain medicine program. Anesth Analg. 2008 Mar;106(3):786–94, table of contents.

[243] Jastrowski Mano KE, Khan KA, Ladwig RJ, Weisman SJ. The impact of pediatric chronic pain on parents' health-related quality of life and family functioning: reliability and validity of the PedsQL 4.0 Family Impact Module. J Pediatr Psychol. 2011 Jun;36(5):517–27.

[244] Palermo TM. Impact of recurrent and chronic pain on child and family daily functioning: a critical review of the literature. J Dev Behav Pediatr. 2000 Feb;21(1):58–69.

[245] Sleed M, Eccleston C, Beecham J, Knapp M, Jordan A. The economic impact of chronic pain in adolescence: methodological considerations and a preliminary costs-of-illness study. Pain. 2005 Dec 15;119(1–3):183–90.

[246] Groenewald CB, Essner BS, Wright D, Fesinmeyer MD, Palermo TM. The economic costs of chronic pain among a cohort of treatment-seeking adolescents in the United States. J Pain. 2014 Sep;15(9):925–33.

[247] Hechler T, Ruhe AK, Schmidt P, Hirsch J, Wager J, Dobe M, et al. Inpatient-based intensive interdisciplinary pain treatment for highly impaired children with severe chronic pain: randomized controlled trial of efficacy and economic effects. Pain. 2014 Jan;155(1):118–28.

[248] Evans JR, Benore E, Banez GA. The Cost-effectiveness of intensive interdisciplinary pediatric chronic pain rehabilitation. J Pediatr Psychol. 2016 Sep;41(8):849–56.

[249] Eccleston C, Palermo TM, Williams AC de C, Lewandowski Holley A, Morley S, Fisher E, et al. Psychological therapies for the management of chronic and recurrent pain in children and adolescents. Cochrane database Syst Rev. 2014;(5):CD003968.

[250] Odell S, Logan DE. Pediatric pain management: the multidisciplinary approach. J Pain Res. 2013;6:785–90.

[251] Palermo TM, Eccleston C, Lewandowski AS, Williams AC de C, Morley S. Randomized controlled trials of psychological therapies for management of chronic pain in children and adolescents: an updated meta-analytic review. Pain. 2010 Mar;148(3):387–97.

[252] Simons LE, Sieberg CB, Pielech M, Conroy C, Logan DE. What does it take? Comparing intensive rehabilitation to outpatient treatment for children with significant pain-related disability. J Pediatr Psychol. 2013 Mar;38(2):213–23.

[253] Banez GA, Frazier TW, Wojtowicz AA, Buchannan K, Henry DE, Benore E. Chronic pain in children and adolescents: 24–42 month outcomes of an inpatient/day hospital interdisciplinary pain rehabilitation program. J Pediatr Rehabil Med. 2014;7(3):197–206.

[254] Kajiume T, Sera Y, Nakanuno R, Ogura T, Karakawa S, Kobayakawa M, et al. Continuous intravenous infusion of ketamine and lidocaine as adjuvant analgesics in a 5-year-old patient with neuropathic cancer pain. J Palliat Med. 2012 Jun;15(6):719–22.

[255] Schwartzman RJ, Patel M, Grothusen JR, Alexander GM. Efficacy of 5-day continuous lidocaine infusion for the treatment of refractory complex regional pain syndrome. Pain Med. 2009 Mar;10(2):401–12.

[256] Demant DT, Lund K, Finnerup NB, Vollert J, Maier C, Segerdahl MS, et al. Pain relief with lidocaine 5% patch in localized peripheral neuropathic pain in relation to pain phenotype: a randomised, double-blind, and placebo-controlled, phenotype panel study. Pain [Internet]. 2015 Nov;156(11):2234–44. Available from: http://www.ncbi.nlm.nih.gov/pubmed/26090758

[257] Campbell JN. How does topical lidocaine relieve pain. Pain. 2012;153(2):255–6.

[258] Peppin JF, Albrecht PJ, Argoff C, Gustorff B, Pappagallo M, Rice FL, et al. Skin matters: a review of topical treatments for chronic pain. part two: treatments and applications. Pain Ther. 2015 Jun;4(1):33–50.

[259] Davies PS, Galer BS. Review of lidocaine patch 5% studies in the treatment of postherpetic neuralgia. Drugs. 2004;64(9):937–47.

[260] Gammaitoni AR, Alvarez NA, Galer BS. Safety and tolerability of the lidocaine patch 5%, a targeted peripheral analgesic: a review of the literature. J Clin Pharmacol. 2003 Feb;43(2):111–7.

[261] Argoff CE, Galer BS, Jensen MP, Oleka N, Gammaitoni AR. Effectiveness of the lidocaine patch 5% on pain qualities in three chronic pain states: assessment with the Neuropathic Pain Scale. Curr Med Res Opin. 2004;20(Suppl 2):S21–8.

[262] Barbano RL, Herrmann DN, Hart-Gouleau S, Pennella-Vaughan J, Lodewick PA, Dworkin RH. Effectiveness, tolerability, and impact on quality of life of the 5% lidocaine patch in diabetic polyneuropathy. Arch Neurol. 2004 Jun;61(6):914–8.

[263] Galer BS, Jensen MP, Ma T, Davies PS, Rowbotham MC. The lidocaine patch 5% effectively treats all neuropathic pain qualities: results of a randomized, double-blind, vehicle-controlled, 3-week efficacy study with use of the neuropathic pain scale. Clin J Pain. 2002;18(5):297–301.

[264] Galer BS, Rowbotham MC, Perander J, Friedman E. Topical lidocaine patch relieves postherpetic neuralgia more effectively than a vehicle topical patch: results of an enriched enrollment study. Pain. 1999 Apr;80(3):533–8.

[265] Herrmann DN, Barbano RL, Hart-Gouleau S, Pennella-Vaughan J, Dworkin RH. An open-label study of the lidocaine patch 5% in painful idiopathic sensory polyneuropathy. Pain Med [Internet]. 2005;6(5):379–84. Available from: http://www.ncbi.nlm.nih.gov/pubmed/16266359

[266] Katz NP, Gammaitoni AR, Davis MW, Dworkin RH, Lidoderm Patch Study Group. Lidocaine patch 5% reduces pain intensity and interference with quality of life in patients with postherpetic neuralgia: an effectiveness trial. Pain Med. 2002 Dec;3(4):324–32.

[267] Meier T, Wasner G, Faust M, Kuntzer T, Ochsner F, Hueppe M, et al. Efficacy of lidocaine patch 5% in the treatment of focal peripheral neuropathic pain syndromes: a randomized, double-blind, placebo-controlled study. Pain. 2003 Nov;106(1–2):151–8.

[268] Wolff RF, Bala MM, Westwood M, Kessels AG, Kleijnen J. 5% lidocaine medicated plaster in painful diabetic peripheral neuropathy (DPN): a systematic review. Swiss Med Wkly. 2010 May 29;140(21–22):297–306.

[269] Devers A, Galer BS. Topical lidocaine patch relieves a variety of neuropathic pain conditions: an open-label study. Clin J Pain. 2000 Sep;16(3):205–8.

[270] Burch F, Codding C, Patel N, Sheldon E. Lidocaine patch 5% improves pain, stiffness, and physical function in osteoarthritis pain patients. A prospective, multicenter, open-label effectiveness trial. Osteoarthritis Cartilage. 2004 Mar;12(3):253–5.

[271] Galer BS, Sheldon E, Patel N, Codding C, Burch F, Gammaitoni AR. Topical lidocaine patch 5% may target a novel underlying pain mechanism in osteoarthritis. Curr Med Res Opin. 2004 Sep;20(9):1455–8.

[272] Gammaitoni AR, Galer BS, Onawola R, Jensen MP, Argoff CE. Lidocaine patch 5% and its positive impact on pain qualities in osteoarthritis: results of a pilot 2-week, open-label study using the neuropathic pain scale. Curr Med Res Opin. 2004;20(Suppl 2):S13–9.

[273] Gimbel J, Linn R, Hale M, Nicholson B. Lidocaine patch treatment in patients with low back pain: results of an open-label, nonrandomized pilot study. Am J Ther. 2005;12(4):311–9.

[274] Chaplan SR, Bach FW, Shafer SL, Yaksh TL. Prolonged alleviation of tactile allodynia by intravenous lidocaine in neuropathic rats. Anesthesiology. 1995 Oct;83(4):775–85.

[275] Boas RA, Covino BG, Shahnarian A. Analgesic responses to i.v. lignocaine. Br J Anaesth. 1982 May;54(5):501–5.

[276] Kastrup J, Petersen P, Dejgård A, Angelo HR, Hilsted J. Intravenous lidocaine infusion—a new treatment of chronic painful diabetic neuropathy? Pain. 1987 Jan;28(1):69–75.

[277] Sörensen J, Bengtsson A, Bäckman E, Henriksson KG, Bengtsson M. Pain analysis in patients with fibromyalgia. Effects of intravenous morphine, lidocaine, and ketamine. Scand J Rheumatol. 1995;24(6):360–5.

[278] Moulin DE, Clark AJ, Gilron I, Ware MA, Watson CPN, Sessle BJ, et al. Pharmacological management of chronic neuropathic pain - consensus statement and guidelines from the Canadian Pain Society. Pain Res Manag. 2007;12(1):13–21.

[279] Mailis A, Taenzer P. Evidence-based guideline for neuropathic pain interventional treatments: spinal cord stimulation, intravenous infusions, epidural injections and nerve blocks. Pain Res Manag. 2012;17(3):150–8.

[280] Chabal C, Jacobson L, Russell LC, Burchiel KJ. Pain response to perineuromal injection of normal saline, epinephrine, and lidocaine in humans. Pain. 1992 Apr;49(1):9–12.

[281] Stracke H, Meyer UE, Schumacher HE, Federlin K. Mexiletine in the treatment of diabetic neuropathy. Diabetes Care. 1992 Nov;15(11):1550–5.

[282] Galer BS, Miller K V, Rowbotham MC. Response to intravenous lidocaine infusion differs based on clinical diagnosis and site of nervous system injury. Neurology. 1993 Jun;43(6):1233–5.

[283] Attal N, Rouaud J, Brasseur L, Chauvin M, Bouhassira D. Systemic lidocaine in pain due to peripheral nerve injury and predictors of response. Neurology. 2004 Jan 27;62(2):218–25.

[284] Viola V, Newnham HH, Simpson RW. Treatment of intractable painful diabetic neuropathy with intravenous lignocaine. J Diabetes Complications. 2006;20(1):34–9.

[285] Carroll I, Gaeta R, Mackey S. Multivariate analysis of chronic pain patients undergoing lidocaine infusions: increasing pain severity and advancing age predict likelihood of clinically meaningful analgesia. Clin J Pain. 2007 Oct;23(8):702–6.

[286] Galer BS, Harle J, Rowbotham MC. Response to intravenous lidocaine infusion predicts subsequent response to oral mexiletine: a prospective study. J Pain Symptom Manage. 1996 Sep;12(3):161–7.

[287] Xu J, Yang J, Lin P, Rosenquist E, Cheng J. Intravenous therapies for complex regional pain syndrome: a systematic review. Anesth Analg. 2016 Mar;122(3):843–56.

[288] Rosen N, Marmura M, Abbas M, Silberstein S. Intravenous lidocaine in the treatment of refractory headache: a retrospective case series. Headache. 2009 Feb;49(2):286–91.

[289] Williams DR, Stark RJ. Intravenous lignocaine (lidocaine) infusion for the treatment of chronic daily headache with substantial medication overuse. Cephalalgia. 2003 Dec;23(10):963–71.

[290] Marks DM, Newhouse A. Durability of benefit from repeated intravenous lidocaine infusions in fibromyalgia patients: a case series and literature review. Prim care companion CNS Disord. 2015;17(5).

[291] Pain Infusion Clinic Standard [Internet]. 2014. Available from: https://www.cpsbc.ca/files/pdf/NHMSFP-Pain-Infusion-Clinic.pdf

[292] Jamison RN. Nonspecific treatment effects in pain medicine. Pain Clin Updat. 2011;19(2):1–7.

[293] Haanstra TM, Kamper SJ, Williams CW, Spriensma AS, Lin C-WC, Maher CG, et al. Does adherence to treatment mediate the relationship between patients' treatment outcome expectancies and the outcomes pain intensity and recovery from acute low back pain? Pain. 2015;156:1530–6.

[294] Bialosky JE, Bishop MD, Cleland JA. Individual expectation: an overlooked, but pertinent, factor in the treatment of individuals experiencing musculoskeletal pain. Phys Ther. 2010 Sep;90(9):1345–55.

[295] Crow R, Gage H, Hampson S, Hart J, Kimber A, Thomas H. The role of expectancies in the placebo effect and their use in the delivery of health care: a systematic review. Health Technol Assess. 1999;3(3):1–96.

[296] Iles RA, Davidson M, Taylor NF, O'Halloran P. Systematic review of the ability of recovery expectations to predict outcomes in non-chronic non-specific low back pain. J Occup Rehabil. 2009 Mar;19(1):25–40.

[297] Ozegovic D, Carroll LJ, David Cassidy J. Does expecting mean achieving? The association between expecting to return to work and recovery in whiplash associated disorders: a population-based prospective cohort study. Eur Spine J. 2009 Jun;18(6):893–9.

[298] Goossens MEJB, Vlaeyen JWS, Hidding A, Kole-Snijders A, Evers SMAA. Treatment expectancy affects the outcome of cognitive-behavioral interventions in chronic pain. Clin J Pain. 2005;21(1):18-26-72.

[299] Peerdeman KJ, van Laarhoven AIM, Keij SM, Vase L, Rovers MM, Peters ML, et al. Relieving patients' pain with expectation interventions: a meta-analysis. Pain. 2016 Jun;157(6):1179–91.

[300] Hanssen MM, Peters ML, Vlaeyen JWS, Meevissen YMC, Vancleef LMG. Optimism lowers pain: evidence of the causal status and underlying mechanisms. Pain. 2013 Jan;154(1):53–8.

[301] Geers AL, Helfer SG, Kosbab K, Weiland PE, Landry SJ. Reconsidering the role of personality in placebo effects: dispositional optimism, situational expectations, and the placebo response. J Psychosom Res. 2005 Feb;58(2):121–7.

[302] Geers AL, Wellman JA, Fowler SL, Helfer SG, France CR. Dispositional optimism predicts placebo analgesia. J Pain. 2010 Nov;11(11):1165–71.

[303] Gepstein R, Arinzon Z, Adunsky A, Folman Y. Decompression surgery for lumbar spinal stenosis in the elderly: preoperative expectations and postoperative satisfaction. Spinal Cord. 2006 Jul;44(7):427–31.

[304] Di Blasi Z, Harkness E, Ernst E, Georgiou A, Kleijnen J. Influence of context effects on health outcomes: a systematic review. Lancet (London, England). 2001 Mar 10;357(9258):757–62.

[305] Verheul W, Sanders A, Bensing J. The effects of physicians' affect-oriented communication style and raising expectations on analogue patients' anxiety, affect and expectancies. Patient Educ Couns. 2010 Sep;80(3):300–6.

[306] Tates K, Meeuwesen L. Doctor-parent-child communication. A (re)view of the literature. Soc Sci Med. 2001 Mar;52(6):839–51.

[307] Coakley R, Schechter N. Chronic pain is like… The clinical use of analogy and metaphor in the treatment of chronic pain in children. Pediatr Pain Lett. 2013;15(1):1–8.

[308] Horvath P. Treatment expectancy as a function of the amount of information presented in therapeutic rationales. J Clin Psychol. 1990 Sep;46(5):636–42.

[309] Hyland ME. Using the placebo response in clinical practice. Clin Med. 2003;3(4):347–50.

[310] Bensing JM, Verheul W. The silent healer: the role of communication in placebo effects. Patient Educ Couns. 2010 Sep;80(3):293–9.

[311] Finniss DG, Benedetti F. Mechanisms of the placebo response and their impact on clinical trials and clinical practice. Pain. 2005 Mar;114(1–2):3–6.

[312] Fields HL, Levine JD. Biology of placebo analgesia. Am J Med. 1981 Apr;70(4):745–6.

[313] de la Fuente-Fernández R, Ruth TJ, Sossi V, Schulzer M, Calne DB, Stoessl AJ. Expectation and dopamine release: mechanism of the placebo effect in Parkinson's disease. Science. 2001 Aug 10;293(5532):1164–6.

[314] Meissner K, Distel H, Mitzdorf U. Evidence for placebo effects on physical but not on biochemical outcome parameters: a review of clinical trials. BMC Med. 2007;5:3.

[315] Wager TD, Scott DJ, Zubieta JK. Placebo effects on human mu-opioid activity during pain. Proc Natl Acad Sci U S A. 2007 Jun 26;104(26):11056–61.

[316] Benedetti F. Mechanisms of placebo and placebo-related effects across diseases and treatments. Annu Rev Pharmacol Toxicol. 2008;48:33–60.

[317] Scott DJ, Stohler CS, Egnatuk CM, Wang H, Koeppe RA, Zubieta JK. Placebo and nocebo effects are defined by opposite opioid and dopaminergic responses. Arch Gen Psychiatry. 2008 Feb;65(2):220–31.

[318] Eippert F, Finsterbusch J, Bingel U, Büchel C. Direct evidence for spinal cord involvement in placebo analgesia. Science. 2009 Oct 16;326(5951):404.

[319] Finniss DG, Nicholas MK, Benedetti F. Placebo analgesia—understanding the mechanisms and implications for clinical practice. Rev pain. 2009 Oct;3(2):15–9.

[320] Lewis DW, Winner P, Wasiewski W. The placebo responder rate in children and adolescents. Headache. 2005 Mar;45(3):232–9.

[321] Simmons K, Ortiz R, Kossowsky J, Krummenacher P, Grillon C, Pine D, et al. Pain and placebo in pediatrics: a comprehensive review of laboratory and clinical findings. Pain. 2014 Nov;155(11):2229–35.

[322] Benedetti F. Placebo and the new physiology of the doctor-patient relationship. Physiol Rev. 2013 Jul 1;93(3):1207–46.

[323] Zubieta JK, Bueller JA, Jackson LR, Scott DJ, Xu Y, Koeppe RA, et al. Placebo effects mediated by endogenous opioid activity on mu-opioid receptors. J Neurosci. 2005 Aug 24;25(34):7754–62.

[324] Benedetti F, Amanzio M. Mechanisms of the placebo response. Pulm Pharmacol Ther. 2013 Oct;26(5):520–3.

[325] Werdehausen R, Kremer D, Brandenburger T, Schlösser L, Jadasz J, Küry P, et al. Lidocaine metabolites inhibit glycine transporter 1: a novel mechanism for the analgesic action of systemic lidocaine? Anesthesiology. 2012 Jan;116(1):147–58.

Chapter 6

Analgesics Use in Dentistry

Shaip Krasniqi and Armond Daci

Additional information is available at the end of the chapter

http://dx.doi.org/10.5772/66600

Abstract

Pain is a protective warning sign activated by tissue damage during different pathological processes. The clinical manifestation of pain is individual, multifactorial and very complex and requires the implementation of sound pharmacological approaches. The treatment of odontogenic pain is focused not only in the relief of pain but also in the suppression of causes of pain, mainly the inflammation. Acting as inhibitors of pain mechanism, analgesics are used for symptomatic treatment of pain. There are several groups of analgesic drugs used in dentistry practice and most frequent are nonsteroidal anti-inflammatory drugs (NSAIDs) and aniline analgesics. The contemporary strategies for the treatment of odontogenic pain are focused in analgesic drug combinations, which are more effective and have a better safety profile. Ibuprofen and acetaminophen agents are considered gold standard of dental analgesia for mild to moderate intensity of pain, while in moderate to severe pain the use of individual opioid analgesics or combination of opioid and nonopioid analgesics is recommended. The treatment of pain in children and elderly patients is associated with some limitations accompanied with safety concerns and dose reduction. Treatment of pain in dentistry is focused in achieving the satisfactory level of analgesia at low doses possible.

Keywords: dental pain, analgesics, NSAIDs, dentistry, opioids

1. Introduction

Pain has accompanied humans since their appearance on earth. Different natural remedies with analgesic properties date back to ancient Egypt and Greeks, including Dioscorides and Hippocrates who prescribed the use of willow bark with salicylic acid as the main ingredient. In the late nineteenth century, three prototypes of today's modern nonopioid antipyretic analgesics were discovered: acetaminophen and aspirin (formulated in 1895 by Frederick Bayer and Felix Hoffman) and phenazon, which still make up about 50% of the market of antipyretic analgesics worldwide [1]. Opiates such as morphine, which are derived from the opium poppy, were also used for thousands of years. Later on codeine, as a naturally methylated morphine, was isolated in France in 1830 by Jean-Pierre Robiquet. In 1937, German scientists Max Bockmuhl and Gustav Ehrhart synthesized methadone [2].

Pain is a subjective symptom signaling a requirement to act urgently and is usually associated with other subjective feelings such as anxiety, anger and discomfort. The expression of nature and intensity of pain is a subject of different patient-related characteristics. There are several patient factors having an impact in the patient's interpretation of pain, such as gender, age, physiological factors and drug abuse history, neuropathic and other disease and psychological profile of individual humans [3].

Dental pain (toothache or odontalgia) is a common subjective complaint of dental patients following the different interventional procedures and dental diseases. Dental pain presents one of the most common causes (approximately 12%) of patients seeking emergency treatment in dental healthcare in the United States [4].

Odontogenic pain is a complex cascade process initiated from dental tissue damage and accompanied with heterogeneous neuronal stimuli as a consequence of neurovascular, neuroinflammation and morphologic reactions [5].

The development of new analgesics is a very dynamic process and nowadays clinicians have a greater range of agents in order to select the most efficient and safe analgesic therapy. Taking into consideration the period 1960–2009, 59 analgesics have been introduced and their use still remains important [6].

Analgesics are considered one of the most important drugs groups in dental practice considering the prescription rate, clinical efficacy, cost-effectiveness and safety profile of this drug group. According to this level of importance in dental clinical practice, there are different approaches to develop treatment algorithm and guidelines for dental pain treatment in order to rationalize the use of analgesics. The rationalization of analgesics use is an ongoing challenge, since some analgesics are over-the-counter (OTC) drugs and can be taken without medical prescription.

The management of dental pain in clinical practice is a complex part of dental care and requires high-level knowledge of analgesic pharmacology and implementing the standards of rational use.

There is a valuable evidence for significant relationship between nonrational use of analgesics and diminution of drug therapy, increased adverse drug reactions and socioeconomic consequences [7, 8].

Nevertheless, prescription of analgesic drugs for dental indications is often accompanied with challenges, which diminish the treatment success and increase the potential risk for serious adverse effects.

http://dx.doi.org/10.5772/66600

There are several reasons for the decrease in clinical efficacy of analgesic therapy, including the lack of real assessment and monitoring of pain by dentistry doctor, nonadequate quantification of subjective pain experienced by patients, lack of updated pharmacological knowledge of dental pain treatments, experience scarcity in safety profile of analgesic and insufficient knowledge regarding analgesic combinations. There is evidence that prescription errors with analgesic medicaments are substantially high and are a major cause of manifestations of analgesics side effects [9]. The percentage of analgesic-related prescription errors, as reported by Smith et al., is relatively high, with 29% in adult patients and in pediatric patients it is even higher at 59%. From total prescription percentage, 14% were serious or severe analgesic prescription errors with high harmful potential for patients, mainly in pediatric patients [10].

The prescription of analgesic drugs and treatment of dental pain is more complex when it is accompanied with other health disorders and diseases. In these cases, quantification of pain and its evaluation and treatment is a convoluted clinical challenge. The main complex challenges are patients with diabetes and other chronic diseases, patients with renal and hepatic insufficiency and patients with opioid addictive disorders [11, 12].

Pain has an impact in the quality of life of patients with complaints for prolonged experience of pain, it increases healthcare costs and it is a risk for progress to chronic pain with negative reflection in health and mental status of patients [13]. The experience of prolonged pain brings healthcare workers under more complex situations and the selection of appropriate pain treatment is more difficult [14].

Rational prescription of analgesics in dentistry involves the selection of appropriate pain reliever, right clinical indication, selection of adequate dosage and route of administration and implementation of cost-effectiveness and risk-benefits standards.

Hence, information with the objective of elaborating an analgesic's utilization patterns is considered as of high relevance in order to optimize the pain treatment in dentistry.

2. Dental indications for analgesic use

Odontogenic pain due to periapical and pulpal disease is considered as the most frequent in dental health settings [15] and it is a warning sign and subjective perception of altered pulpodentinal tissue and periapical tissue. These two can be distinguished one from the other and this perception has an impact on the appropriate selection of analgesic drugs.

According to the course of clinical manifestation of the dental pain, it can be classified as acute or chronic and/or with and without malignant disease. Acute pain lasts from several hours to a number of days, while chronic pain can be present for several months and, if primary dental care is not applied, pain can last for years.

Acute pain is usually a reflection symptom of several clinical conditions such as dental trauma, inflammatory conditions of dental tissue and other related tissue structures, including the temporomandibular and masticatory muscle damages. There are several painful dental conditions indicating the analgesic use.

The characteristic of odontogenic pain is so-called referred pain, which means that the damage located in one part of dental tissue can be projected to another dental tissue. Dental referred pain is a complex clinical phenomenon, which requires a highly experienced dentist to diagnose and locate the primary source of pain [16].

The majority of clinical indications of analgesic prescriptions relate to the treatment of acute and chronic dental pain and adjunctive intraoperative and postoperative pain. Moreover, in dental practice associated procedures such as dental extractions require the use of pain reliever therapy [17].

In addition to the understanding of primary mechanism of pain, the dental clinician needs to quantify the perceived intensity of pain. These are preconditions to develop an effective strategy for the selection of efficacious and safe analgesic treatment. According to anticipated pain intensity, the dental pain can be mild, moderate and severe. This classification of dental pain intensity is crucial in the selection procedure of analgesic therapy for satisfactory relief of pain. In patients with mild dental pain, the first lines of analgesics are the nonsteroidal anti-inflammatory drugs (NSAIDs). NSAIDs can be prescribed in over-the-counter doses and in some cases in combination with other analgesics such as paracetamol [18].

The drug of choice from NSAIDs group for the treatment of mild odontogenic pain is ibuprofen 200 mg or naproxen 200–225 mg individual dose. In patients with persistent mild dental pain, the combination of ibuprofen or naproxen with paracetamol is more effective than individual NSAID agents. Where NSAIDs are contraindicated, the appropriate choice is 500–1000 mg of paracetamol.

Acetyl salicylic acid is not the drug of choice for treatment of dental pain due to its interference with platelet aggregation and patients with heart disease receiving this drug should be treated with precautions.

In patients with moderate dental pain, the analgesic of choice is a NSAID used in pharmacological full doses. NSAIDs can be individually administered or in combination with aniline derivatives, such as mefenamic acid and meclofenamic acid. In some patients where NSAIDs are not effective in combination with paracetamol, a weak opioid analgesic can be considered. The individual dose of ibuprofen is 400 mg, while that of the naproxen is 500–550 mg. In patients where pain is not controlled effectively, the addition of full dose of paracetamol is recommended. If pain is still present, the addition of weak opioid agents in full doses is advised, i.e., codeine 30 mg, hydrocodone 5 mg [19].

In patients with severe dental pain, the pharmacological treatment consists usually of combinations of strong opioid analgesics with high doses of NSAID agents, with or without aniline derivatives. In such patients, treatment of pain should be under close supervision of the dental doctor due to a higher probability of adverse drug reactions. The first choice of drug is hydrocodone 10 mg, oxycodone 5 mg, codeine 60 mg, or tramadol 50–75 mg. Due to high potential of abuse, tramadol is not the drug of choice for the treatment of severe odontogenic pain. In patients with unsatisfactory level of pain control, the combination of full dose opioid agents and NSAIDs is recommended [20].

http://dx.doi.org/10.5772/66600

2.1. Factors influencing the analgesic selection

There are several factors that play a crucial role in the selection of analgesic drugs in dental pain treatment including:

1. Pathophysiological pain mechanism. This is a predictive factor in analgesic choice. Mechanisms include cancer metastases, postoperative dental pain, nerve root infiltration, nerve root infiltration, neuropathic pain, etc.
2. Patient age. The selection of analgesic is also determined by patient age. The administration of analgesics in children and elderly patients differs from adults patients. The use of a number of analgesics in children is limited due to unmaturated metabolism processes. The elderly usually require a restriction of analgesic dose due to decreased potential of metabolism and/or excretion with reflection in pharmacokinetics and pharmacodynamic of drugs.
3. Route of administration. This is determined by the general health condition of the patient, patient's characteristics of disease, bioavailability and pharmaceutical formulation of the analgesic. Oral use of analgesics is recommended where it is possible. Controlled release of pharmaceutical formulations is more suitable for chronic pain than fast release forms.
4. Patients-related features. There are several conditions, which may affect the success of analgesic treatment in dental patients. The placebo effect should be considered carefully by dental doctors. Initially, the dental doctors should address the potential renal and hepatic toxic effect, including the gastrointestinal disturbances which may impact the pharmacokinetic and safety profile.

Experienced dental clinicians select a safe and effective analgesic therapy using individual drugs or different analgesic combinations to treat dental pain based on individual conditions. This selection in dental practice is not always simple due to numerous confounding factors related to the mechanism and clinical manifestation of pain [21].

3. Utilization pattern of analgesic use

Drug utilization studies are useful quantitative tools for feedback information of analgesic use and for identifying the measures for quality improvement of dental pain therapy. There is an increase in the rate of prescription of analgesics. The most popular analgesic drug group is NSAIDs, followed by acetaminophen, while opioid analgesics are reserved for high intensity dental pain. There is an increase in the prescribing of opioid analgesics or their combination with nonopioid analgesics in nontraumatic dental condition-related visits with more severe pain in the emergency departments [22, 23]. In one recent published study with a large cohort of patients, opioids such as hydrocodone (78%), followed by oxycodone (15.4%), propoxyphene (3.5%) and codeine (1.6%) were reported to be the most frequently prescribed analgesics after surgical extraction of teeth which requires dental care.

However, recently different studies reported a drop by 5.6% in the prescribing of opioids [24, 25]. Taking this into consideration, more should be done to prevent opioid abuse and dentists play an important role in this regard, helping to minimize opioid abuse by careful patient education and appropriate prescribing practice [26]. In mild to moderate acute dental pain, acetaminophen and NSAIDs are the most appropriate choices. COX-2 inhibitors may be considered for patients at risk of gastrointestinal disease or those taking blood thinners such as warfarin. Also, prescribers must be aware to decrease the use of maximum recommended doses and advocate shorter duration of treatment [27]. Ibuprofen was found to dominate over other analgesics [28–31]. This also applies to pediatric dentistry, whereby ibuprofen and paracetamol predominate in prescription rates [32].

However, there are controversial studies, which show that diclofenac or paracetamol may offer improved benefits. Moreover, in patients undergoing third molar surgery, nimesulide followed by diclofenac, ketoprofen and ibuprofen were the most prescribed NSAIDs.

In general, this difference in prescribing may be influenced by different practitioners in different countries, less reported side effects of medications and their effectiveness in different indications [33, 34].

3.1. Prescription and nonprescription analgesics in dental use

The use of analgesics in general practice is regulated by marketing authorization instructions of drug regulatory agencies of the respective states. The number of analgesics in over-the-counter (OTC) drug group is permanently increasing and the consequence of this is the loss of active monitoring from health professionals.

Pain is a common factor for seeking dental advice but may also occur after different interventions. The dentist is responsible to create strategies for the management of different types of pain from the dental, oral, facial, or postoperative procedures. Nonopioid analgesics are available as "over-the-counter" medications and in U.S.A, 16 millions of these drugs are prescribed annually. There are fewer indications for opioids compared to nonopioid analgesics due to their side effects profile; these should be used with caution only in case of severe pain [21].

There are several OTC analgesics and the most used are ibuprofen, acetylsalicylic acid (aspirin), acetaminophen, ketoprofen and, recently, naproxen sodium. The main characteristic used to classify these analgesics within the OTC group is the dosage [35]. NSAIDs, including ibuprofen and naproxen, are used as nonprescription OTC analgesics in doses of 200–400 mg (1200 mg/d) and 440 mg (660 mg/d for maximum of 10 days), respectively. Also, acetaminophen is widely used as an OTC product which is used also in combination with hydrocodone, oxycodone, codeine and propoxyphene. Maximum doses of acetaminophen should not exceed 4000 mg and particular attention is paid to alcohol users, in whom this drug can cause hepatotoxicity [36, 37]. In general, ibuprofen is normally safe and effective for patients who use OTC analgesic, but it has also been shown that in a small percentage of patients who use OTC analgesics maximum doses are exceeded. More sophisticated research analyses are needed in this area to improve our understanding of dosing patterns of nonprescription

http://dx.doi.org/10.5772/66600

analgesics. This requires improved patient education about nonprescription analgesic use and prevention of possible adverse events [38, 39]. In OTC NSAID analgesic users, more caution is necessary in the elderly or in patients with rheumatoid arthritis who are already taking NSAIDs, or low dose aspirin, ACEI or diuretics. The shortest duration of treatment is required and the lowest effective doses of NSAIDs are crucial in their efficacy and safety [40]. Due to this, close medical supervision is advisable.

4. Nonsteroidal anti-inflammatory drugs (NSAIDs), opioids and their mechanism of action

NSAIDs exhibit their analgesic effect due to the inhibition of prostaglandin synthesis at the peripheral nerve endings, while opioids demonstrate their effect in central nervous system through its depression [41]. NSAIDs mechanism of action is through the inhibition of prostaglandin and thromboxane (eicosanoids) biosynthesis by inhibition of cyclooxygenase activity (COX-1 discovered by John Vane or COX-2 from Daniel Simmons) in reversible or irreversible fashion and dose-dependent manner competition of arachidonic acid. In the past four decades, many new drugs such as piroxicam, flurbiprofen, diclofenac, naproxen, ibuprofen, etoricoxib and celecoxib were introduced based on their COX activity. Their mechanism of action depends on whether they inhibit COX-1, COX-2, or both, which are responsible for the synthesis of different prostaglandins found in pathological situations (COX-2 is more expressed in inflammatory conditions). However, this inhibition also results in the loss of some protective effects of prostaglandins with respect to the gastrointestinal (COX-1), cardiovascular, platelet and renal function [42]. Taking this into consideration, COX-1 inhibitors are more prone to cause gastrointestinal bleeding, which can be prevented by a switch to COX-2 inhibitors. However, short-term use of the latter is recommended based on their cardiovascular side effects which results from the imbalance of PGI_2 as antithrombic mediator and as one of the most important prostanoid in regulating homeostasis of the cardiovascular system and also TXA_2 as prothrombic mediator [43–45]. Recently, there has been an increasing interest in their effects extended beyond COX enzymes and fascinating results have been shown in different pathologies such as cancer through major cellular signaling pathways, which mediate inflammatory response [46, 47].

Opioid mechanism of action is mediated via their affinity for μ, κ, δ and opioid receptor like-1 (ORL-1) which are G-protein-coupled opioid receptors acting on GABAergic neurotransmission, in CNS and throughout the body, by acting as agonists, weak agonists and partial agonists. These responses are mainly mediated from Gi proteins by closing N-type voltage-operated calcium channels and opening calcium-dependent inwardly rectifying potassium channels, which result in hyperpolarization and reduction in neuronal excitability. Another mediated effect is the decrease of intracellular cAMP, which modulates the release of substance P, a nociceptive neurotransmitter [48].

These receptors are activated also by endogenous ligands such as endorphins. It is shown that their action is also dose mediated by showing better efficacy when the dose increased.

However, side effects should be taken into consideration. Most significant opioid effects are mediated through μ and κ receptors including for morphine and other semisynthetic and synthetic drugs such as meperidine, methadone, hydrocodone, oxycodone, fentanyl, buprenorphine, pentazocine and tramadol.

5. Principles of dental pain management

5.1. In adult patients

Pain management in dental practice is usually an unpredicted challenge and is highly related to individual patient response to pain, the expectations of the patient, pathophysiological mechanism of pain and selection of analgesic drugs. Pain relief is a very important precondition during interventional dental treatment and ensures a trustful and comfortable relationship between patients and the dental doctor [49].

Almost all dental procedures are accompanied by pain of different intensity, nature and length and treatment of pain pre- or postdental intervention is an integral part of dental treatment [27]. Efficient pain treatment during dentistry healthcare is mandatory for the achievement of desirable clinical outcome and successful dental clinical treatment. Usually in the preparation phase of patient, before the initiation of dentistry interventions, the use of local anesthesia ensures the control of patient pain [50].

The clinical evidence shows that local anesthesia results in the relief of pain during intraoperative dental period and shortly for postoperative pain and dental doctor should consider effective pain management during all stages of dental treatment. As the dental pathological process usually involves inflammation, the effect of local anesthesia is reduced due to prostaglandins interference with tetrodotoxin-resistant receptors, which diminishes the nerve responses to local anesthesia [51].

For effective dental pain management, dental doctors should address attention to disease, patient and finally to available nonpharmacological and pharmacologically effective treatment options.

The dental doctor should initially assess the pathological process of dental tissue in order to understand the mechanism of disease and to predict the health status of the patient. It is very important to define the etiology of the pathological process, especially to determine the eventual inflammatory response [52].

There is reported evidence that premedication with NSAIDs drugs such as ibuprofen or indomethacin significantly increases the level of alveolar nerve block anesthesia in dental interventions (78 and 62%) compared to placebo (32%) [53]. During the process of soft tissue trauma, a pain response occurs and this warrants the measures for pain treatment.

In dental operative procedure, preoperative administration of medication, including analgesic drugs, is recommended in order to diminish postoperative pain and to reduce the need for postoperative analgesic.

An effective strategy for dental pain treatment is based on the dynamic process of creation of a logical treatment map, which is built by the methodology of conceptualization to visualize the relationship between patient symptoms, dental interventions, therapeutic treatment and patient's needs and expectations.

Furthermore, there is available misleading information showing that naproxen sodium has a superior analgesic efficacy compared with ibuprofen at postdose interval from 1 to 12 h [28, 54, 55]. The important analgesic agents for use in dentistry are also para-aminophenol derivative such as paracetamol (acetaminophen). Administration of individual paracetamol is recommended in mild form of dental pain only when the NSAIDs are contraindicated. Otherwise, there is clinical evidence showing that ibuprofen in doses 200–512 mg versus paracetamol 600–1000 mg is superior in relief of postoperative pain. The novel strategy for pain treatment is the use of combination containing ibuprofen and paracetamol. This combination is more effective than the effect of individual analgesic when taken at 6 h after dental intervention.

The evidence shows that the most frequent doses of respective analgesics prescribed in clinical practice are 400 mg for ibuprofen and 1000 mg for paracetamol [56]. For more intensive pain when the administration of individual NSAID analgesic or combination of NSAID and paracetamol are not effective, the administration of an opioid and NSAIDs is recommended. The analgesic effect achieved by this drug combination is higher than the doubling of dose of either analgesic administered alone [57].

There are several possibilities of combinations of nonnarcotic and narcotic analgesics, which might be effective for the treatment of dental pain. The mostly used analgesic combinations in dental pain management are acetaminophen-codeine (300 mg + 30 mg), oxycodone-ibuprofen (5 mg + 400 mg), or hydrocodone-acetaminophen (5 mg + 325 mg or 7.5 mg + 500 mg) [58]. The main paradigm for treatment of dental pain is the appropriate selection of effective analgesic, at lower possible dose with the lowest probability for side effects (**Table 1**).

Type of pain in dentistry	**Analgesic drug**	**Dosing (Adults)**	**Adverse effects**
Acute dental pain	Ibuprofen Ketoprofen Diclofenac Flurbiprofen Naproxen Sodium Acetaminophen Celecoxib Codeine/ Acetaminophen	200–400 mg every 6–8 h 25–75 mg tbl every 6–8 h 50 mg tbl. 3 times daily 50–100 mg tab every 8 h 500 mg, followed by 250 mg every 6–8 h 500–1000 mg 3 times daily 200 mg 2 times daily 30–60/325–650 mg every 4–6 h	Gastric ulceration-bleeding, diarrhea, hepatotoxicity, allergy, skin rashes, urticaria, cardiovascular-MI, atherothrombosis, CHF, ischemic stroke; Opioid side effects-respiratory depression, dependence, etc.
Postoperative pain Periodontal surgery Orthodonic tooth movement Pain from pulpal or periapical tissues	Ibuprofen Ibuprofen/ Acetaminophen Naproxen	200–400 mg every 6–8 h (OTC) 400/1000 mg every 6–8 h 220 mg every 12 h (OTC)	NSAIDs associated side effects, however, OTC doses are better tolerated

Type of pain in dentistry	Analgesic drug	Dosing (Adults)	Adverse effects
Dental surgery—impacted third molar surgery and Dental surgery—dental root canal treatment	Diclofenac/ Paracetamol Ibuprofen/ Paracetamol	100/1000 mg single oral dose with 8 h observation 600/1000 mg 30 minutes before procedure or after surgery	Nausea, drowsiness headache
After third molar extraction Oral surgical or endodontic treatment Temporomandibular disorders Nontraumatic dental Conditions with severe pain	Hydrocodone Oxycodone Codeine Tramadol	10 mg every 4–6 h 5 mg every 6 h 60 mg every 6 h 50–75 mg 4–6 h	Nausea, sedation, dizziness, constipation, addiction, sleep disorders
Intensive dental pain	Oxycodone/ Ibuprofen Oxycodone/ Acetaminophen Hydrocodone/ Acetaminophen	5/400 mg every 6 h 5/500 mg every 6 h 5/325 mg or 7.5/500 mg every 4–6 h	Nausea, sedation, dizziness, constipation, addiction, sleep disorders

Table 1. General use of analgesic drugs in the different types of pain in dentistry.

5.2. Elderly patients

The strategy for dental pain treatment in elderly patients is generally the same as treatment of pain in general adult population with some differences due to age-related changes principally in physiology and pharmacokinetics in this group of patients. Clinical practice shows that elderly patients are more prone to feel the pain than adult patients and frequently are undertreated.

In the management of dental pain the clinician should consider several factors:

- Age-related pharmacokinetic changes with reduced capacities of absorption, distribution, metabolism and excretion of drugs in general and analgesics in particular. This is the main reason why it is recommended that in elderly patients the dose of drugs should be reduced generally at three-fourths of dose of adult patients [59].

- Decreased pharmacodynamic capacities of drugs due to age-related physiological changes expressed as alterations in receptor affinity, receptors number and postreceptor signaling pathways, which have an impact in the development of drug tolerance and dependency [60].

- Multiple comorbidities, which require a higher number of drugs (polypharmacy) for pharmacological treatment with increased risk of drug interactions and side effects.

- The frequency and intensity of pain reported by elderly patients might be reduced and not correspond with real pain assessment, especially when they suffer from dementia and other neurodegenerative diseases.

- Patient adherence to drug therapy of elderly patients is usually decreased and support from family and nursing health care personnel should be considered.

http://dx.doi.org/10.5772/66600

The strategy of dental pain relief in elderly patients should be based on several principles and initially we should select the available nonpharmacological measure for pain treatment. If nonpharmacological options are ineffective we need to carefully select the appropriate analgesic drug considering the risk/benefit ratio. After selection of appropriate analgesic the initiation of therapy should start with dose titration starting with lowest dose increasing slowly to effective safe dose. The analgesic therapy should be monitored closely by dental clinicians in order to achieve a successful pain relief and to prevent the possible side effects. The course of analgesic therapy should be as short as possible and also need to be stopped in case of any sign of infectivity and persistency of pain.

For pain relief in elderly patients, the recommended analgesic drug is paracetamol. In case of hepatic or renal functional disorders, dose adaptation is recommended, while in terminal hepatic insufficiency, the administration of paracetamol is contraindicated, in this case the use of NSAIDs is preferred, but these patients need close monitoring. NSAID should be given to elderly patients in the lowest effective dose and in short periods of time in order to avoid the possible side effects of these analgesic drugs. In case of severe dental pain, the use of opioid analgesic is indicated. Usually, oral opioids in the lowest possible doses, such are tramadol and some others, are used. In order to use the opioid analgesic drugs in the lowest doses, the combination of paracetamol and tramadol or codeine is recommended. In elderly patients with intensive dental pain, the strong opioid of choice is morphine [61].

5.3. Children

In clinical pediatric care, effective pain management is a standard routine approach and is mandatory in the modern concept of health care. It is accepted that the basic mechanism of pain in infants and children is substantially similar to adults with some exception in neonates related to some differences in physiological mechanism of pain, which is characterized with slower and less precise conduction of pain but without significant differences in pain perception [62].

Modern pain management for children addressing the medical conditions and surgical interventions and postoperative period has substantially advanced over the last two decades.

Advanced pain management strategy is based on two main directions, including the interventional pharmacological and nonpharmacological approach. The interventional pharmacological approach consists of the use of NSAIDs and other analgesics administered via different routes of administration (i.v. bolus administration, continuous infusion, rectal, transdermal and other routes of administration); local anesthetics, epidural anesthesia and peripheral nerve blockade. Nonpharmacological measures consist of health education of children and psychological approach to release the perception of fear and other behavioral problems in children patients, breathing techniques, hypnosis, transcutaneous electrical nerve stimulation, guided imagery, acupuncture, relaxation and other techniques to relieve the pain [63].

Pain management strategy in children consists of several principles, which reflect the differences between children and adult pain treatments. The strategy of pain relief should focus on the prevention of pain and this ensures better treatment success before painful procedures.

Usually this starts with preparing the child and the family in advance, in order to reduce fear and anxiety before intervention and applying patient-controlled analgesia (PCA). In case of major surgical interventions the treatment of predicted pain after treatment in children can continue with oral analgesics depending on patient needs.

Dental clinicians should assess the pain intensity using the appropriate children pain scale. It is recommended to use the FLACC scale for pain measurement in pediatric patients aged 1 month to 3 years, while for children above 3–7 years the Wong-Baker pain rating scale is used (**Figure 1**), which has demonstrated to be more sensitive compared to visual analogue scale. For children above 7 years, the Visual Analogue/Numerical Rating Scale is used. A universal measuring tool does not exist but according to a systematic review FACES scale demonstrated to be effective in children from 3 to 12 years in which gradient of emotions cartoons are chosen by children based on their level of pain. There is also another measurement, such as Oucher pain scale, which does not differ much from the others, but it is more specific in different racial face expressions such as Caucasian, African American, Hispanic, First Nations Boy and Girl and Asian Boy and Girl [64–69].

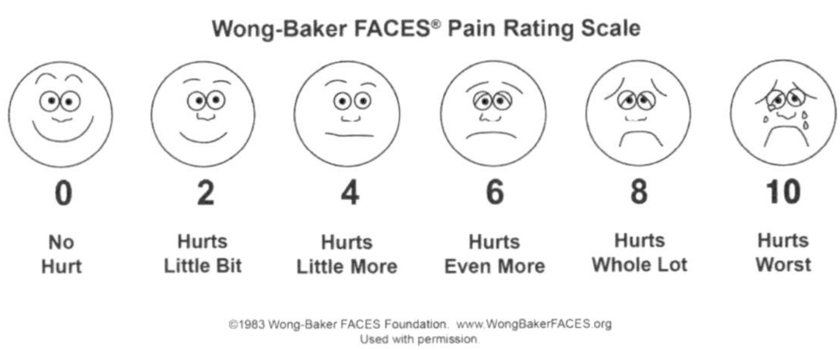

Figure 1. Wong-Baker faces pain rating scale explains to the person that each face is for a person who has no pain (hurt), some, or a lot of pain by asking the person to choose that best describes how much pain he has.

Multimodal and multiapproach therapy is the cornerstone of pain management in children. This technique uses different analgesia and nonpharmacological complementary approach in order to enhance the pain control and minimize drug-induced adverse effects. This method supports the use of combined nonopioid (NSAIDS, other analgesic agents, local anesthetics, alpha$_2$-adrenergic agonists, voltage-gated calcium channel alpha-$_2$ delta-proteins) and opioid analgesics and other agents in smaller doses in order to prevent the clinical manifestations of drugs side effects [70]. Dosage calculations of analgesics for children are based on mg/kg body weight administered by intravenous, oral and rectal route, while intramuscular injections should be avoided. It is recommended that severe pain is treated by infusions, PCA and other routes of continuous analgesic administration.

Pain treatment options in neonates and premature infants should avoid the use of opioid analgesics. However, in cases when there is no other option, opioid analgesics should be closely monitored in intensive care units. In this group of infants, opioids are more prone to develop dependency and depression of cardiorespiratory functions.

http://dx.doi.org/10.5772/66600

The mainstream in pharmacological pain treatment consists of administration of NSAIDs, paracetamol. Usually it is recommended to use paracetamol (infant dose is 10–15 mg/kg/dose every 6–8 h, pediatric oral dose 10–15 mg/kg/dose every 4 h), ibuprofen (10 mg/kg/dose every 6 h) and diclofenac (1 mg/kg/tds or 1.5 mg/kg/bd, maximum daily dose is 3 mg/kg). While naproxen (2 years or older: 5 mg/kg orally twice a day; 12 years or older: 220 mg orally every 8–12 h) is indicated more in inflammatory diseases. In modalities of analgesic therapy combinations the dosage of individual analgesics are decreased.

For more intensive pain the use of opioids is recommended. Codeine (0.5–1 mg/kg every 4–6 h) is a weak opioid analgesic and to increase the analgesic effect it is often combined with paracetamol. However, FDA alerts about odeine use in children and it should be used with careful monitoring only in patients from which benefits outweigh the risks [71]. Another opioid analgesic for treatment of mild to severe dental pain in children is tramadol (1–1.5 mg/kg). For severe dental pain, the use of morphine (0.2–0.5 mg/kg q4–6 h) is recommended. Other alternatives to morphine are also considered, including fentanyl, hydromorphone, methadone and other opioid agents.

Other approaches to pain treatment of dental pain in children include the use of regional analgesia such as local anesthetic instillation, wound anesthetic infiltration, topical regional analgesia (lignocaine gel), peripheral nerve block and other methods. Dental pain management in children is complex and further improvements are needed to improve the efficacy and safety of pain treatment [72].

5.4. Analgesic use in renal and hepatic insufficiency

There is an increased risk for renal dysfunction in patients undergoing analgesic treatment, although moderate use is not associated with increased risk of renal disease or dysfunction [73]. Patients with renal failure should be carefully considered due to the increased risk of side effects in dental treatment and also when analgesic therapy is indicated. This requires consultation with the nephrologists or hepatologists for the grade of the disease and an important monitoring for clinical parameters which need to be observed. Regarding medication, dose adjustments need to be considered as an important step to reduce side effects or toxicity. For NSAIDs dose reduction or avoidance is also indicated in more advanced stages of renal failure. In aspirin, acetaminophen and ibuprofen treatment indications prolongation of dosing interval is recommended; however, dose reduction is recommended for diclofenac and naproxen. When the GFR is <10 mL/min avoidance need to be considered, excluding acetaminophen in intervals of 8–12 h. On the other side narcotic analgesics (morphine, fentanyl, codeine) are metabolized by the liver and usually do not require dose adjustment [74, 75]. But special caution should also be exercised in patients with end-stage renal disease without dialysis whereby the use of opioids such as codeine, dihydrocodeine, dextropropocyphene and hydrocodone is not recommended (tramadol may be used with caution). Also, only short-term treatment must be prescribed for morphine, diamorphine, or dose reduction in fentanyl by 25–50% or methadone 50–70% with specialist advice on prescribing and special care in the elderly due to highly variable pharmacokinetics [76, 77].

Due to pharmacokinetic changes in the elderly and reduced renal and metabolism capacity, acetaminophen is the drug of choice for the control of mild to moderate pain in doses of 500–1000 mg every 4 h. Moreover the overuse of this drug is related with side effects including acute liver failure, hepatotoxicity and in rare cases nephrotoxicity. Taking this into consideration, chronic dosing needs to be avoided in patients with decreased liver function or cirrhosis [78, 79]. In cirrhotic patients, NSAIDs should be avoided or used with extreme caution due to increased risk of gastrointestinal bleeding and risk of hepatotoxicity or acute hepatic decompensation or risk of renal failure.

For opioids, low dose of tramadol is considered as second choice in this group of patients after acetaminophen [80].

Opioid side effects are more common in hepatic impairment due to prolongation of their effects. Conversely, fentanyl and methadone pharmacokinetic is less affected by hepatic impairment. Fentanyl is recommended more than methadone. And also hydromorphone, morphine and oxicodone are other choices that are recommended with caution [81]. Consultation with specialist and also titration should be done slowly, monitoring of drug concentrations and adverse effects are crucial steps in the use of analgesics in dental management for patients with impairment of renal or hepatic functions (**Table 2**).

Population	Analgesic drug	Dosing	Adverse effects
Elderly	Acetaminophen (First choice in mild to moderate pain)	500–1000 mg every 8 h (maximum 3 g)(reduce maximum dose 50–70% for adults with reduced hepatic function or alcohol abusers)	Gastric ulceration-bleeding; Abdominal pain; Hepatotoxicity and acute liver failure; Acute renal failure; Allergy; Skin, Rashes; Urticaria, Cardiovascular-Myrocardial infection, atherothrombosis, Chronic heart failure; Ischemic Stroke; More sensitive for opioids induced side effects. More pronounced drug interaction associated adverse effects.
	NSAIDs (Ibuprofen, Naproxen, Flurbiprofen, Ketorolac, Celecoxib)	Lowest effective dose for the shortest Possible time (It is recommended to use NSAIDss with PPIs to avoid gastrointestinal bleeding, or use celecoxib in patients with no significant risk factors for cardiovascular events)	
	Opioids (Oxycodone, Hydrocodone, Tramadol) (moderate to severe pain)	Oxycodone 2.5 mg every 6 h Hydrocodone 5 mg every 6 h Tramadol 25 mg daily with increase every 2–3 days with 25 mg up to 100 mg. (It recommended 25–50% dose reduction from recommended dosage in adults and shortest possible time)	
Children	Acetaminophen Ibuprofen (age 2–12) Naproxen (age 2–12)	10–15 mg/kg every 4–6 h 5–7 mg/kg every 8–12 h 5–10 mg/kg every 8–12 h	Acetaminophen hepatotoxicity in liver disorders Gastric irritation, ulceration, bleeding and perforation and clotting impairment from NSAIDs Codeine associated nausea, sedation, constipation, dependency.
	Codeine/Acetaminophen (3 days or less and only with careful monitoring and only in patients which benefits outweighs the risks)	0.5–1 mg/kg every 4–6 h	

http://dx.doi.org/10.5772/66600

Population	Analgesic drug	Dosing	Adverse effects
	Morphine (Only in severe dental pain)	0.2–0.5 mg/kg every 4–6 h	
Renal and hepatic insufficiency	Acetaminophen	500–1000 mg every 6–8 h (no need for adjustment in renal insufficiency, reduce dose up to 2 g daily n cirrhosis	Coagulopathies from liver disease; Acute renal injury; Hepatotoxicity; NSAIDs and Opioid-associated side effects.
	Ibuprofen	200–600 mg every 4–6 h (no need for adjustment in renal insufficiency, avoid or use with caution in hepatic insufficiency)	
	Dihidrocodeine	10–30 mg every 4–6 h (decrease dose 25% in renal insufficiency)	
	Fentanyl	12 mcg/h transdermal patch (only if patients have been taking other strong narcotic pain medicines for at least a week)	

Table 2. Use of analgesic drugs in dentistry in special populations.

6. Analgesic clinical efficacy and safety in dental pain management

Evidence-based medicine strongly supports the evaluation of analgesic efficacy and safety. The majority of this research uses the third-molar extraction model of acute dental pain to determine relief of pain intensity over time with different available analgesics. The clinical efficacy of dental analgesics is focused on comparison of individual analgesics and placebo and monotherapy analgesics with combined therapy.

Efficacy and safety of analgesic drugs is shown to be enhanced through the use in combination due to the reduction of single drug component. Usually, the choice of analgesic is based on personal preference. In systematic reviews for dental and general surgical randomized controlled trials with naproxen, diclofenac and rofecoxib, they were shown to be superior compared to placebo and also COX-2 inhibitors demonstrated equipotent efficacy relative to NSAIDs.

Moreover in dental and orthopedic pain, valdecoxib, celecoxib, ibuprofen and acetaminophen alone or with oxycodone demonstrated superiority of COX-2 inhibitors compared to acetaminophen, but not to ibuprofen alone. Also, oral ibuprofen is significantly superior to placebo and when the doses were maximal the effect were enhanced.

When compared to diclofenac, ibuprofen was less efficacious even after showing a reduction by at least 50% of pain for 100% of patients participated. Acetaminophen was also proven to be similarly efficacious in general and orthopedic surgery and less effective in dental surgery compared to NSAIDs. When it is combined with opioids such as codeine or oxycodone, it was shown to be superior compared to placebo; however, it was more prone to side effect. The same was proven with tramadol alone.

In general, NSAIDs demonstrate higher efficacy in dental pain and are considered as the main alternative and drug of choice for dental pain. However, even though opioids are relatively less effective, they may be considered when NSAIDs are contraindicated and also different combination could be administered for some patients that require adequate pain relief [82].

Common reported adverse events of NSAIDs are dyspepsia, gastric ulceration-bleeding, diarrhea from COX-1 inhibitors, cardiovascular disease (congestive heart failure, atherothrombosis, myocardial infarction, ischemic stroke), reduced renal perfusion, or nephrotic syndrome accompanied with edema, acute kidney failure in rare cases from COX-2 inhibitors. Ibuprofen use in normal doses is one of the drugs with least risk or alternative option as selective COX-2 inhibitors. Acetaminophen adverse effects resulting from their higher dosage, chronic use, or in patient with liver disease includes liver toxicity, prolongation of prothrombine time, urticaria or skin rashes and acute renal tubular necrosis. Severe hepatotoxicity was reported in patients with risk factors such as HIV, hepatitis C and chronic alcohol users. In postoperative pain, a single dose usage and rational prescribing is demonstrated to be safe.

Moreover, narcotic analgesics have more frequent adverse effects and many patients abandoned treatment which make them poor choice in dental pain. When contemplating surgery, it is recommended to suppress NSAID medication from 1–2 to 4–5 days, which also depends on the drug type and dose regimen. Analgesic combination, which contains NSAIDs, is recommended to be used with caution only in short course for the acute dental pain [41, 83–86]. These above-mentioned side effects usually tend not to occur with the occasional use of NSAIDs, which makes these drugs safe in dental practice. NSAID usage for more than 10 days should be consulted with the practitioner. Even though they are considered relatively safe within the recommended dosage for use of up to 10 days, cautions should be exercised in NSAIDs-exacerbated respiratory disease, asthma, patients with prior myocardial infarction who are receiving antithrombotic therapy and those with a history of renal disease [87, 88].

Strategies to lower risk events for gastrointestinal toxicity from NSAIDs include the use of the lowest dose, switch to acetaminophen or COX-2 inhibitors, or antiulcer cotherapy use (PPI, H2-blockers, antacids, prostaglandins). Cardiovascular-related adverse effects have resulted in rofecoxib and valdecoxib being withdrawn from the market. However, uses were for a long period of time and dose dependent or even in short course of treatments for 10 days after bypass surgery. Currently, celecoxib, etoricoxib, lumiraxocib and parecoxib, with better cardiovascular risk profiles, are still in the market. Hence, NSAIDs may increase the risk for myocardial infarction, in particular those with more COX-2 selectivity such as diclofenac. Taking this into consideration, avoiding COX-2 inhibitors and following treatment with antiulcer drugs is recommended in high risk patients [82]. Ibuprofen and naproxen are considered the safest NSAIDs. Overall risk from analgesic used in dentistry is low and importantly when they are used in acute dental pain. Moreover, the most serious safety concerns about the use of opioids are the side effect profile which includes respiratory depression, dependence, sedation, euphoria, constipation, cognitive dysfunction, pruritus, nausea and immunologic and endocrine effects, which are more prone from μ receptor activity. Dependence is another challenge and this occurs more in severe acute, chronic and terminal pain for longer than a week and after repeated administration. Furthermore, tolerance to opioids is developed when higher doses are used.

Selective κ agonist such as nalbuphine is shown to be safer even though this should never be given to a patient who is dependent. Important care is recommended for codeine metabolism from CYP2D6 ultrarapid metabolizers, which are more prone to morphine-induced side effects or for CYP2D6 deficient or patient who are on inhibitors of this cytochrome may not produce analgesic effect of hydrocodone and oxycodone. Methadone has potential to cause cardiac arrhythmia. Due to this pretreatment and periodic cardiograms are recommended for patients suspected for drug interactions or increasing methadone dosing. Important care should also be taken with conversion of one opioid to another from opioid conversion tables (for example, morphine to methadone). Regarding treatment of withdrawal, partial agonists such as buprenorphine is recommended [19, 89].

Recently, there have been important developments in the investigation of lower addictive potential opioids such as tamper-resistant extended release, also opioid abuse screening tools, genetic testing and fMRIs for patients at risk of opioid abuse while maintaining treatments for patients with appropriate management.

Even though recent research has shown that a number of potential predictors for personalization of therapy exist, there is still insufficient evidence for opioid prescribing from patient's characteristics. Data-based personalized prescribing of opioids for optimization of analgesic effectiveness and mitigate risks of opioid-related mortality and abuse is highly desirable with the potential to benefit patients by raising world clinical care and optimizing cost effectiveness of opioid analgesic therapy [90].

7. Analgesic monotherapy versus combined therapy in dental practice

Analgesic monotherapy and combined therapy is shown in different clinical situations such as reducing pain in surgical procedures, periodontal and endodontic procedures which is documented also from different clinical trials. Many NSAIDs which are used in dental pain includes ibuprofen, aspirin, diflunisal, etodolac, mefenamic acid, ketoprofen, ketorolac and flubiprofen. Ibuprofen is the most commonly used in acute pain and is often prescribed as the first choice analgesic associated with its anti-inflammatory actions in the dentistry practice. Paracetamol acts in the central nervous system and it possesses analgesic and antipyretic effects. It is the first choice for patients who cannot tolerate NSAIDs. Higher doses such as 1000 mg are more favorable in the context of its efficacy and were comparable with ibuprofen.

There is strong evidence that combined analgesics therapy lead to greater efficacy and fewer adverse events compared with monotherapy of analgesics in higher doses. Different randomized controlled trials that compared combinations of several analgesics (NSAIDs and acetaminophen) revealed that the combination of acetaminophen with different NSAID drugs was more effective than either acetaminophen or individual NSAID alone [18, 91, 92].

Currently there are many combinations of paracetamol with other NSAIDs such as ibuprofen, ketoprofen and diclofenac and they have resulted in providing superior analgesia than using the drug alone. Otherwise in the patients with moderate to severe pain induced by postoperative pain, the combination of lower doses of ibuprofen with paracetamol has not shown benefits when compared with ibuprofen used alone. This is an indication that dosage choice is an important factor regarding its related combinations [93–95].

Naproxen is indicated in toothache and its pain relief efficacy is comparable with ibuprofen. It is comparable with etodolac, but less effective in swelling when compared with diclofenac when they were used in oral surgical procedures, including postoperative third molar surgery or orthodontic pain [96–98]. Diclofenac is used in moderate to severe pain following third molar extraction and it could be used in an intravenous form in risk population groups such as the elderly and renal insufficiency, postoperative anticoagulation which uses ketorolac as the only choice for the moderate to severe acute pain. Very similar effects were shown when transdermal diclofenac patches were used compared to oral administration [99, 100].

Due to safety concerns COX-2 selective inhibitors have been introduced as a safe alternative in dentistry practice with superior analgesic and inflammatory conditions in periodontal diseases and after oral surgery procedures. Etoricoxib and celecoxib groups were shown to be comparable to ibuprofen on its efficacy in the dental pulpal pain or postoperative pain relief, third molar surgery but superior toacetaminophene [101–103].

Their use is favorable in patients with upper-GI-complications, in the aspirin user for cardiovascular comorbidities, or those allergic to aspirin and perioperative settings due to their lack of properties over blood clotting. But they are limited to be used in such short periods including postoperative periods due to their cost effectiveness compared to other NSAIDs. Also, their long-term uses in the painful temporo mandibular joint disorders and chronic orofacial pain in the patients without cardiovascular risk factors could be considered as another therapeutic option [41, 104].

8. Significant drug interactions of analgesics

NSAIDs display major interactions when used alongside anticoagulant and antiplatelet effects of warfarin and clopidrogel, which results in enhancement of their effects and increased risk of bleeding. In this situation acetaminophen is an appropriate choice at the lowest possible dose, in short-term treatment only. Ibuprofen use in patients taking cardioprotective aspirin does not interfere with its antiplatelet activity, even though there are studies that demonstrate reduced cardioprotective benefits and increase gastrointestinal risk, in contrast to diclofenac or acetaminophen which did not influence effects of aspirin on platelet function [86]. Moreover, patients taking daily aspirin for cardiovascular disease prevention should avoid chronic use of ibuprofen and FDA recommends taking ibuprofen in intervals of more than 8 h before or more than 30 min after the immediate release of aspirin to reduce potential interaction in platelet function [40]. Concurrent use of NSAIDs with warfarin or corticosteroid may increase gastrointestinal risk. They also increase the risk of gastrointestinal ulceration in concomitant use with biphosphonates. Effects of antidiabetic sulfonylureas are increased with coadministration of NSAIDs.

http://dx.doi.org/10.5772/66600

A decrease of renal extraction of methotrexate is shown with the use of NSAIDs, which can bring to its toxicity. Also, the serum concentrations of lithium are raised and non-NSAID analgesic should be recommended. Additionally, fluconazole was shown to increase celecoxib concentration due to its metabolism inhibition.

Interactions with lesser significance are NSAIDs use with ACE inhibitors, diuretics, Ca-channel bBlockers and beta-blockers which results in diminished antihypertensive effects. However, short-term use does not pose a major risk in healthy individuals, but in hypertensive patients and especially in the elderly if the treatment will be continued for a long term a careful selection and close monitoring is required. Antacids were shown to decrease NSAIDs effects. NSAIDs are also found to interact with SSRIs (selective serotonin reuptake inhibitors) to increase the risk of bleeding including also upper gastrointestinal and postoperative bleeding [37, 105, 106]. Acetaminophen has very few drug interactions. Carbamazepine as metabolic inducer may decrease drug levels of acetaminophen. Its combination with alcohol or drugs that harm the liver may increase the risk for liver toxicity.

Dental practitioners should be aware of these interactions and use analgesic drug therapy within the limit of dosage or interval of use and in carefully considered combinations. Furthermore, they should avoid them when there is increased risk for toxicity [81, 107]. Narcotic analgesic interactions include antipsychotics (phenotiazines) which enhance their hypotensive effect and also CYP2D6 inhibitors (cimetidine, chlorpheniramine, fluoxetine and quinidine), which inhibit their effects including hydrocodone. Inhibitors or inducers of CYP3A4 cause clinical significant interactions when used with morphine, oxycodone and methadone by mediating opioid toxicity or impairment of pain treatment. Also, SSRIs and MAOIs effects are more associated with meperidine, methadone, tramadol, buprenorphine, oxycodone, hydrocodone, pentazocine and fentanyl, which may also result in the cause of the serotonin syndrome. Barbiturates may enhance their sedative effects. Also an increase of meperidine metabolism is induced by phenytoine. Taking this into consideration physicians should recognize and monitor patients carefully for drug interactions and possibly try to avoid polypharmacy [89, 108, 109].

9. Challenges of dental pain management

Safe and effective dental pain management strategy requires an understanding of several factors. Pain is perceived differently by individual patients, depending on their biogenetic profile, gender, age, sociocultural attitudes, comedical and psychiatric conditions and several other factors [110]. Due to ethical consideration there are limited scientific data for drug efficacy in dental pain management and this is why it is important to challenge the work of clinicians in daily clinical practice. Dental clinicians assign a comprehensive practice that involves the pharmacological, biological and psychosocial aspects of pain management in order to ensure effective low risk pain treatment. Therefore, they need to implement and coordinate the extrapolated evidence base, knowledge, personal clinical experience and close monitoring of patients to achieve the effective balance of pain treatment in dental patients [11].

In general more attention should be paid by dental practitioners to reducing opioid drug abuse and monitoring of prescription and nonprescription uses of analgesics, improvement of drug choice alone or in combination, new analgesic alternatives and adjustment in course of treatment according to clinical needs. Also, individualization of therapy and dosage needs to be done carefully in the risk groups mentioned above, coupled with the need for adequate monitoring of drug interactions.

Author details

Shaip Krasniqi[1] and Armond Daci[2*]

*Address all correspondence to: armond.daci@uni-pr.edu

1 Faculty of Medicine, Institute of Pharmacology and Toxicology and Clinical Pharmacology, University of Prishtina "Hasan Prishtina", Prishtina, Kosovo

2 Department of Pharmacy, Faculty of Medicine, University of Prishtina, Prishtina, Kosovo

References

[1] Brune K, Hinz B. History of Analgesics. In Encyclopedia of Pain. Berlin Heidelberg: Springer; 2013, pp. 1490–6. DOI: 10.1007/978-3-642-28753-4_1766

[2] Brune K. The early history of non-opioid analgesics. Acute Pain. 1997;1(1):33–40. DOI: 10.1016/S1366-0071(97)80033-2#_blank#Persistent link using digital object identifier

[3] Fainsinger RL, Nekolaichuk C, Lawlor P, Hagen N, Bercovitch M, Fisch M, Galloway L, Kaye G, Landman W, Spruyt O, Zhukovsky D. An international multicentre validation study of a pain classification system for cancer patients. European Journal of Cancer. 2010;46(16):2896–904. DOI: 10.1016/j.ejca.2010.04.017 DOI:10.1016/j.ejca.2010.04.017#doilink

[4] Anderson R, Thomas DW. 'Toothache stories': a qualitative investigation of why and how people seek emergency dental care. Community Dental Health. 2003;20(2):106–11.

[5] Trowbridge HO. Review of dental pain—histology and physiology. Journal of Endodontics. 1986;12(10):445–52. DOI: 10.1016/S0099-2399(86)80197-2 DOI:10.1016/S0099-2399(86)80197-2#_blank#Persistent link using digital object identifier

[6] Kissin I. The development of new analgesics over the past 50 years: a lack of real breakthrough drugs. Anesthesia & Analgesia. 2010;110(3):780–9. DOI: 10.1213/ANE.0b013e3181cde882

[7] Compton WM, Jones CM, Baldwin GT. Relationship between nonmedical prescription-opioid use and heroin use. New England Journal of Medicine. 2016;374(2):154–63. DOI: 10.1056/NEJMra1508490

[8] Scott NL, Miner JR. The safe and rational use of analgesics: non-opioid analgesics. Current Emergency and Hospital Medicine Reports. 2016;4(2):66–70. DOI: 10.1007/s40138-016-0102-5

[9] Van Doormaal JE, Van Den Bemt PM, Mol PG, Zaal RJ, Egberts AC, Haaijer-Ruskamp FM, Kosterink JG. Medication errors: the impact of prescribing and transcribing errors on preventable harm in hospitalised patients. Quality and Safety in Health Care. 2009;18 (1):22–7. DOI: 10.1136/qshc.2007.023812

[10] Smith HS, Lesar TS. Analgesic prescribing errors and associated medication characteristics. The Journal of Pain. 2011;12(1):29–40. DOI: 10.1016/j.jpain.2010.04.007 DOI:10.1016/j.jpain.2010.04.007#doilink

[11] Savage SR, Kirsh KL, Passik SD. Challenges in using opioids to treat pain in persons with substance use disorders. Addiction Science & Clinical Practice. 2008;4(2):4.

[12] Nielsen FE, Gram-Hansen P, Christensen JH, Sørensen HT, Klausen IC, Ravn L. Reduced consumption of analgesics in patients with diabetes mellitus admitted to hospital for acute myocardial infarction. Pain. 1991;47(3):325–8. DOI: 10.1016/0304-3959(91)90223-K DOI:10.1016/0304-3959(91)90223-K#_blank#Persistent link using digital object identifier

[13] Casey CY, Greenberg MA, Nicassio PM, Harpin RE, Hubbard D. Transition from acute to chronic pain and disability: a model including cognitive, affective and trauma factors. Pain. 2008;134(1):69–79. DOI: 10.1016/j.pain.2007.03.032 DOI:10.1016/j.pain.2007.03.032#doilink

[14] McCarberg BH, Billington R. Consequences of neuropathic pain: quality-of-life issues and associated costs. The American Journal of Managed Care. 2006;12(9 Suppl): S263–8.

[15] Nalliah RP, Allareddy V, Elangovan S, Karimbux N, Lee MK, Gajendrareddy P, Allareddy V. Hospital emergency department visits attributed to pulpal and periapical disease in the United States in 2006. Journal of Endodontics. 2011;37(1):6–9. DOI: 10.1016/j.joen.2010.09.006 DOI:10.1016/j.joen.2010.09.006#doilink

[16] Murray GM. Referred pain, allodynia and hyperalgesia. The Journal of the American Dental Association. 2009;140(9):1122–4. DOI: 10.14219/jada.archive.2009.0339

[17] Hargreaves KM, Hutter JW. Endodontic pharmacology. In Cohen S, Burns R, eds. Pathways of the Pulp. St Louis: Mosby; 2002, pp. 665–82.

[18] Ong CK, Seymour RA, Lirk P, Merry AF. Combining paracetamol (acetaminophen) with nonsteroidal antiinflammatory drugs: a qualitative systematic review of analgesic efficacy for acute postoperative pain. Anesthesia & Analgesia. 2010;110(4):1170–9. DOI: 10.1213/ANE.0b013e3181cf9281

[19] Becker DE. Pain management: part 1: managing acute and postoperative dental pain. Anesthesia Progress. 2010;57(2):67–79. DOI: 10.2344/0003-3006-57.2.67

[20] Cairns BE, Kolta A, Whitney E, Craig K, Rei N, Lam DK, Lynch M, Sessle B, Lavigne G. The need for further research. Journal of the Canadian Dental Association. 2014;80:e49.

[21] Hargreaves K, Abbott PV. Drugs for pain management in dentistry. Australian Dental Journal. 2005;50(4 Suppl 2):S14–22.DOI: 10.1111/j.1834-7819.2005.tb00378.x

[22] Okunseri C, Okunseri E, Thorpe JM, Xiang Q, Szabo A. Medications prescribed in emergency departments for nontraumatic dental condition visits in the United States. Medical Care. 2012;50(6):508. DOI: 10.1097/MLR.0b013e318245a575 DOI:10.1097%2FMLR.0b013e318245a575#pmc_ext

[23] Okunseri C, Okunseri E, Xiang Q, Thorpe JM, Szabo A. Prescription of opioid and nonopioid analgesics for dental care in emergency departments: findings from the National Hospital Ambulatory Medical Care Survey. Journal of Public Health Dentistry. 2014;74(4):283–92. DOI: 10.1111/jphd.12055 DOI:10.1111%2Fjphd.12055#pmc_ext

[24] Levy B, Paulozzi L, Mack KA, Jones CM. Trends in opioid analgesic–prescribing rates by specialty, US, 2007–2012. American Journal of Preventive Medicine. 2015;49(3):409–13. DOI: 10.1016/j.amepre.2015.02.020 DOI:10.1016/j.amepre.2015.02.020#doilink

[25] Baker JA, Avorn J, Levin R, Bateman BT. Opioid prescribing after surgical extraction of teeth in Medicaid patients, 2000–2010. Journal of the American Medical Association. 2016;315(15):1653–4. DOI: 10.1001/jama.2015.19058.

[26] Denisco RC, Kenna GA, O'Neil MG, Kulich RJ, Moore PA, Kane WT, Mehta NR, Hersh EV, Katz NP. Prevention of prescription opioid abuse: the role of the dentist. The Journal of the American Dental Association. 2011;142(7):800–10. DOI: 10.14219/jada.archive.2011.0268

[27] Donaldson M, Goodchild JH. Appropriate analgesic prescribing for the general dentist. General Dentistry. 2009;58(4):291–7.

[28] Kulkarni MD, Baig MS, Hussaini SA, Doifode SM. Drug utilization pattern in OPD of government dental college and hospital, Aurangabad. International Journal of Basic & Clinical Pharmacology. 2013;2:69–70. DOI: 10.5455/2319-2003.ijbcp20130113

[29] Haliti NR, Haliti FR, Koçani FK, Gashi AA, Mrasori SI, Hyseni VI, Bytyqi SI, Krasniqi LL, Murtezani AF, Krasniqi SL. Surveillance of antibiotic and analgesic use in the Oral Surgery Department of the University Dentistry Clinical Center of Kosovo. Therapeutics and Clinical Risk Management. 2015;11:1497. DOI: 10.2147/TCRM.S87595 DOI:10.2147%2FTCRM.S87595#pmc_ext

[30] Pise ND, Kaikade SB. Drug utilization evaluation of analgesics in tertiary care dental hospital in Dhule district. International Journal of Biomedical Research. 2016;7(6):344–5. DOI: 10.7439/ijbr.v7i6.3324

[31] Moore PA, Nahouraii HS, Zovko JG, Wisniewski SR. Dental therapeutic practice patterns in the US II. Analgesics, corticosteroids and antibiotics. General Dentistry. 2005;54(3):201–7.

[32] Paudel KR, Sah NK, Jaiswal AK. Prevalence of pharmacotherapy in the department of paediatric dentistry. Kathmandu University Medical Journal. 2010;8(2):190–4. DOI: 10.3126/kumj.v8i2.3556

[33] Levrini L, Carraro M, Rizzo S, Salgarello S, Bertelli E, Pelliccioni GA, Garau V, Bandettini M, Caputi S, Lörincz A, Szûcs A. Prescriptions of NSAIDs to patients undergoing third molar surgery. Clinical Drug Investigation. 2008;28(10):657–68. DOI: 10.2165/00044011-200828100-00006

[34] Datta P, Datta PP. Drug utilization pattern in Oral Medicine Department of Saveetha Dental College, Tamil Nadu, India. National Journal of Medical Research. 2015;5(4):272–4.

[35] Analgesics in Dentistry. Available at: https://www.netcegroups.com/964/Course_55041.pdf 2013.

[36] Dionne RA, Berthold CW. Therapeutic uses of non-steroidal anti-inflammatory drugs in dentistry. Critical Reviews in Oral Biology & Medicine. 2001;12(4):315–30. DOI: 10.1177/10454411010120040301

[37] Hersh EV, Pinto A, Moore PA. Adverse drug interactions involving common prescription and over-the-counter analgesic agents. Clinical Therapeutics. 2007;29(11):2477–97. DOI: 10.1016/j.clinthera.2007.12.003 DOI:10.1016/j.clinthera.2007.12.003#_blank#-Persistent link using digital object identifier

[38] Heard KJ, Ries NL, Dart RC, Bogdan GM, Zallen RD, Daly F. Overuse of non-prescription analgesics by dental clinic patients. BMC Oral Health. 2008;8(1):1. DOI: 10.1186/1472-6831-8-33

[39] Lavonas EJ, Fries JF, Furst DE, Rothman KJ, Stergachis A, Vaida AJ, Zelterman D, Reynolds KM, Green JL, Dart RC. Comparative risks of non-prescription analgesics: a structured topic review and research priorities. Expert Opinion on Drug Safety. 2012;11 (1):33–44. 10.1517/14740338.2012.629782

[40] Moore N, Pollack C, Butkerait P. Adverse drug reactions and drug–drug interactions with over-the-counter NSAIDs. Therapeutics and Clinical Risk Management. 2015;11:1061. DOI: 10.2147/TCRM.S79135 DOI:10.2147%2FTCRM.S79135#pmc_ext

[41] Poveda Roda R, Bagán JV, Jiménez Soriano Y, Gallud Romero L. Use of nonsteroidal antiinflammatory drugs in dental practice: a review. Medicina Oral, Patología Oral y Cirugía Bucal (Internet). 2007;12(1):10–8.

[42] Botting RM. Inhibitors of cyclooxygenases: mechanisms, selectivity and uses. Journal of Physiology and Pharmacology. 2006;57:113.

[43] Kawabe JI, Ushikubi F, Hasebe N. Prostacyclin in vascular diseases-recent insights and future perspectives. Circulation Journal. 2010;74(5):836–43. DOI: 10.1253/circj.CJ-10-0195

[44] Kearney PM, Baigent C, Godwin J, Halls H, Emberson JR, Patrono C. Do selective cyclo-oxygenase-2 inhibitors and traditional non-steroidal anti-inflammatory drugs increase

the risk of atherothrombosis? Meta-analysis of randomised trials. British Medical Journal. 2006;332(7553):1302–8. DOI: http://dx.doi.org/10.1136/bmj.332.7553.1302

[45] Dogne JM, Hanson J, Supuran C, Pratico D. Coxibs and cardiovascular side-effects: from light to shadow. Current Pharmaceutical Design. 2006;12(8):971–5.DOI: http://dx.doi.org/10.2174/138161206776055949

[46] Ng K, Meyerhardt JA, Chan AT, Sato K, Chan JA, Niedzwiecki D, Saltz LB, Mayer RJ, Benson AB, Schaefer PL, Whittom R. Aspirin and COX-2 inhibitor use in patients with stage III colon cancer. Journal of the National Cancer Institute. 2015;107(1):dju345. DOI: 10.1093/jnci/dju345

[47] de Pedro M, Baeza S, Escudero MT, Dierssen-Sotos T, Gómez-Acebo I, Pollán M, Llorca J. Effect of COX-2 inhibitors and other non-steroidal inflammatory drugs on breast cancer risk: a meta-analysis. Breast Cancer Research and Treatment. 2015;149(2):525–36. DOI: 10.1007/s10549-015-3267-9

[48] Al-Hasani R, Bruchas MR. Molecular mechanisms of opioid receptor-dependent signaling and behavior. The Journal of the American Society of Anesthesiologists. 2011;115 (6):1363–81. DOI: 10.1097/ALN.0b013e318238bba6.

[49] Walton RE, Reader AF Local anesthesia. In Walton RE, Torabinejad M, eds. Principles and Practice of Endodontics, 3rd ed. Philadelphia: W.B. Saunders Company; 2002, pp. 99–117.

[50] Malamed SF. Handbook of Local Anesthesia, 6th Edition. Published by Mosby, MO, USA. 2012, pp 432.

[51] Henry MA, Hargreaves KM. Peripheral mechanisms of odontogenic pain. Dental Clinics of North America. 2007;51(1):19–44. DOI: 10.1016/j.cden.2006.09.007

[52] Rood JP, Pateromichelakis S. Inflammation and peripheral nerve sensitisation. British Journal of Oral Surgery. 1981;19(1):67–72. DOI: 10.1016/0007-117X(81)90023-8 DOI:10.1016/0007-117X(81)90023-8#_blank#Persistent link using digital object identifier

[53] Parirokh M, Ashouri R, Rekabi AR, Nakhaee N, Pardakhti A, Askarifard S, Abbott PV. The effect of premedication with ibuprofen and indomethacin on the success of inferior alveolar nerve block for teeth with irreversible pulpitis. Journal of Endodontics. 2010;36 (9):1450–4. DOI: 10.1016/j.joen.2010.05.007 DOI:10.1016/j.joen.2010.05.007#doilink

[54] Kalyvas DG, Tarenidou M. Influence of nonsteroidal anti-inflammatory drugs on osseointegration. Journal of Oral Science. 2008;50(3):239–46. DOI: 10.2334/josnusd.50.239

[55] Kiersch TA, Halladay SC, Koschik M. A double-blind, randomized study of naproxen sodium, ibuprofen and placebo in postoperative dental pain. Clinical Therapeutics. 1992;15(5):845–54.

[56] Bailey E, Worthington HV, van Wijk A, Yates JM, Coulthard P, Afzal Z. Ibuprofen and/or paracetamol (acetaminophen) for pain relief after surgical removal of lower wisdom

teeth. Cochrane Database of Systematic Reviews 2013; 12:1–55. DOI:10.1002/14651858.CD004624.pub2.

[57] Wideman GL, Keffer M, Morris E, Doyle Jr RT, Jiang JG, Beaver WT. Analgesic efficacy of a combination of hydrocodone with Ibuprofen in postoperative pain. Clinical Pharmacology and Therapeutics. 1999;65(1):66–76. DOI: 10.1016/S0009-9236(99)70123-2

[58] Wynn RL. Narcotic analgesics for dental pain: available products, strengths and formulations. General Dentistry. 2000;49(2):126–8.

[59] Cusack BJ. Pharmacokinetics in older persons. The American Journal of Geriatric Pharmacotherapy. 2004;2(4):274–302. DOI: 10.1016/j.amjopharm.2004.12.005 DOI:10.1016/j.amjopharm.2004.12.005#_blank#Persistent link using digital object identifier

[60] Guay DR, Artz MB, Hanlon JT, Schmader KE. The Pharmacology of Aging. Brocklehurst's Textbook of Geriatric Medicine and Gerontology. New York, NY: Churchill Livingstone; 2003, pp. 155–61.

[61] Huanga AR, Mallet L. Prescribing opioids in older people. Maturitas. 2013;74(2):123–9. DOI: 10.1016/j.maturitas.2012.11.002.

[62] Anand KJ. Consensus statement for the prevention and management of pain in the newborn. Archives of Pediatrics & Adolescent Medicine. 2001;155(2):173–80. DOI: 10.1001/archpedi.155.2.173

[63] Shim YS, Kim AH, Jeon EY, An SY. Dental fear & anxiety and dental pain in children and adolescents: a systemic review. Journal of Dental Anesthesia and Pain Medicine. 2015;15 (2):53–61. DOI:http://dx.doi.org/10.17245/jdapm.2015.15.2.53

[64] Khatri A, Kalra N. A comparison of two pain scales in the assessment of dental pain in East Delhi children. ISRN Dentistry. 2012; 247351:1–8. DOI: 10.5402/2012/247351

[65] Azarpazhooh A, Chong V, Chuk M, Dosanjh A, Lee Y, Norsen H, Toth K. The dental utility of pain-assessment tools: an evidence-based report. Community Dentistry 2011. retrieved from: https://www.dentistry.utoronto.ca/system/files/w3_2011.pdf

[66] Shindova M, Belcheva A. Pain assessment methods among pediatric patients in medical and dental research. Medical Biology Studies, Clinical Studies, Social Medicine and Health Care. 2016; 6(1):16–23.

[67] Manworren RC, Hynan LS. Clinical validation of FLACC: preverbal patient pain scale. Pediatric Nursing. 2003 ;29(2):140.

[68] Garra G, Singer AJ, Taira BR, Chohan J, Cardoz H, Chisena E, Thode HC. Validation of the Wong-Baker FACES pain rating scale in pediatric emergency department patients. Academic Emergency Medicine. 2010;17(1):50–4. DOI: 10.1111/j.1553-2712.2009.00620.x

[69] Hjermstad MJ, Fayers PM, Haugen DF, Caraceni A, Hanks GW, Loge JH, Fainsinger R, Aass N, Kaasa S, European Palliative Care Research Collaborative (EPCRC). Studies

comparing Numerical Rating Scales, Verbal Rating Scales and Visual Analogue Scales for assessment of pain intensity in adults: a systematic literature review. Journal of Pain and Symptom Management. 2011;41(6):1073–93. DOI: 10.1016/j.jpainsymman.2010.08.016 DOI:10.1016/j.jpainsymman.2010.08.016#doilink

[70] Yaster M. Multimodal analgesia in children. European Journal of Anaesthesiology (EJA). 2010;27(10):851–7. DOI: 10.1097/EJA.0b013e328338c4af

[71] Weaver JM. New FDA black box warning for codeine: how will this affect dentists? Anesthesia Progress. 2013;60(2):35.

[72] Coric A, Banozic A, Klaric M, Vukojevic K, Puljak L. Dental fear and anxiety in older children: an association with parental dental anxiety and effective pain coping strategies. Journal of Pain Research. 2014;7:515–21. DOI: 10.2147/JPR.S67692.

[73] Rexrode KM, Buring JE, Glynn RJ, Stampfer MJ, Youngman LD, Gaziano JM. Analgesic use and renal function in men. Journal of the American Medical Association. 2001;286 (3):315–21. DOI: 10.1001/jama.286.3.315.

[74] Hamid MJ, Dummer CD, Pinto LS. Systemic conditions, oral findings and dental management of chronic renal failure patients: general considerations and case report. Brazilian Dental Journal. 2006;17(2):166–70. DOI:10.1590/S0103-64402006000200016

[75] Cerveró AJ, Bagán JV, Soriano YJ, Roda RP. Dental management in renal failure: patients on dialysis. Medicina Oral, Patología Oral y Cirugía Bucal. 2008;13(7):E419–26.

[76] Murtagh FE, Chai MO, Donohoe P, Edmonds PM, Higginson IJ. The use of opioid analgesia in end-stage renal disease patients managed without dialysis: recommendations for practice. Journal of Pain & Palliative Care Pharmacotherapy. 2007;21(2):5–16.

[77] Niscola P, Scaramucci L, Vischini G, Giovannini M, Ferrannini M, Massa P, Tatangelo P, Galletti M, Palumbo R. The use of major analgesics in patients with renal dysfunction. Current Drug Targets. 2010;11(6):752–8. DOI: 10.2174/138945010791170879

[78] Ouanounou A, Haas DA. Pharmacotherapy for the elderly dental patient. Journal (Canadian Dental Association). 2015;80:f18.

[79] Mazer M, Perrone J. Acetaminophen-induced nephrotoxicity: pathophysiology, clinical manifestations and management. Journal of Medical Toxicology. 2008;4(1):2–6. DOI: 10.1007/BF03160941

[80] Martínez SR, Serna JT, Silvestre FJ. Dental management in patients with cirrhosis. Gastroenterología y Hepatología (English Edition). 2016;39(3):224–32.DOI: 10.1016/j.gastre.2016.02.020 DOI:10.1016/j.gastre.2016.02.020#doilink

[81] Smith H, Bruckenthal P. Implications of opioid analgesia for medically complicated patients. Drugs & Aging. 2010;27(5):417–33. DOI: 10.2165/11536540-000000000-00000

[82] Ong CK, Seymour RA. An evidence-based update of the use of analgesics in dentistry. Periodontology 2000. 2008;46(1):143–64.

[83] Cicconetti A, Bartoli A, Ripari F, Ripari A. COX-2 selective inhibitors: a literature review of analgesic efficacy and safety in oral-maxillofacial surgery. Oral Surgery, Oral Medicine, Oral Pathology, Oral Radiology and Endodontology. 2004;97(2):139–46. DOI: 10.1016/j.tripleo.2003.08.032 DOI:10.1016/j.tripleo.2003.08.032#doilink

[84] Au AH, Choi SW, Cheung CW, Leung YY. The efficacy and clinical safety of various analgesic combinations for post-operative pain after third molar surgery: a systematic review and meta-analysis. Plos One. 2015;10(6):e0127611. DOI: 10.1371/journal.pone.0127611

[85] Guggenheimer J, Moore PA. The therapeutic applications of and risks associated with acetaminophen use: a review and update. The Journal of the American Dental Association. 2011;142(1):38–44. DOI: 10.14219/jada.archive.2011.0026 DOI:10.14219/jada.archive.2011.0026#doilink

[86] Branco FP, Pinheiro ML, Volpato MC, De Andrade ED. Analgesic choice in dentistry. Part I: the mechanism of action. Brazilian Journal of Oral Sciences. 2005;4(14):762–65.

[87] Pinheiro ML, Cristina M andrade VE, Branco PF. Analgesic choice in dentistry Part II: the toxicity. Brazilian Journal of Oral Sciences. 2005; 4(14):880–83.

[88] Aminoshariae A, Kulild JC, Donaldson M. Short-term use of nonsteroidal anti-inflammatory drugs and adverse effects: an updated systematic review. The Journal of the American Dental Association. 2016;147(2):98–110. DOI: 10.1016/j.adaj.2015.07.020 DOI:10.1016/j.adaj.2015.07.020#doilink

[89] Trescot AM. Opioid pharmacology and pharmacokinetics. In Controlled Substance Management in Chronic Pain. Springer International Publishing, USA. 2016, pp. 45–62. DOI:14 10.1007/978-3-319-30964-4_4

[90] Bruehl S, Apkarian AV, Ballantyne JC, Berger A, Borsook D, Chen WG, Farrar JT, Haythornthwaite JA, Horn SD, Iadarola MJ, Inturrisi CE. Personalized medicine and opioid analgesic prescribing for chronic pain: opportunities and challenges. The Journal of Pain. 2013;14(2):103–13. DOI: http://dx.doi.org/10.1016/j.jpain.2012.10.016 DOI:10.1016/j.jpain.2012.10.016#doilink

[91] Dionne R. Additive analgesia without opioid side effects. Compendium of Continuing Education in Dentistry (Jamesburg, NJ: 1995). 2000;21(7):572–4.

[92] Paudel KR. Therapeutic practice preference in dentistry: antibiotics, analgesics and antiseptics. Asian Journal of Medical Sciences (E-ISSN 2091-0576; P-ISSN 2467-9100). 2014;4(4):17–23.

[93] Spivakovsky S. Will adding acetaminophen (paracetamol) to ibuprofen be more effective in relieving postoperative pain on symptomatic necrotic teeth? Evidence-Based Dentistry. 2012;13(4):105. DOI: 10.1038/sj.ebd.6400889

[94] Alexander L, Hall E, Eriksson L, Rohlin M. The combination of non-selective NSAID 400 mg and paracetamol 1000 mg is more effective than each drug alone for treatment of acute pain. A systematic review. Swedish Dental Journal. 2013;38(1):1–4.

[95] Bailey E, Worthington H, Coulthard P. Ibuprofen and/or paracetamol (acetaminophen) for pain relief after surgical removal of lower wisdom teeth, a Cochrane systematic review. British Dental Journal. 2014;216(8):451–5. DOI: 10.1038/sj.bdj.2014.330

[96] Akbulut N, Üstüner E, Atakan C, Çölok G. Comparison of the effect of naproxen, etodolac and diclofenac on postoperative sequels following third molar surgery: a randomised, double-blind, crossover study. Medicina Oral, Patologia Oral Y Cirugia Bucal. 2014;19(2): e149. DOI: 10.4317/medoral.19518 DOI:10.4317%2Fmedoral.19518#pmc_ext

[97] Kara İM, Polat S, İnce F, Gümüş C. Analgesic and anti-inflammatory effects of oxaprozin and naproxen sodium after removal of impacted lower third molars: a randomized, double-blind, placebo-controlled crossover study. Journal of Oral and Maxillofacial Surgery. 2010;68(5):1018–24. DOI: 10.1016/j.joms.2009.09.094 DOI:10.1016/j.joms.2009.09.094#doilink

[98] Polat O, Karaman AI, Durmus E. Effects of preoperative ibuprofen and naproxen sodium on orthodontic pain. The Angle Orthodontist. 2005;75(5):791–6.

[99] Christensen K, Daniels S, Bandy D, Ernst CC, Hamilton DA, Mermelstein FH, Wang J, Carr DB. A double-blind placebo-controlled comparison of a novel formulation of intravenous diclofenac and ketorolac for postoperative third molar extraction pain. Anesthesia Progress. 2011;58(2):73–81. DOI: 10.2344/0003-3006-58.2.73

[100] Bhaskar H, Kapoor P. Comparison of transdermal diclofenac patch with oral diclofenac as an analgesic modality following multiple premolar extractions in orthodontic patients: a cross over efficacy trial. Contemporary Clinical Dentistry. 2010;1(3):158. DOI: 10.4103/0976-237X.72783

[101] Tschoppe P, Kielbassa AM. The role of COX-2 in dentistry. Past or future? Swiss Monthly Record for Dentistry=Swiss Monthly magazine of dentistry and stomatology/SSO. 2005;116(9):880–6.

[102] May N, Epstein J, Osborne B. Selective COX-2 inhibitors: a review of their therapeutic potential and safety in dentistry. Oral Surgery, Oral Medicine, Oral Pathology, Oral Radiology and Endodontology. 2001;92(4):399–405. DOI: 10.1067/moe.2001.115127 DOI:10.1067/moe.2001.115127#doilink

[103] Madani ZS, Moghadamnia AA, Panahi A, Mir AP. Analgesic effect of etoricoxib compared to ibuprofen on post endodontic pain. Oral Health and Dental Management. 2013;12:511. DOI: 10.4172/2247-2452.1000511

[104] Murnion BP. Combination analgesics in adults. Australian Prescriber. 2010;33(4). DOI:10.18773/austprescr.2010.056

[105] Der Khatchadourian Z, Moreno-Hay I, de Leeuw R. Nonsteroidal anti-inflammatory drugs and antihypertensives: how do they relate? Oral Surgery, Oral Medicine, Oral Pathology and Oral Radiology. 2014;117(6):697–703. DOI: 10.1016/j.oooo.2014.02.028 DOI:10.1016/j.oooo.2014.02.028#doilink

[106] Hersh EV, Moore PA. Adverse drug interactions in dentistry. Periodontology 2000. 2008;46(1):109–42. DOI: 10.1111/j.1600-0757.2008.00224.x

[107] Moore PA, Hersh EV. Principles of pain management in dentistry. The ADA Practical Guide to Substance Use Disorders and Safe Prescribing. 2015;5:31.

[108] Kotlinska-Lemieszek A, Klepstad P, Haugen DF. Clinically significant drug–drug interactions involving opioid analgesics used for pain treatment in patients with cancer: a systematic review. Drug Design, Development and Therapy. 2015;9:52–55. DOI: 10.2147/DDDT.S86983 DOI:10.2147%2FDDDT.S86983#pmc_ext

[109] Weinstock RJ, Johnson MP. Review of top 10 prescribed drugs and their interaction with dental treatment. Dental Clinics of North America. 2016;60(2):421–34. DOI:http://dx.doi.org/10.1016/j.cden.2015.11.005 DOI:10.1016/j.cden.2015.11.005#doilink

[110] Kim H, Neubert JK, San Miguel A, Xu K, Krishnaraju RK, Iadarola MJ, Goldman D, Dionne RA. Genetic influence on variability in human acute experimental pain sensitivity associated with gender, ethnicity and psychological temperament. Pain. 2004;109(3):488–96. DOI: 10.1016/j.pain.2004.02.027 DOI:10.1016/j.pain.2004.02.027#doilink

Chapter 7

Headache of Analgesic Abuse as a Cause of New Pain Pathways Development

Silvia Ussai and Alessandro Rizzardo

Additional information is available at the end of the chapter

http://dx.doi.org/10.5772/67244

Abstract

Medication-overuse headache (MOH) is a worldwide health problem with a prevalence of 1–2%. It is a severe form of headache where the patients often have a long history of unsuccessful headache treatments. MOH is characterized by chronic headache and the overuse of different headache medications. Through the years, withdrawal of the overused medication has been recognized as the treatment of choice. However, currently, there is no clear consensus regarding the optimal strategy for the management of MOH. Treatment approaches are based on expert opinion rather than scientific evidence. This chapter focuses on an overall discussion of medication abuse as a novel pain pathway in headaches.

Keywords: headache treatment, migraine, medication-overuse headache, pain pathways, chronic headache

1. Introduction

Headache is one of the first causes for pain consultation in primary care settings and one of the major complaints of pain made at the neurology clinic [1]. Overall it is estimated that 4% of the general population suffer from migraine, representing at least 280,000,000 people requiring treatment only for just one cause of cephalea [2]. If the number of all other headache causes is added to the total number of migraine patients, the number of people requiring treatment for headaches represents almost one-sixth of the global population.

Due to the high number of patients as well as the varied causes of headaches, cephalea treatments are varied ranging from mild, over-the-counter painkillers such as paracetamol [3], to high complex molecules, intended to act as neuromodulators and prevent pain crisis, such as topiramate [4], and sometimes further requiring nonopioid and opioid analgesics such as ketoprofen [5] and codeine [6]. With so many people suffering from headaches and having such a varied set of available drugs for treatment, it is no surprise that the problem of overuse and abuse of such treatments exists, leading to the appearance of secondary adverse effects such as the development of new pain pathways, among a certain group of patients. To understand the complexity of a problem like this, it is necessary to gain a deep knowledge of headache physiopathology, pharmacological options, and treatment guidelines, in order to identify the reasons leading to cephalea treatment overuse, and the arising of such a tricky problem such as the development of new pain pathways.

2. Classification of headaches

Although the concept of cephalea has mostly remained the same since it was first used to describe this type of disorder, its classification has been evolving continuously in line with modern physiopathological and pharmacologic concepts. The term cephalea or cephalalgia denotes pain located anywhere in the head and neck, regardless of the etiology; however, such a vast subject requires a very detailed classification scheme to determine which would be the best treatment for each type. Headaches are divided into two major groups: primary headaches and secondary headaches. Primary headaches are those appearing spontaneously with no association to any other disease or medical condition, while secondary headaches are those appearing in close temporal relation to another condition known to produce cephalea [7]. The main difference between both groups is whether or not an association is found with another cause, thus primary headaches have an intrinsic physiopathology while secondary cephalea is the consequence of another disease, trauma, or medical condition.

Primary cephalalgia is divided into four major categories:

(1) Migraine

(2) Tension-type headache

(3) Trigeminal autonomic cephalalgias

(4) Other primary headache disorders [8]

While secondary cephalea has eight:

(1) Headache attributed to trauma or injury to the head and/or neck

(2) Headache attributed to cranial or cervical vascular disorder

(3) Headache attributed to nonvascular intracranial disorder

(4) Headache attributed to a substance or its withdrawal

(5) Headache attributed to infection

(6) Headache attributed to disorder of homoeostasis

http://dx.doi.org/10.5772/67244

(7) Headache or facial pain attributed to disorder of the cranium, neck, eyes, ears, nose, sinuses, teeth, mouth, or other facial or cervical structure

(8) Headache attributed to psychiatric disorder [9]

From the above-mentioned cephalea types, migraine and tension-type headaches represent up to 80% of all cases [10]; however, it is important to recognize all other types of cephalea so as to avoid misdiagnosis and treatment errors since these could be the first steps toward the overuse and abuse of headache treatment drugs.

3. Headache physiopathology

A detailed description of the physiopathology of each type of headache goes far from the reach of this chapter, thus the discussion will be focused on the most common subtypes; migraine and tension-type headache as well as on a common feature for each cephalea type: the pain pathway.

3.1. Physiopathology of migraine

Despite being the most common cause of headache, the underlying pathogenesis of migraine is not known and every day, new data is being made available which aid in the clarification of the possible processes behind such a major public health problem.

Once considered a cephalalgia of vascular origin involving intracranial blood vessel dilatation, recent data reveals that the physiopathology of migraine is much more complex; abnormal modulation of brain nociceptive systems [12], brain excitability, recurrent activation, and sensitization of the trigeminovascular pathway [13] all work together not only to produce but also to prolong the migraine.

The integration of the above-mentioned factors is shown in **Figure 1**, where the interaction and upregulation of each element over the other is made clear.

Moreover, **Figure 1** demonstrates why there are so many available migraine treatments, as each one has to work on a very narrow cluster of the whole pathogenic chain and why the effect of a particular therapy may diminish over time due to the upregulation and potentiation between different pathological events associated with migraine.

The good news behind such a complex physiopathology is the high number of therapeutic targets available to work with, rendering the therapeutic options almost infinite. Although the ideal treatment would be one that could act over all the mechanisms, or at least the most important one, unfortunately, such a treatment is far from being available, and current knowledge points to what seems to be the convergence point of all migraine pathogenic mechanisms: serotonin [14]. Abnormally low levels of this important neurotransmitter seem to be the cause of at least two of the pathological aspects: blood vessel dilation and brain hyperexcitability; hence, it is not surprising to find that there is a remarkable therapeutic effect by serotonin agonists on migraine.

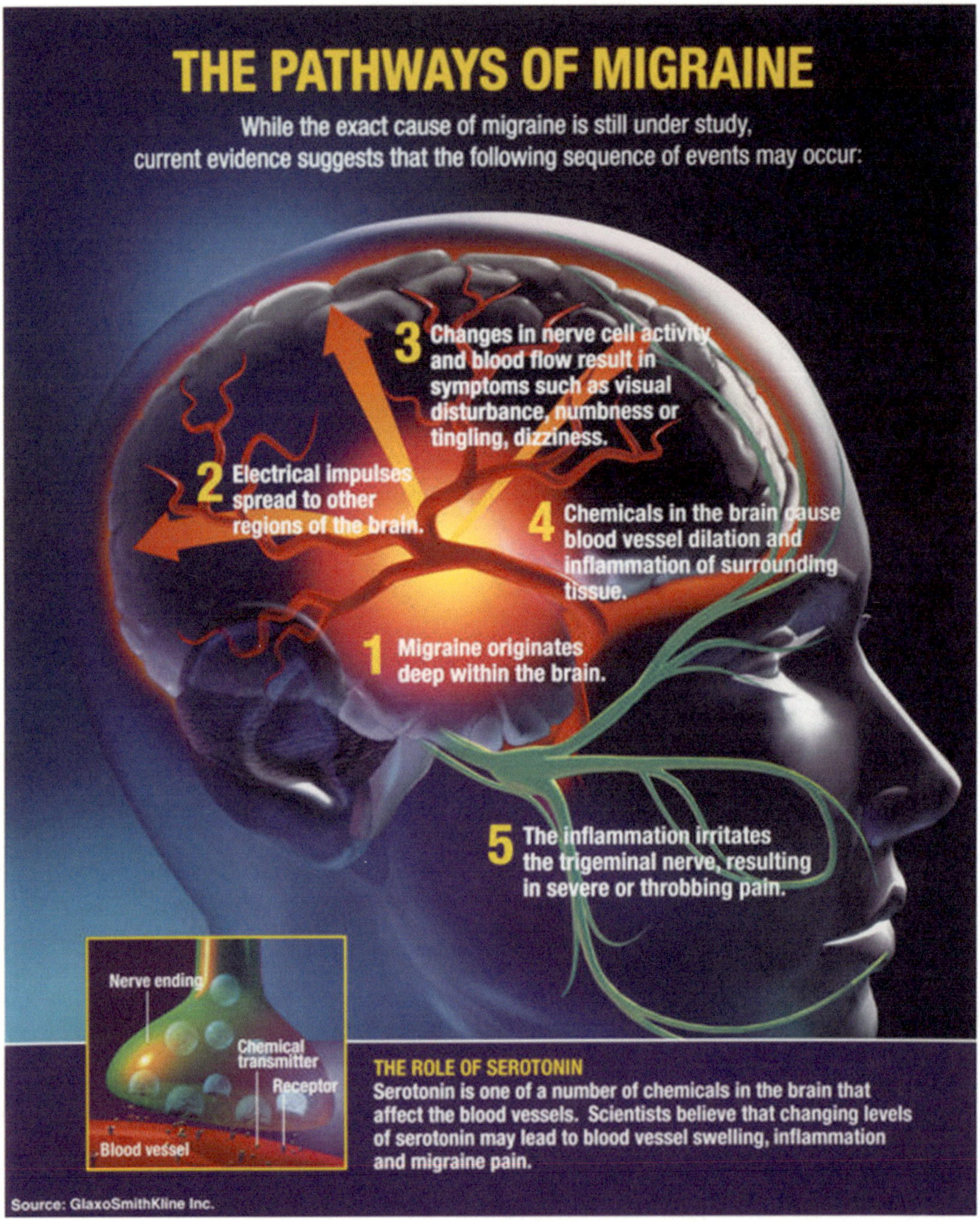

Figure 1. The pathways of migraine [11].

3.2. Physiopathology of tension-type headaches

Even though migraine represents a major public health concern and is the leading cause of headache, tension-type headache should not be underestimated since it represents the second most common cause of cephalalgia with a prevalence of 46.9% in the general population [15], and provides the potential for a great field of study as tension-type headaches may be present in an acute scenario (known as episodic tension-type headache) or chronically, being called in such cases chronic tension-type headache. The most interesting fact regarding this dual presentation profile is that in some people tension-type headache remains acute and sporadic while some others progress toward a chronic condition. At the initial stage, both episodic and chronic tension-type headaches share a common pathophysiological pattern associated with scalp and head muscles chronically contracting as well as certain neck movements [16], these are usually identified as the triggers and are the targets for therapy in the past; however, recent investigations have shown that chronic muscle contraction alone is not enough to cause a pain crisis, but it also includes the presence of central nervous system factors such as a hypersensitivity to pain stimuli which causes a tension-type headache to evolve from just a simple contraction [17] to a chronic disorder affecting quality of life [18].

It is possible that at the very beginning all tension-type headaches begin this way but when there is increased excitability of the central nervous system generated by repetitive and sustained pericranial myofascial input [19] permanency occurs and upregulation creates a cycle of chronic tension-type headache, with lower stimuli requirements needed to trigger the next pain crisis. At the molecular level, chronic tension-type headache has been associated with low serotonin levels [20] acting as an upregulator in the case of migraine, on the other hand, there is the recent description of nitric oxide playing a role in both migraine and tension-type headaches, acting as a cranial and extracranial blood vessel dilator as well as a central nervous system sensitizer, these findings have led to a hypothesis about a common pain pathway shared by all primary chronic cephalalgias or at least between the two major groups, migraine and chronic tension-type headache [21].

4. Headache pain pathway

It is a well-known fact that cerebral tissue has no pain receptors, making it impossible to generate painful stimuli directly from the brain; most head and neck tissues such as bone, muscle, skin, and even blood vessels share a common innervation pattern where nociceptive C and A-delta fibers from the first root of the trigeminal nerve are involved as seen in **Figure 2**.

The aforementioned common innervation pattern may cause headache to arise from almost any head structure from muscles to meningeal membranes progressing to a chronic condition based on preexisting genetic, biochemical, and behavioral characteristics of each individual. Once the pain has become chronic, at least two molecular events have been identified as responsible (totally or partially) for pain upregulation: low serotonin levels and high nitric oxide, both of them upregulating pain pathways in at least two major headache groups: migraine and chronic tension-type cephalalgia [23]. Based on the above, positive strides can be made toward the development of new drugs intended not only to treat pain but also to prevent it [24] since the existence of both a common neurologic pain pathway as well as shared molecular features among major primary headache groups provides that possibility; moreover, it could be possible to treat different primary headache types with a single drug working on key, shared points of the pain pathway [25]; however, more extensive research as well as a deeper understanding of different pain pathway integration is needed to achieve such goals; primary headache treatments still focus on two main targets: pain control and crisis prevention.

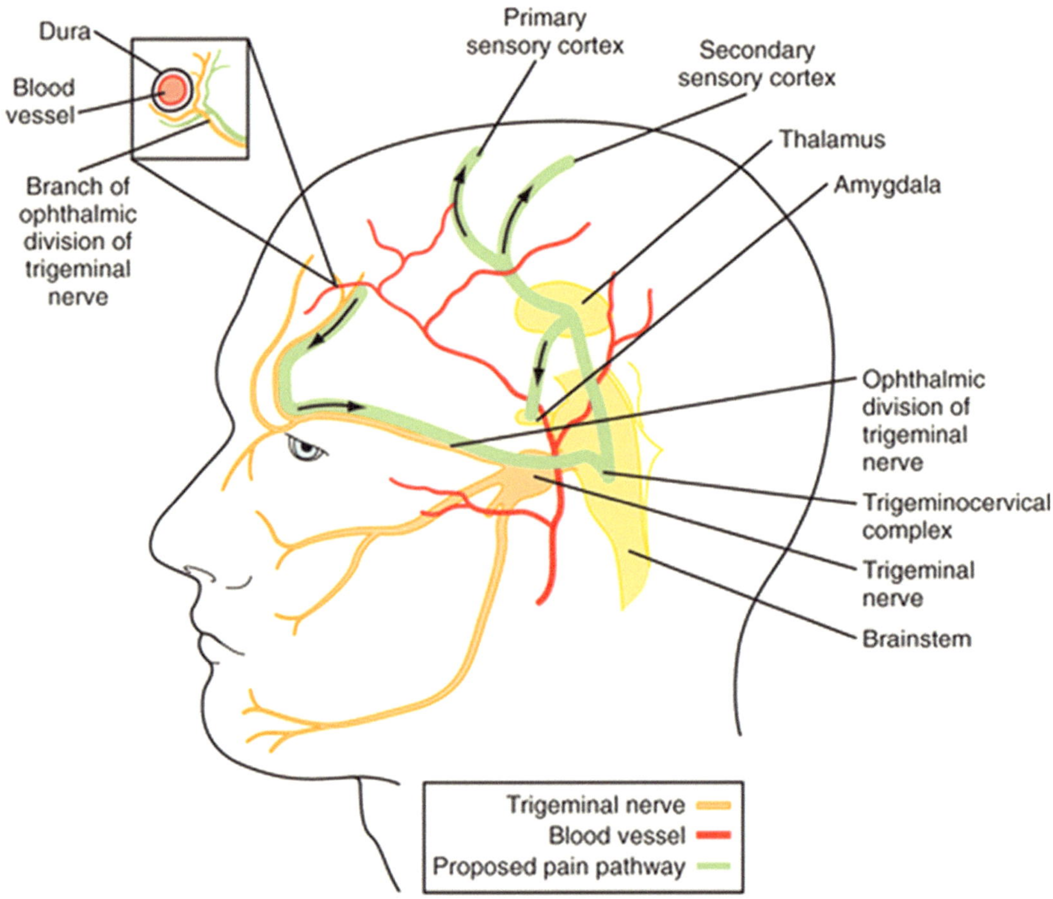

Figure 2. Blood vessel innervation pattern and migraine associate pain pathways [22].

5. Pharmacological options for headache treatment

It is a well-known fact that prevention of a medical condition is usually the best approach because it tends to be easier, cheaper, and cost effective; hence the aim of primary headache treatment should be focused on such a target. However, at this moment, prevention strategies for primary headache are not 100% reliable and the failure rates are high [26] leading to the use of palliative measures in order to relieve patients' suffering derived mainly from migraine and tension-type headache.

In this regard, current pharmacological approaches include two major groups of action: pain relief and brain modulation, each one aimed to act on a particular stage. Although pain relief should be the last resort and be used only when modulation and prevention have failed, this is the main therapeutic approach in real life, treating the problem once it has fully showed up; the reason behind such behavior could be related to the ancient approach toward headache based on pain relief, used for decades when primary headache was not known as it is today and no other therapeutic option was available; and although there may be numerous and powerful effective pain killers and analgesics available, this option should be restricted only to cases where prevention has failed; always giving priority to novel, preventive therapies offering patients a better quality of life [27]. With the everyday increase in knowledge on primary headache pathophysiology, neurochemistry, and pain pathways, modern, current treatments of primary headaches intended to act as brain modulators have gained popularity because they are more expensive than conventional pain killers, such drugs are able to give patients a better quality of life, decreasing the negative impact of headache on both personal and work commitments [28]. Novel migraine and tension-type headache treatments exert their action in several ways but with a common goal: reduction of pain crisis by downregulating sensitized brain pathways, which usually act as a trigger or maintain the headache pain crisis, leading to an overall reduction of acute primary headache and thus a drop in the requirements for over-the-counter (OTC) painkillers and prescription analgesic use.

According to the U.S. Headache Consortium the scope of modern migraine treatment must be to:

- *Reduce attack frequency and severity*
- *Reduce disability*
- *Improve quality of life*
- *Prevent headache*
- *Avoid headache medication escalation*
- *Educate and enable patients to manage their disease* [29]

It is clear that the use of OTC painkillers and analgesics are a last resort and is considered to be a damage control strategy, leading the way not only to better control of the migraine but also to a reduction in headache medication overuse [30].

Hence, the aforementioned medications may be extrapolated for use with tension-type and cluster headaches due to them having similar pathological pathways and neurotransmitters shared by the three major causes of primary headache.

The modern approach toward current headache management is shown in **Figure 3**.

After careful analysis of **Figure 3**, one can deduce that primary headaches still remain a diagnostic and therapeutic challenge, where a misdiagnosis or improper drug selection could lead to treatment failure, with unexpected consequences not only by reducing the patient's quality of life but also due to the possible development of complications, thus it is mandatory to have a clear idea of available treatments and their mechanisms of action in order to properly select one or another option when necessary.

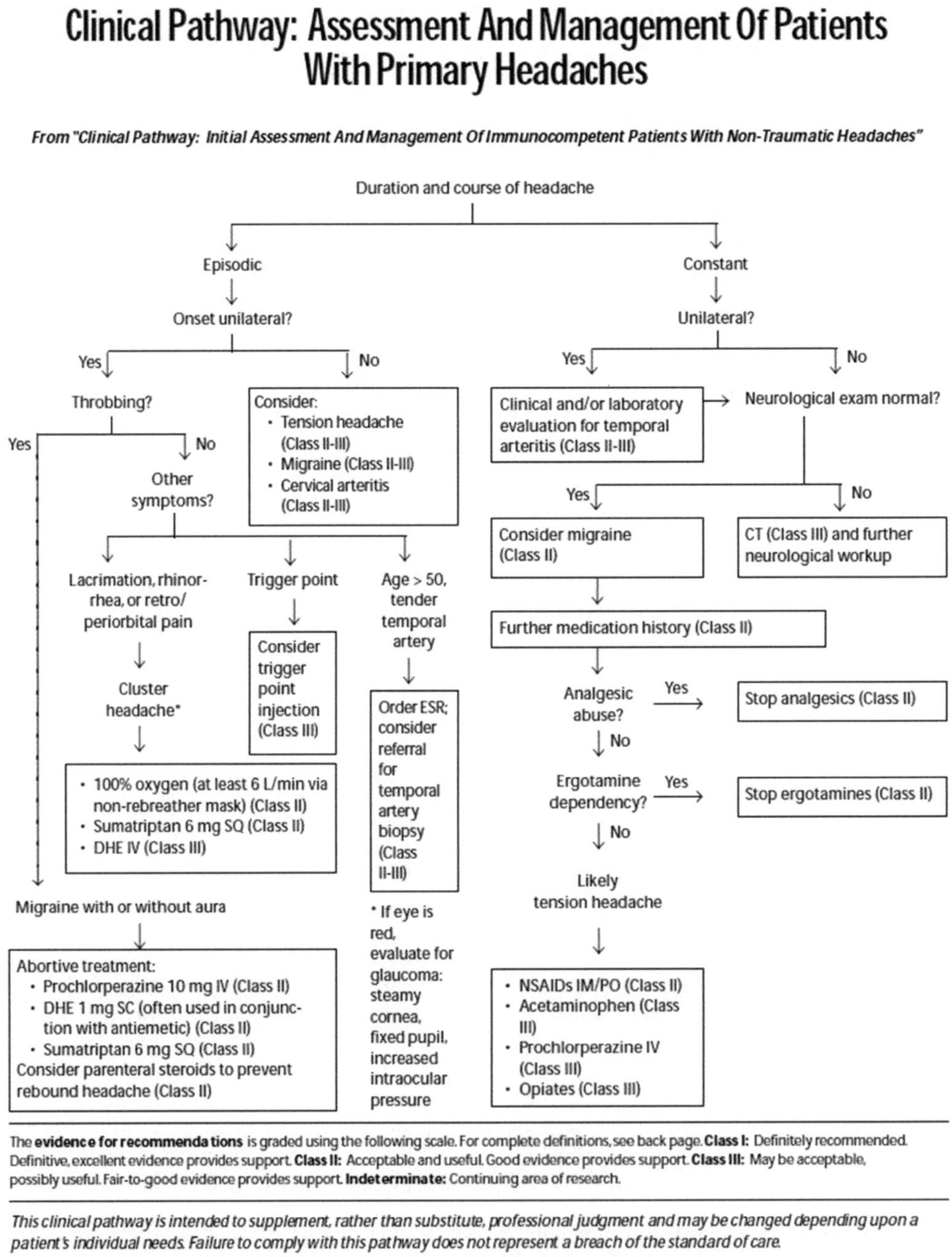

Figure 3. Assessment and management of patients with primary headaches [31].

http://dx.doi.org/10.5772/67244

5.1. Comparison of the mechanism of action of different primary headache treatments

Due to the complex underlying pathologic mechanisms regarding primary headaches, common pain pathways, as well as the different drugs types and mechanisms of action, it is best to evaluate the most effective treatment for a particular patient by using a comparison chart because even though general guidelines may be helpful, primary headache treatment still needs to be individualized and adapted to the particular requirements of each patient. Modern therapeutic options for primary headaches as well as their primary and complementary mechanisms of action and indications are summarized in **Table 1**.

Preventive and abortive treatments			
Drug*	**Drug class**	**Mechanism of action**	**Indication**
Amitriptyline [32] (Nortriptyline)	**Tricyclic antidepressants**	**Primary:** Serotonin reuptake inhibitor **Secondary:** Still not properly known	**Migraine** (prevention) **Tension-type headache** (prevention) [33]
Sumatriptan [34] (Rizatriptan, Naratriptan, Eletriptan, Donitriptan, Almotriptan, Frovatriptan, Avitriptan, Zolmitriptan)	**Triptans**	**Primary:** Selective Intracranial Blood Vessels constrictor acting as 5-HT1B and 5-HT1D serotonin receptors agonists **Secondary:** Blockage of sensitized neural pathways [35]	**Migraine** (Pain crisis abortive medication) **Cluster headache** (Pain crisis abortive medication)
Ergotamine (Dihydroergotamine)	**Ergopeptine**	**Primary:** Constriction of intracranial extra cerebral blood vessels working as 5-HT1B receptor agonist and 5-HT1D serotonin receptor blocker **Secondary:** Inhibition of trigeminal neurotransmission	**Migraine** (Long lasting pain crisis) [36]
Propranolol [37] (Nadolol, Timolol, Metoprolol, Atenolol)	**Beta blockers**	**Primary:** Inhibition of intracranial extra cerebral blood vessels dilation through Beta adrenergic receptors blockage	**Migraine** (prevention) **Cluster Headache** (prevention)
Valproic Acid - valproate -	**Antiepileptic drug** *not chemically related to other anticonvulsivant*	**Primary:** Under investigation, it's presumed that valproate may decrease nerve impulse transmission in previous sensitized pain pathways [38]	**Migraine** (Pain crisis abortive medication) [39] **Cluster Headache** (Preventive) [40]
Topiramate	**Anticonvulsant**	**Primary:** Modification of several receptor-gated and voltage-sensitive ion channels, including voltage-activated Na^+ and Ca^{2+} channels and non-NMDA receptors [41] **Secondary:** Modulation of gamma-aminobutyric acid- (GABA-) and/ or glutamate-mediated neurotransmission [42]	**Migraine** (prevention) [43] **Cluster headache** (Adjunctive treatment) [44] **Tension-type headache** (Prevention) [45]

Preventive and abortive treatments			
Drug*	**Drug class**	**Mechanism of action**	**Indication**
Rescue treatments (pain control)			
Acetylsalicylic acid - Aspirin-**	**NSAIDs**	**Primary:** COX-1 and COX-2 inhibition	**Tension-type headache** (Rescue) [46]
Paracetamol**	**Mild analgesic**	**Primary:** - Suppression of signal towards the dorsal horn from the peripheral nerves by blocking TRPA1-receptors (peripheral pain pathway blockage) [47] - Inhibition of the reuptake of the endogenous cannabinoid/ vanilloid anandamide by neurons down regulating TRPV1 nociceptor stimulation (central pain pathway blockage) [48]	**Tension-type Headache** (Rescue) **Migraine** (Rescue) [49]+
Ibuprofen** (Ketoprofen)	**NSAIDs**	**Primary:** COX-2 inhibition [50]	**Tension-type headache** (Rescue) [51] **Migraine** (Rescue) [52]
Butorphanol	**Opiates**	**Primary:** Binding to central opioids receptors, down regulating central pain stimuli transmission [53]	**Migraine** (Rescue)++

*The model drug is shown as the main drug even when there are other molecules sharing the same mechanism of action (shown below the main category group in brackets).

**Even when each one has good therapeutic effect using alone, recent investigations suggest that combination of fixed doses of paracetamol, NSAIDs, and caffeine is more effective that any single drug alone [54].

+Some studies show that the addition of metoclopramide to paracetamol potentiates its effects on migraine patients [49].

++Despite the well-known analgesic effect of opiates, there is no strong clinical trials supporting their use in migraine, thus its use must be considered when all other available therapies have failed [55].

Table 1. Comparison of different primary headache available treatments.

Different options are available to stop migraine attacks: acute, symptomatic treatment. According to recent clinical evidence, the common approach to treating a migraine attack is based on early intervention when the pain is still mild, which can result in shortening the time to achieve a pain-free response. A proper clinical approach, individual considerations for each patient and a quick view of the guidelines may help to provide the best treatment for specific case [56].

5.2. Acute, sporadic headache treatment

Many people in the general population have experienced at least one headache crisis which is usually of no major concern since it may be treated with OTC painkillers with no further complications or sequelae. In fact, sporadic headaches need no medical attention and most cases are resolved by the patients themselves [57].

The most popular treatments for this type of acute, primary headache include paracetamol, when pain intensity is mild to moderate, and aspirin or any other NSAIDs such as ibuprofen, for high intensity headaches; it usually requires no more than a single dose to control the crisis [58]. From this perspective, acute sporadic headache treatment represents no problem at all

http://dx.doi.org/10.5772/67244

since the risk of complications derived from treatment use and abuse are low or even null; however, many tension-type headaches begin as sporadic ones and with time they progress to a classic chronic cephalalgia. On the other hand, many undiagnosed migraine patients with low intensity crisis make it through the year with a very low frequency of intense attacks (less than one a month) and may handle their headache as a sporadic one with relative success in its initial stages [59] but sooner or later, a chronic pattern will develop, requiring medical assistance, with treatment optimization and monitoring in order to avoid headache treatment abuse-related problems. Since paracetamol, aspirin, ibuprofen, and various other OTC drugs are effective, safe treatments for acute headache crisis [60], there are no major concerns regarding the risks and so the use of such medication must not be discouraged because it is not a threat for patients; however, the underdiagnosis of migraine as well as tension-type headaches must be addressed. Many undiagnosed patients are left to deal with, on their own, against complex headaches which do require professional counseling in order to obtain proper relief and avoid headache overuse treatment-related problems, which are much more difficult to manage.

5.3. Chronic headache treatment

It is clear that a common, acute headache crisis presents no danger neither for the patient nor public health; however, when headache crises become more frequent requiring regular self-medication, often with poor outcomes and when such crises are accompanied by other symptoms such as auras or nausea, it becomes compulsory on the part of the physician to evaluate the patient for more complex etiologies, more than just a sporadic headache, in this case, a thorough medical consultation is mandatory in order to properly assess the patient, providing a diagnosis and a treatment intended not only to relieve pain but also to prevent recurrences. As stated previously, a high percentage of migraine sufferers have had no formal diagnosis of the disease [61], while some others progress from acute crisis of the tension-type headache to a chronic pattern when sensitization pathways become activated [62]; in both cases, symptoms may develop so subtly that patients are not fully aware of the disease state and may remain on the same self-medicating strategy for years despite the poor outcome. Even worse, this increases the chances of developing complications associated with improper management of chronic cephalea and treatment abuse. In this regard, the best strategy to conquer this problem is education. Beyond pharmacological treatment, it is important to inform the general public about primary headaches and how such entities may be easily confused with a banal headache and explain why their insidious evolution may render them undiagnosed for a long period of time; it is mandatory to educate patients about their diseases, giving emphasis to how important preventive medications are as primary therapy intended to reduce the likelihood of pain crises and increase their quality of life, leaving analgesics and OTC painkillers as a last resort when prevention has failed [63].

Implementation of education programs about headaches from school and on to the general public can be a key strategy to address the problem of underdiagnosis, misdiagnosis, and improper management of headaches [64]. The aim of such programs must be to encourage people to seek medical advice when certain headache patterns show up and this will help direct them to specialized physicians who will provide the appropriate care and counseling [65, 66]. Unfortunately, due to an increase in the access to over-the-counter treatments, low income, lack of medical secure coverage, and unawareness about migraine, tension-type headaches, and other primary cephalalgias, the trend is moving toward self-medication instead of professional counseling [67] which has led to the improper use or even abuse of headache medications; however, once a headache patient has reached regular medical care, efforts must be made in order to enhance doctor-patient communication and provide as much information as possible to the patient [68] since having an in-depth knowledge of these diseases will lead to better management [69]; once patients are aware of a medical condition such as primary headaches, they act as multipliers among their families, relatives, friends, and coworkers [70], making it easier to catch public interest on a public health problem like migraine and other primary headaches. It remains clear that education and information play a key role in addressing chronic primary headache; however, once a patient has grasped these important concepts and the physician has given a diagnosis, it is necessary to utilize the right tools in order to correctly estimate the impact of headache on their quality of life [71] and to choose the right treatment for each individual case; otherwise, using standardized protocols even in the medical community may present the danger of improper treatment and abuse of certain medications [72]. To accomplish such a delicate task, health care providers rely on many tools such as MIDAS (Migraine Disability Assessment Score) intended to objectively evaluate headache frequency, pain intensity, and associated symptoms so as to measure not only the impact of headache on quality of life but also to assess treatment outcomes leading to a personal, tailored treatment regimen for each patient [73]. Once the diagnosis has been achieved and the impact on both quality of life and productivity is assessed [74], the precise treatment can then be chosen for each patient. It is important to note that the main goal of chronic primary headache treatment is to lower as much as possible the number of pain crises (preventive treatment), the secondary objective is to end a possible a crisis once it has evolved and has been triggered (abortive treatment), and finally, rescue patients once a crisis has stopped (rescue treatment). Long-term treatment options for each step of therapy have widened, providing physicians with a variety of drugs acting on different key points in the pathological chain as seen in **Table 1**. Everyday there is the development of a more complex therapeutic arsenal against migraine as well as other primary headaches. Gaining the proper knowledge of all available treatment options may be a challenge to even the most expert specialists; thus, this report has rendered the task easier by providing an organized list of all available therapeutic options summarized in **Tables 2** and **3**.

First-line preventive medications for migraine			
Drug name	**FDA-approved**	**Formulation**	**Dosage**
Onabotulinum toxin A	Yes	Injection	Dose: Varies (FDA official dose is 155 units via 31 injections every 3 months)
Anticonvulsants			
Topiramate	Yes	Oral	Total dose varies from 25 or 50 mg/day up to 400 mg/day
Valproic or divalproex sodium	Yes	Oral	Usual dose: 500–1000 mg/day in divided doses
B-blockers			
Propranolol	Yes	Oral	60–120 mg/day
Metoprolol	No	Oral	25–100 mg/day
Atenolol	No	Oral	25–50 mg/day
Nebivolol	No	Oral	2.5–10 mg/day

http://dx.doi.org/10.5772/67244

First-line preventive medications for migraine			
Drug name	**FDA-approved**	**Formulation**	**Dosage**
Tricyclic antidepressants			
Amitriptyline **Nortriptyline**	No	Oral	Stating dose: 10 mg at bedtime, titrate up to 25–50 mg at night. Maximum dose: 150 mg/day
Doxepin	No	Oral	Starting dose: 10 mg at bedtime, titrate up to 25–50 mg/day. Maximum dose: 150 mg/day
Protriptyline	No	Oral	5–20 mg/day
NSAIDs*			
Naproxen	No	Oral	500–550 mg/day; maximum dose 1000–1100 mg/day
Calcium channel blocker			
Verapamil	No	Oral	120 mg/day slow-release tablet, titrate to 240 mg/day

Table reproduced and adapted from the original source [75].

*Other NSAIDs are useful as well.

Table 2. First-line migraine preventive medications.

Second-line migraine preventive therapy*			
Drug name	**FDA-approved**	**Formulation**	**Dosage**
Antiseizure medications			
Gabapentin	No	Oral	Usual dose: 600–2400 mg/day Some patients do well on low doses (100–300 mg/day)
Pregabalin	No	Oral	25 mg bid to 150 tid
Muscle relaxants			
Cyclobenzaprine	No	Oral	5–10 mg/day
Tizanidine	No	Oral	Usual dose: 2–4 mg every night; patients start with ¼ to ½ tablet. May be increased to 12 mg/day
Antidepressants			
Desvenlafaxine	No	Oral	50–100 mg/day
Duloxetine	No	Oral	30–60 mg/day
Venlafaxine	No	Oral	75–225 mg/day
Natural agent			
Purified butterbur	No	Oral	100–150 mg/day

Table reproduced and adapted from the original source [76].

*Polypharmacy also is commonly used as second-line treatment of migraine (i.e., amitriptyline with propranolol or amitriptyline with valproic acid).

Table 3. Second line migraine preventive medications.

With the above information in mind it makes it easier to decide what the best options are for each patient; however, migraine treatment as well as the treatment for chronic tension-type and other primary cephaleas must be chosen considering each particular patient condition, available treatments at their location, exposure to triggers, and so on [77]. Usually this type of initial approach is enough to achieve adequate control of symptoms but if unsuccessful, it becomes mandatory to prioritize which attributes from each drug are better for a particular patient in order to choose the best mix of pharmacologic therapy [78]. In this regard, when precise medical treatment has been chosen, it is very important to measure its impact [79], not doing so could run the risk of the patient receiving a useless treatment over a long period of time leading to further problems regarding that particular treatment as well as future therapies. In this sense, it is also important to address the patient's expectations of the treatment in order to be able to provide not only a good outcome but also to gauge what the patient is expecting from treatment regarding tolerability, effectiveness, side effects, and other aspects of therapy; otherwise, there is a high risk of noncompliance which may lead patients toward self-medication and all the implied risk attributed to it. In addition, it is necessary to be aware of the adverse effects because even though the therapeutic action is good enough to improve the quality of life, the development of adverse side effects may lead to therapy discontinuation. A summary of the main adverse side effects associated with the main treatment categories are summarized in **Tables 4–6**.

Medications for abortive therapy	
Drug name	**Possible side effects**
Ergot Dihydroergotamine mesylate	Nausea, numbness of fingers and toes
Triptans Sumatriptan succinate* Zolmitriptan* Rizatriptan* Naratriptan+ Almotriptan malate*× Frovatriptan succinate+ Eletriptan hydrobromide*	**Side effects for all the triptans are similar** **This class of drugs is well tolerated but the more common side effects may include:** Nausea, headache, sleepiness, dry mouth, dizziness, fatigue, hot/cold sensations, chest pain, and flushing Other potential side effects that rarely occur include: Head, jaw, chest and arm discomfort/tightening/tingling; throat discomfort, muscle cramps, and flushing

*Short-acting.
+Long-acting.
×FDA approved for teens ages 12–18.
Table reproduced and adapted from the original source [80].

Table 4. Side effects of main first-line migraine abortive drugs.

It remains clear that proper treatment selection, impact evaluation, and limiting the side effects are all challenging tasks requiring highly specialized medical staff with adequate experience; otherwise, the outcome may not be satisfactory leading to possible therapy discontinuation,

http://dx.doi.org/10.5772/67244

self-medication, and the use of alternative treatments whose effectiveness and safety may not be well known. Unfortunately, there are still many cases worldwide of misdiagnosis, erroneous management, and self-medication due to lack of specialized medical assistance. All these factors are a "recipe for disaster" since many headache rescue treatments are available over the counter and thousands, perhaps millions of people try to fight alone against migraine, tension-type headache, and other primary cephaleas, lacking proper advice, leading to one of the worst complications of primary cephalalgias: drug overuse and abuse.

Medications for preventive therapy		
Drug name	**Possible major side effects**	**Instructions when used for headaches**
Nonsteroidal anti-inflammatories Naproxen sodium	GI** upset, GI bleeding, nausea, vomiting, rash and change in liver function, rebound headache	Is take twice a day, every day, for headache prevention
Tricyclic antidepressants Imipramine HCl	Dizziness, drowsiness, dry mouth, weakness, weight gain	Frequently started at low dosages and slowly increased
Amitriptyline HCl	Fatigue, dry mouth, weight gain and constipation	Frequently started at low dosages and slowly increased to a therapeutic level; taken by night, EKG*** optional
Antihistamines Cyproheptadine HCl	May induce sleep or may shorten migraine attack, weight gain, drowsiness	Usually started at low dosages and slowly increased; often taken at bedtime
Selective serotonin receptor inhibitors (SSRIs)* Fluoxetine HCl	Nausea, dry mouth, increased appetite, agitation	Usually started at low dosages and slowly increased; usually taken at morning
Beta blockers Atenolol Propranolol	Fatigue, depression, weight gain, memory disturbance, faintness and diarrhea, decreased performance in athletes	Depending on the form, may be taken one to three times a day
Calcium channel blockers Verapamil Diltiazem HCl	Constipation and dizziness; hair loss	Frequently started at low dosages and slowly increased. Taken twice a day; usually the first dose is taken in the morning
Anticonvulsants Valproic acid	Nausea, drowsiness, weight gain, tremors and rare liver failure; may cause birth defects	Frequently started at low dosages and slowly increased. Periodic blood tests required
Topiramate	Rare: Glaucoma, kidney stone at high doses (>150 mg), weight loss, word finding difficulties	Frequently started at low dosages and slowly increased; may be taken 2 to 3 times/daily
Gabapentin	Generally well tolerated	Usually started at low dosages and slowly increased; may be taken 2–3 times/daily

Table reproduced and adapted from the original source [80].

*Other SSRIs include citalopram, escitalopram, fluvoxamine, paroxetine, sertraline.

**GI, gastrointestinal.

***EKG, electrocardiogram.

Table 5. Side effects of main first-line migraine preventive drugs.

Over-the-counter medications for symptomatic relief		
Drug name	**Symptoms relieved**	**Precautions and possible side effects**
Nonsteroidal anti-inflammatories		
Aspirin	Relief of fever and pain	Do not use in children under 14 years of age due to the potential for Reye's Syndrome Side effects may include: heartburn, gastrointestinal (GI) bleeding, bronchospasm or constriction that causes narrowing of the airways, anaphylaxis and peptic ulcer
Acetaminophen	Relief of fever and pain	Few side effects, if taken as directed, although they may include: changes in blood counts and liver functions
Ibuprofen	Relief of fever, pain and inflammation	Side effects may include gastrointestinal upset, GI bleeding, nausea, vomiting, rash and changes in liver function
Naproxen Sodium	Headache pain relief	Side effects may include GI upset, GI bleeding, nausea, vomiting, rash and changes in liver function

Table reproduced and adapted from the original source [80].

Table 6. Side effects of main migraine rescue drugs.

6. Primary cephalea treatment overuse and abuse statistics worldwide

Once a patient receives the diagnosis of migraine or any other primary headache, treatments usually become supervised by a medical team and patients are directed on what to do and what not to do regarding pharmacological therapy and although this group of patients carries a certain risk for medication abuse or overuse, usually there are no major concerns unless the patient abandons regular control and supervised treatment. Unfortunately, up to 50% of migraine patients remain undiagnosed [81] and even worst, up to 82% of patients with a diagnosis of nonmigraine headache actually meet the major migraine criteria [82] leading to improper handling and medication.

Regarding chronic tension-type headaches, up to 40% of patients have not received a formal diagnosis and are not aware of what disease they are suffering from [83]; they often think they have a benign condition causing the self-medication of migraine rescue drugs (OTC painkillers and analgesics) to become a trend, leading to the worsening of their underlying disorder.

On the other hand, a group of patients with a formal diagnosis of a primary headache disorder abandon follow-up due to lack of insurance, discouraging results or moving away to an area with no specialists with experience on headache treatment, keeping their treatment as something they do on their own, usually increasing dosing and dose intervals, leading to preventive and abortive medication overuse [84]. Aside from the above mentioned, there is another group of existing patients suffering from *chronic daily headache* affecting up to 5% of

http://dx.doi.org/10.5772/67244

the general population [85], self-medicating with over-the-counter painkillers and analgesics to deal with pain crisis, increasing the risk of evolution toward chronic headache [86] due to central nervous system sensitization [87].

Even when not included in the International Headache Society Classification of Headache, chronic daily headache is a common disorder defined by some authors as *"a disorder where patients suffer very frequent headaches (15 or more days/month), including those headaches", furthermore, "Chronic Daily Headache (CDH) may be divided into two main groups; Primary CDH is not related to any structural or systemic illness. Population based studies suggest that Chronic Tension Type Headache is the leading cause of primary CDH, on the other hand, Secondary CDH occurs 15 or more times a month or has some identifiable underlying cause* [88]" (secondary CDH is summarized in **Table 7**).

Chronic daily headache
Primary chronic daily headache
Headache duration >4 hours
Chronic migraine (previously transformed migraine)
Chronic tension-type headache
New daily persistent headache
Hemicrania continua
Headache duration <4 hours
Cluster headache
Paroxysmal hemicranias
Hypnic headache
Idiopathic stabbing headache
Secondary chronic daily headache
Posttraumatic headache
Cervical spine disorders
Headache associated with vascular disorders (arteriovenous malformation, arteritis including giant cell arteritis, dissection, and subdural hematoma)
Headache associated with nonvascular intracranial disorders [intracranial hypertension, infection (EBV, HIV), neoplasm]
Other (temporomandibular joint disorder, sinus infection)

Abbreviations: EBV, Epstein-Barr virus; HIV, human immunodeficiency virus.
Table reproduced and adapted from the original source [89].

Table 7. Chronic daily headache causes.

Among all these patients *"thirty-five percent overused simple analgesics, 22% ergotics, 12.5% opioids, and 2.7% triptans; the remaining 27.8% have overused different combinations"* [28]. The major concern about these statistics is that although treatments may be helpful in the initial stages, their chronic, unsupervised use and abuse tends to lead toward pain chronification; increasing the number of pain crises, intensity of pain, and resistance to regular analgesic dosing. Moreover, relapsing after medication withdrawal is still a major issue regarding both preventive and rescue primary headache treatments [90]. How many patients progress toward chronification will vary depending on the abused medication, according to Bigal *"available data suggest that opioids induce migraine chronification (progression), and the effect is dose dependent (critical dose around 8 days of exposure per month) and more pronounced in men. Barbiturates also induce migraine progression, and the effect is dose dependent (critical dose around 5 days of exposure per month) and more pronounced in women. Triptans induce migraine progression only in those with high migraine frequency at baseline (10–14 days per month), but not overall. NSAIDs protect against migraine progression unless individuals have 10 or more headache days per month (when they become inducers, rather than protective). Finally, caffeine-containing over-the-counter products increase risk of progression"* [91], thus each available drug used must be monitored individually in order to avoid overuse and abuse-related complications. Why and how primary headaches progress to chronification because of treatment abuse is still partially unknown and a field of very active research.

7. Underlying pathways for headache chronification following treatment abuse

It is a well-known fact that chronic exposure to pain treatment [92] as well suffering from chronic pain, especially chronic headache, increase the risk of chronic pain development due to *"reduced endogenous inhibition of pain, implying that an individual's processing of pain-related information changes with the onset of the syndrome"* [93]; however, the underlying mechanisms behind it still remain partially unknown.

Among the painful syndromes, chronic headache is one of those most commonly associated with long lasting analgesic consumption, termed medication overuse headache (MOH) when it occurs, a pathological entity "defined by the International Headache Society as a headache induced by the overuse of analgesics, triptans, or other acute headache compounds whose detailed pathophysiology is still unknown" [94]. Current knowledge indicates that it can take up to 25 years for a chronic pain condition to develop after the use of chronic analgesics MOH [95] with strong evidence to support that chronic use of analgesics is a good predictor of an increased occurrence of both migraine and nonmigrainous headaches within the next 11 years, with a combined risk ratio of 19.6%, which is extremely high when compared to only 3.1% for patients who do not overuse analgesic treatments [96]. But analgesics are not the only medications involved in MOH, ergots and triptans also play a key role in MOH, with a shorter interval between initial treatment and development of induced chronic headache. *"The delay between first intake and these attacks is the shortest for triptans (1–2 years), longer for ergots (3–5 years)"* [97] and the longest for analgesics as it was previously mentioned. In this regard, the risk of induced chronic headache is lower for triptans (i.e., sumatriptan) than for ergotamine [98], which is good news for patients since triptans are the drug of choice before ergotamine. The problem when trying to establish a prevention/treatment strategy for drug-induced headache

http://dx.doi.org/10.5772/67244

as well as MOH arises from the fact that different drugs are involved in their development; hence, there is no single way to explain the related mechanisms or physiopathology. Even more complex is the attempt to establish the diagnosis of MOH or drug-induced headache since most of the time the clinical profile of the primary entity is the same as the induced one, making it very difficult to establish a difference among them and even worse, to determine when the primary headache has ended and MOH appeared. A single approach to establish such differences is symptom improvement with treatment withdrawal [99]; the headache was drug induced and not of a primary origin and once the trigger (the drug) has ceased, symptoms should improve.

Figure 4 shows a schema of what happens during drug-induced headache and how the diagnosis may be addressed regardless of the underlying molecular mechanisms.

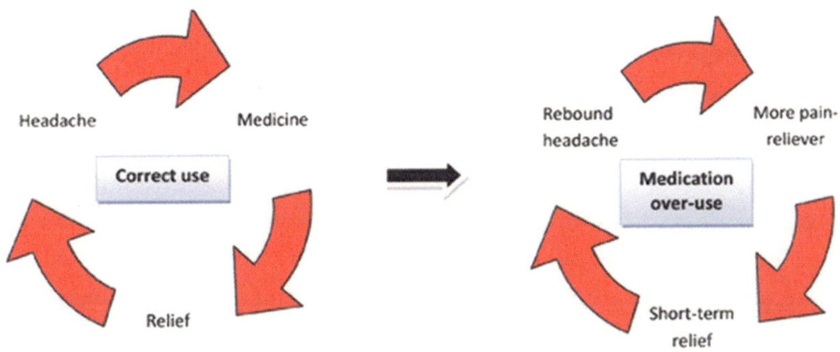

Figure 4. Drug-induced headache vicious circle [100].

Of note, opioids have been found to be one of the most problematic drugs found to induce chronic headache, regardless of the purpose of their use whether it be chronic headache or any other chronic pain condition such as back pain, oncologic pain, and so on. The underlying mechanism seems to be *"the activation of toll-like receptor-4 on glial cells, resulting in a pro- inflammatory state that manifests clinically as increased pain"* [101], such activation may explain not only the development of MOH but also of the transformation to migraine [102].

Another hypothesis sustained by preclinical research is the presence of neuroadaptive changes related to chronic use of opiates; such changes *"include increased expression of calcitonin gene-related peptide (CGRP) in trigeminal primary afferent neurons. Centrally, they include increased excitatory neurotransmission at the level of the dorsal horn and nucleus caudalis. Critically, these neuroadaptive changes persist for long periods of time and the evoked release of CGRP is enhanced following morphine pretreatment* [103]; *all these changes lead to Induced Hyperalgesia* [101, 104] *and thus Headache Chronification."*

But opiates are not the only molecules associated with MOH, there is also strong evidence suggesting that combined analgesics as well as joined ergotamine-caffeine preparations may induce a metabolic decrease in several brain areas, especially the orbitofrontal cortex leading to a decrease in intrinsic pain downregulation circuits and the development of chronic headaches such as MOH and modified migraine (MM) [105]. Such metabolic changes may be associated with the sensitization of the trigeminal and somatic nociceptive systems; another possible path leading to MOH was demonstrated by Ayzenberg et al. on triptan-induced MOH [106].

Furthermore, the mechanisms stated earlier may be connected to others both centrally and peripherally by a complex net of interactions currently unknown but feasible such as "*upregulation of calcitonin gene–related peptide, substance P, and nitric oxide synthase in trigeminal ganglia; expansion of receptive field and decreased nociceptive threshold of central trigeminal neurons; decrease in diffuse noxious inhibitory control; and increased susceptibility to develop cortical spreading depression (CSD). These changes indicate an increase in excitability of cortical and trigeminal neurons. The neuronal hyperexcitability may be the result of derangement of a central, possibly serotonin (5-HT)-dependent, modulating control system. Experiments with animals with low 5-HT showed that the processes of CSD and trigeminal nociception are enhanced in this condition*" [107] as it has been demonstrated by Bongsebandhu et al. in animal models.

The available information clearly supports the theory that analgesics and painkillers play an active role in the chronification of headache, which is a real concern for the medical community considering the high number of available over-the-counter analgesics. Furthermore, primary therapies such as triptans are also involved in MOH development after chronic use and there is even weaker evidence to explain the underlying pathways that cause this occurrence. At the moment the most probable mechanism of triptan-induced MOH is "*induction of neural adaptations that result in a state of latent sensitization, which might increase sensitivity to migraine triggers*" [108], in addition, "*triptan administration promotes increased expression of neuronal nitric oxide synthase in dural afferents, which is critical for enhanced sensitivity to environmental stress, which is a biological basis for increased frequency of headache following*" [109].

Certainly, current knowledge regarding MOH and other types of headache chronification caused by the use of therapy is still lacking although the results from many research reports are available. However, until a deeper scientific understanding is available regarding this relatively new entity, it becomes necessary to improve the diagnostic criteria and methods, enhance treatment protocols, and provide proper monitoring not only to chronic primary headache patients but also to each one suffering from a chronic pain condition.

Until a more precise and wider scope of information is available, prevention remains the best, most cost-effective option used to prevent headache treatment abuse-related complications. When the disorder of MOH and drug-induced headache presents, the main treatment must be treatment withdrawal and even then the discussion on what is the best withdrawal method (stationary vs. ambulatory) still remains inconclusive [110]; as a preventive strategy, drug combinations must be avoided as much as possible and high-risk patients who develop MOH must be regularly evaluated to ensure that no late complications are showing up during long-term treatment.

http://dx.doi.org/10.5772/67244

Author details

Silvia Ussai[1,2,3]* and Alessandro Rizzardo[3]

*Address all correspondence to: ussai.silvia@gmail.com

1 Bocconi University, MIHMEP, Milan, Italy

2 iRhythmia Research Centre, Bolzano, Italy

3 SIMED Medical Center, Gorizia, Italy

References

[1] Ramadan, N. M., et al. "Evidence-based guidelines for migraine headache in the primary care setting: pharmacological management for prevention of migraine." St Paul, MN: US Headache Consortium; 2000

[2] Diener, H., Limmrotha, V. "Medication-overuse headache: a worldwide problem" The Lancet Neurology 4(1) (January 2005): 11–12.

[3] Symon, D. N. K. "Twelve cases of analgesic headache." Archives of Disease in Childhood 78(6) (1998): 555–556.

[4] Evers, S. "Treatment of migraine with prophylactic drugs." Expert Opinion on Pharmacotherapy 9(15) (2008): 2565–2573.

[5] Steiner, T. J., Lange, R. "Ketoprofen (25 mg) in the symptomatic treatment of episodic tension type headache: double-blind placebo-controlled comparison with acetaminophen (1000 mg)." Cephalalgia 18(1) (1998): 38–43.

[6] Boureau, F., et al. "Double-blind comparison of an acetaminophen 400 mg-codeine 25 mg combination versus aspirin 1000 mg and placebo in acute migraine attack." Cephalalgia 14(2) (1994): 156–161.

[7] Headache Classification Committee of the International Headache Society (IHS. "The international classification of headache disorders, (beta version)." Cephalalgia 33(9) (2013): 629–808.

[8] Stovner, L., Hagen, K., Jensen, R., Katsarava, Z., Lipton, R., Scher, A., Steiner, T., Zwart, J.-A. The global burden of headache: a documentation of headache prevalence and disability worldwide. Cephalalgia, 27 (2007): 193–210.

[9] Göbel, H., Petersen-Braun, M., Soyka, D. "The epidemiology of headache in Germany: a nationwide survey of a representative sample on the basis of the headache classification of the International Headache Society." Cephalalgia 14.2 (1994): 97–106.

[10] Edmeads, J., et al. "Impact of migraine and tension-type headache on life-style, consulting behaviour, and medication use: A Canadian population survey." Canadian Journal of Neurological Sciences/Journal Canadien des Sciences Neurologiques 20(02) (1993): 131–137.

[11] The Pathways of Migraine. Help for Headaches & Migraine website. Available from: http://www.helpforheadaches.com/lwfiles/illus-pathways.htm [Accessed: 2016-10-03]

[12] Welch, K. M. A. "Contemporary concepts of migraine pathogenesis." Neurology 61(8 suppl 4) (2003): S2–S8.

[13] Noseda, R., Burstein, R. "Migraine pathophysiology: anatomy of the trigeminovascular pathway and associated neurological symptoms, cortical spreading depression, sensitization, and modulation of pain." Pain® 154 (2013): S44–S53.

[14] Ferrari, M. D., Saxena, P. R. "On serotonin and migraine: a clinical and pharmacological review." Cephalalgia 13(3) (1993): 151–165.

[15] Schwartz, B. S., et al. "Epidemiology of tension-type headache." JAMA 279(5) (1998): 381–383.

[16] Karli, N., et al. "Comparison of pre-headache phases and trigger factors of migraine and episodic tension type headache: do they share similar clinical pathophysiology?." Cephalalgia 25(6) (2005): 444–451.

[17] Bendtsen, L., Jensen, R., Olesen, J. "Decreased pain detection and tolerance thresholds in chronic tension-type headache." Archives of Neurology 53(4) (1996): 373–376.

[18] Langeveld, J. H., et al. "A quality of life instrument for adolescents with chronic headache." Cephalalgia 16(3) (1996): 183–196.

[19] Ashina, S., Bendtsen, L., Ashina, M. "Pathophysiology of tension-type headache." Current Pain and Headache Reports 9(6) (2005): 415–422.

[20] Bendtsen, L. "Central sensitization in tension-type headache—possible pathophysiological mechanisms." Cephalalgia 20(5) (2000): 486–508.

[21] Olesen, J. "The role of nitric oxide (NO) in migraine, tension-type headache and cluster headache." Pharmacology & Therapeutics 120(2) (2008): 157–171.

[22] Headache. Clinical Gate website. Available from: http://clinicalgate.com/77-headache/ [Accessed: 2016-10-03]

[23] Sarchielli, P., et al. "L-Arginine/nitric oxide pathway in chronic tension-type headache: relation with serotonin content and secretion and glutamate content." Journal of the Neurological Sciences 198(1) (2002): 9–15.

[24] Olesen, J., Ashina, M. "Emerging migraine treatments and drug targets." Trends in Pharmacological Sciences 32(6) (2011): 352–359.

[25] Adelman, L. C., et al. "Venlafaxine extended release (XR) for the prophylaxis of migraine and tension-type headache: a retrospective study in a clinical setting." Headache: The Journal of Head and Face Pain 40(7) (2000): 572–580.

[26] Lipton, R. B., et al. "Why headache treatment fails." Neurology 60(7) (2003): 1064–1070.

[27] Lipton, R. B., Silberstein, S. D. "The role of headache-related disability in migraine management Implications for headache treatment guidelines." Neurology 56(suppl 1) (2001): S35–S42.

[28] Colas, R., et al. "Chronic daily headache with analgesic overuse Epidemiology and impact on quality of life." Neurology 62(8) (2004): 1338–1342.

[29] Matchar, D. B., et al. "Evidence-based guidelines for migraine headache in the primary care setting: pharmacological management of acute attacks." 2000. Accessed at www.aan.com/professionals/practice/guidelines.cfm.

[30] Diener, H.-C., Limmroth, V. "Medication-overuse headache: a worldwide problem." The Lancet Neurology 3(8) (2004): 475–483.

[31] Clinical Pathway: Assessment and Management of Patients with Primary Headaches. EBMedicine website. Available from: https://www.ebmedicine.net/topics.php?paction=showTopicSeg&topic_id=116&seg_id=2320 [Accessed: 2016-10-03]

[32] Bendtsen, L., Jensen, R., Olesen, J. "A non-selective (amitriptyline), but not a selective (citalopram), serotonin reuptake inhibitor is effective in the prophylactic treatment of chronic tension-type headache." Journal of Neurology, Neurosurgery & Psychiatry 61(3) (1996): 285–290.

[33] Holroyd, K. A., et al. "Management of chronic tension-type headache with tricyclic antidepressant medication, stress management therapy, and their combination: a randomized controlled trial." JAMA 285(17) (2001): 2208–2215.

[34] Cady, R. K., et al. "Effect of early intervention with sumatriptan on migraine pain: retrospective analyses of data from three clinical trials." Clinical Therapeutics 22(9) (2000): 1035–1048.

[35] Moskowitz, M. A., Cutrer, F. M. "Sumatriptan: a receptor-targeted treatment for migraine." Annual Review of Medicine 44(1) (1993): 145–154.

[36] Tfelt-Hansen, P., et al. "Ergotamine in the acute treatment of migraine." Brain 123(1) (2000): 9–18.

[37] Meyer, J. S., Hardenberg, J. "Clinical effectiveness of calcium entry blockers in prophylactic treatment of migraine and cluster headaches." Headache: The Journal of Head and Face Pain 23(6) (1983): 266–277.

[38] Johannessen, C. U. "Mechanisms of action of valproate: a commentatory." Neurochemistry International 37(2) (2000): 103–110.

[39] Mathew, N. T., et al. "Intravenous valproate sodium (depacon) aborts migraine rapidly: a preliminary report." Headache: The Journal of Head and Face Pain 40(9) (2000): 720–723.

[40] Hering, R., Kuritzky, A. "Sodium valproate in the treatment of cluster headache: an open clinical trial." Cephalalgia 9(3) (1989): 195–198.

[41] White, H. S. "Molecular pharmacology of topiramate: managing seizures and preventing migraine." Headache: The Journal of Head and Face Pain 45(s1) (2005): S48–S56.

[42] Cutrer, F. M. "Antiepileptic drugs: how they work in headache." Headache: The Journal of Head and Face Pain 41(s1) (2001): 3–11.

[43] Brandes, J. L., et al. "Topiramate for migraine prevention: a randomized controlled trial." JAMA 291(8) (2004): 965–973.

[44] Wheeler, S. D., Carrazana, E. J. "Topiramate-treated cluster headache." Neurology 53(1) (1999): 234–234.

[45] Lampl, C., et al. "A prospective, open-label, long-term study of the efficacy and tolerability of topiramate in the prophylaxis of chronic tension-type headache." Cephalalgia 26(10) (2006): 1203–1208.

[46] Steiner, T. J., Lange, R., Voelker, M. "Aspirin in episodic tension-type headache: placebo-controlled dose-ranging comparison with paracetamol." Cephalalgia 23(1) (2003): 59–66.

[47] Claesson, A. "On the mechanism of paracetamol's analgesic activity and a note on related NSAID pharmacology". Manuscript first published on SlideShare.net February 4, 2013.

[48] Högestätt, E. D., Jönsson, B. A., Ermund, A., et al. "Conversion of acetaminophen to the bioactive N-acylphenolamine AM404 via fatty acid amide hydrolase-dependent arachidonic acid conjugation in the nervous system". The Journal of Biological Chemistry 280(36) (2005): 31405–31412.

[49] Derry, S., Andrew Moore, R., McQuay, H. J. "Diclofenac with or without an antiemetic for acute migraine headaches in adults." Cochrane Database Syst Rev. 2012; 2: CD008783.

[50] Vane, J. R., Botting, R. M. "Mechanism of action of anti-inflammatory drugs." Scandinavian Journal of Rheumatology 25(suppl 102) (1996): 9–21.

[51] Dahlöf, C. G. H., Jacobs, L. D. "Ketoprofen, paracetamol and placebo in the treatment of episodic tension-type headache." Cephalalgia 16(2) (1996): 117–123.

[52] Hamalainen, M. L., et al. "Ibuprofen or acetaminophen for the acute treatment of migraine in children a double-blind, randomized, placebo-controlled, crossover study." Neurology 48(1) (1997): 103–107.

[53] Driessen, B., Reimann, W. "Interaction of the central analgesic, tramadol, with the uptake and release of 5-hydroxytryptamine in the rat brain in vitro." British Journal of Pharmacology 105(1) (1992): 147–151.

[54] Diener, H. C., et al. "The fixed combination of acetylsalicylic acid, paracetamol and caffeine is more effective than single substances and dual combination for the treatment of headache: a multicentre, randomized, double-blind, single-dose, placebo-controlled parallel group study." Cephalalgia 25(10) (2005): 776–787.

[55] Snow, V., et al. "Pharmacologic management of acute attacks of migraine and prevention of migraine headache." Annals of Internal Medicine 137(10) (2002): 840–849.

[56] Antonaci, F., et al. "A review of current European treatment guidelines for migraine." The Journal of Headache and Pain 11(1) (2010): 13–19.

[57] Mehuys, E., et al. "Self-medication of regular headache: a community pharmacy-based survey." European Journal of Neurology 19(8) (2012): 1093–1099.

[58] Limmroth, V., et al. "Features of medication overuse headache following overuse of different acute headache drugs." Neurology 59(7) (2002): 1011–1014.

[59] Sheftell, F. D. "Role and impact of over-the-counter medications in the management of headache." Neurologic Clinics 15(1) (1997): 187–198.

[60] Nebe, J., Heier, M., Diener, H. C. "Low-dose ibuprofen in self-medication of mild to moderate headache: a comparison with acetylsalicylic acid and placebo." Cephalalgia 15(6) (1995): 531–535.

[61] Cevoli, S., et al. "Underdiagnosis and undertreatment of migraine in Italy: a survey of patients attending for the first time 10 headache centres." Cephalalgia 29(12) (2009): 1285–1293.

[62] Sandrini, G., et al. "Abnormal modulatory influence of diffuse noxious inhibitory controls in migraine and chronic tension-type headache patients." Cephalalgia 26(7) (2006): 782–789.

[63] Havanka-Kanniainen, H. "Treatment of acute migraine attack: ibuprofen and placebo compared." Headache: The Journal of Head and Face Pain 29(8) (1989): 507–509.

[64] Mannix, L. K., et al. "Impact of headache education program in the workplace." Neurology 53(4) (1999): 868–868.

[65] Schneider, W. J., et al. "A pilot study of a headache program in the workplace: the effect of education." Journal of Occupational and Environmental Medicine 41(3) (1999): 202–209.

[66] Smith, T. R., Nicholson, R. A., Banks, J. W. "Migraine education improves quality of life in a primary care setting." Headache: The Journal of Head and Face Pain 50(4) (2010): 600–612.

[67] Lipton, R. B., Stewart, W. F., Simon, D. "Medical consultation for migraine: results from the American Migraine Study." Headache: The Journal of Head and Face Pain 38(2) (1998): 87–96.

[68] Lang, E., et al. "Effects of recommendations and patient seminars on effectivity of outpatient treatment for headache." Schmerz (Berlin, Germany) 15(4) (2001): 229–240.

[69] Centonze, V., et al. "Patient education and migraine: a pilot study." Functional Neurology 13(2) (1997): 117–123.

[70] Rothrock, J. F., et al. "The impact of intensive patient education on clinical outcome in a clinic-based migraine population." Headache: The Journal of Head and Face Pain 46(5) (2006): 726–731.

[71] Bigal, M. E., et al. "Evaluation of the impact of migraine and episodic tension-type headache on the quality of life and performance of a university student population." Headache: The Journal of Head and Face Pain 41(7) (2001): 710–719.

[72] Bigal, M. E., et al. "Transformed migraine and medication overuse in a tertiary headache centre–clinical characteristics and treatment outcomes." Cephalalgia 24(6) (2004): 483–490.

[73] Stewart, W. F., Lipton, R. B., Kolodner, K. "Migraine disability assessment (MIDAS) score: relation to headache frequency, pain intensity, and headache symptoms." Headache: The Journal of Head and Face Pain 43(3) (2003): 258–265.

[74] Solomon, G. D., Santanello, N. "Impact of migraine and migraine therapy on productivity and quality of life." Neurology 55(9 Suppl. 2) (1999): S29–S35.

[75] Migraine Treatment From A to Z: 2014. Practicalpainmanagement website. Available from: http://www.practicalpainmanagement.com/pain/headache/migraine/migraine-treatment-z- 2014?page=0,3 [Accessed: 2016-10-03]

[76] Migraine Treatment From A to Z: 2014. Practicalpainmanagement website. Available from: http://www.practicalpainmanagement.com/pain/headache/migraine/migraine-treatment-z- 2014?page=0,4 [Accessed: 2016-10-03]

[77] Freitag, F. "Managing and treating tension-type headache." Medical Clinics of North America 97(2) (2013): 281–292.

[78] Dodick, D. W., et al. "Prioritizing treatment attributes and their impact on selecting an oral triptan: results from the TRIPSTAR Project." Current Pain and Headache Reports 8(6) (2004): 435–442.

[79] Willke, R. J., Burke, L. B., Erickson, P. "Measuring treatment impact: a review of patient-reported outcomes and other efficacy endpoints in approved product labels." Controlled Clinical Trials 25(60 (2004): 535–552.

[80] Headache Medications. Cleveland Clinic website. Available from: http://my.clevelandclinic.org/health/diseases_conditions/hic_Overview_of_Headaches_in_Adul ts/hic_headache_medications [Accessed: 2016-10-03]

[81] Lipton, R. B., et al. "Migraine diagnosis and treatment: results from the American Migraine Study II." Headache: The Journal of Head and Face Pain 41(7) (2001): 638–645.

[82] Tepper, S. J., et al. "Prevalence and diagnosis of migraine in patients consulting their physician with a complaint of headache: data from the Landmark Study." Headache: The Journal of Head and Face Pain 44(9) (2004): 856–864.

[83] Kernick, D., Stapley, S., Hamilton, W. "GPs' classification of headache: is primary headache underdiagnosed?." British Journal of General Practice 58(547) (2008): 102–104.

[84] Meskunas, C. A., et al. "Medications associated with probable medication overuse headache reported in a tertiary care headache center over a 15-year period." Headache: The Journal of Head and Face Pain 46(5) (2006): 766–772.

[85] Castillo, J., et al. "Epidemiology of chronic daily headache in the general population." Headache: The Journal of Head and Face Pain 39(3) (1999): 190–196.

[86] Bigal, M. E., et al. "Acute migraine medications and evolution from episodic to chronic migraine: a longitudinal population-based study." Headache: The Journal of Head and Face Pain 48(8) (2008): 1157–1168.

[87] Woolf, C. J. "Central sensitization: implications for the diagnosis and treatment of pain." Pain 152(3) (2011): S2–S15.

[88] Silberstein, S. D., Lipton, R. B. "Chronic daily headache, including transformed migraine, chronic tension-type headache, and medication overuse." Wolff's Headache and Other Head Pain 7 (2001): 247–282.

[89] Wolff's Headache and Other Head Pain. Available from: https://books.google.co.ve/books?hl=es&lr=&id=aJRV199FZcoC&oi=fnd&pg=PA247&dq=migraine+overuse&ots=fyMh7%20Hz-o9&sig=w3HZJbxeHNtxbmun1AKZWqoWUYU#v=onepage&q&f=false[Accessed: 2016-10-03]

[90] Lake, A. E. "Medication overuse headache: biobehavioral issues and solutions." Headache: The Journal of Head and Face Pain 46(s3) (2006): S88–S97.

[91] Bigal, M. E., Lipton, R. B. "Overuse of acute migraine medications and migraine chronification." Current Pain and Headache Reports 13(4) (2009): 301–307.

[92] Mathew, N. T., Kurman, R., Perez, F. "Drug induced refractory headache clinical features and management." Headache: The Journal of Head and Face Pain 30(10) (1990): 634–638.

[93] Edwards, R. R. "Individual differences in endogenous pain modulation as a risk factor for chronic pain." Neurology 65(3) (2005): 437–443.

[94] Evers, S., Marziniak, M. "Clinical features, pathophysiology, and treatment of medication-overuse headache." The Lancet Neurology 9(4) (2010): 391–401.

[95] Diener, H.-C., et al. "Analgesic-induced chronic headache: long-term results of withdrawal therapy." Journal of Neurology 236(1) (1989): 9–14.

[96] Zwart, J.-A., et al. "Analgesic use: a predictor of chronic pain and medication overuse headache: The Head–HUNT Study." Neurology 61(2) (2003): 160–164.

[97] Diener, H.-C., Katsarava, Z. "Medication Overuse Headache*." Current Medical Research and Opinion 17(suppl 1) (2001): s17–s21.

[98] Evers, S., et al. "Sumatriptan and ergotamine overuse and drug-induced headache: a clinicoepidemiologic study." Clinical Neuropharmacology 22(4) (1999): 201–206.

[99] Katsarava, Z., Jensen, R. "Medication-overuse headache: where are we now?." Current Opinion in Neurology 20(3) (2007): 326–330.

[100] The Drugs Don't Work They Just Make You Worse. 2012. Migraine Monologues website. Available from: http://www.migrainemonologues.com/2012/04/drugs-dont-work-they-just- make-you.html [Accessed: 2016-10-03]

[101] Johnson, J. L., et al. "Medication-overuse headache and opioid-induced hyperalgesia: a review of mechanisms, a neuroimmune hypothesis and a novel approach to treatment." Cephalalgia 33 (2012): 52–64.

[102] Wilkinson, S. M., Becker, W. J., Heine, J. A. "Opiate use to control bowel motility may induce chronic daily headache in patients with migraine." Headache: The Journal of Head and Face Pain 41(3) (2001): 303–309.

[103] De Felice, M., Porreca, F. "Opiate-induced persistent pronociceptive trigeminal neural adaptations: potential relevance to opiate-induced medication overuse headache." Cephalalgia 29(12) (2009): 1277–1284.

[104] Parsadaniantz, xS. M., et al. "Opioid and chemokine receptor crosstalk: a promising target for pain therapy?" Nature Reviews Neuroscience 16(2) (2015): 69–78.

[105] Fumal, A., et al. "Orbitofrontal cortex involvement in chronic analgesic-overuse headache evolving from episodic migraine." Brain 129(2) (2006): 543–550.

[106] Ayzenberg, I., et al. "Central sensitization of the trigeminal and somatic nociceptive systems in medication overuse headache mainly involves cerebral supraspinal structures." Cephalalgia 26(9) (2006): 1106–1114.

[107] Bongsebandhu-Phubhakdi, S., Srikiatkhachorn, A. "Pathophysiology of medication-overuse headache: implications from animal studies." Current Pain and Headache Reports 16(1) (2012): 110–115.

[108] De Felice, M., et al. "Triptan-induced latent sensitization: a possible basis for medication overuse headache." Annals of Neurology 67(3) (2010): 325–337.

[109] De Felice, M., et al. "Triptan-induced enhancement of neuronal nitric oxide synthase in trigeminal ganglion dural afferents underlies increased responsiveness to potential migraine triggers." Brain 133(8) (2010): 2475–2488.

[110] Suhr, B., et al. "Drug-induced headache: long-term results of stationary versus ambulatory withdrawal therapy." Cephalalgia 19(1) (1999): 44–49.

Chapter 8

Pharmacovigilance of the Analgesic Therapy

Silvia Ussai

Additional information is available at the end of the chapter

http://dx.doi.org/10.5772/67243

Abstract

Analgesics, the cornerstone for the alleviation of both acute and chronic pain, represent one of the most used classes of medications. While they are essential for the improvement of patients' quality of life, analgesic use is often associated with adverse drug reactions (ADRs) that might affect their usability in particular clinical situations. This indicates that a detailed knowledge of analgesic-derived ADRs is essential for the planning of an efficient pain relief strategy. This chapter reviews the ADRs associated with the two most commonly used analgesic classes, opioid and nonsteroidal anti-inflammatory drugs (NSAID), discussing their common adverse effects and how these can influence their usability in clinical applications. With the publication in recent years of more and more long-term studies, this chapter also provides an overview of the potential risks of long-term analgesic use. This is particularly important for opioid analgesics, whose chronic use can lead to analgesic tolerance and addiction. A full description of potential problems deriving from analgesic use represents the first step in optimizing protocols for its safe application in clinical settings.

Keywords: Opioids, NSAID, ADRs, Analgesics, pharmacovigilance

1. Introduction

Pain relief, both for acute and chronic pain, is an important aspect of modern medicine and healthcare services [1]. Pain is defined as 'an unpleasant sensory and emotional experience associated with actual or potential tissue damage, or described in terms of such damage' by the International Association for the Study of Pain (IASP) [2]: as such, it strongly worsens the quality of life of patients and remains one of the most common reasons for using health care services [1]. Pain relief drugs in the form of analgesics represent one of the most commonly used medications. While analgesics may include different therapeutic active compounds, covering specific pain relief needs, opioid medications and nonsteroidal anti-inflammatory drugs (NSAIDs) remain the most commonly used analgesics [1, 3, 4].

Pain relief management teams have to be aware of the exact nature of the pain itself and its intensity, and must be able to differentiate between acute and chronic pain. These are not only essential factors for pain management itself, but this could also lead to the consideration of possible adverse drug reactions (ADRs) from analgesic use. Indeed, when implementing pain relief management, one must consider the best practice to alleviate pain directly, along with the possibility of having ADRs which would then defeat the purpose of analgesics use itself [5–8]. Additionally, chronic pain is associated with an increased incidence of mental health issues such as anxiety and depression [9]; thus, there is a need to extend the consequences of inefficient pain relief beyond pain management alone.

The proper use of analgesics, that is, targeted drug use against specific types of pain, can avoid or at least minimize ADRs. In this regard, scientific studies reporting on ADRs caused by analgesics become an invaluable tool to predict and prevent ADRs and to evaluate the safety of analgesics in different pain relief practices. While short-term side effects are generally easier to observe, long-term effects, particularly in chronic analgesic users, need specially designed studies or a careful review of previous literature. In the last few years, more literature has been made available that addresses ADRs of both the opioid and NSAID type, allowing for the re-evaluation of the safety of these two medication classes, including their chronic long term use [10–16].

In order to draw attention to analgesic an their risks and to minimize the negative consequences related to their use, the present review comprises a synthesis of the most important safety issues described in scientific literature. This stands as a broad overview of the topic, providing a basic understanding of safety issues associated with analgesics and a starting point for further understanding of the subject at hand.

The ADRs associated with the two most commonly used analgesic classes, opioid and nonsteroidal anti-inflammatory drugs (NSAID), discussing their common adverse effects and how these can influence their usability in clinical applications. In recent years, more and more long-term studies have been published providing an insight into the potential risks of long-term analgesic use, this chapter provides a thorough overview. This is particularly important when discussing opioid analgesics, whose chronic use can lead to analgesic tolerance and even addiction. A full description of the potential problems derived from analgesic use represents the first step in optimizing protocols for its safe application in clinical settings.

2. Opioids

The use of opioids has significantly increased during the last decade and concomitantly the occurrence of related ADRs has become more frequent [3, 17]. Opioids are, by definition, ligands for opioid neuroreceptors, thereby modulating them and their associated responses [3]. With opioid receptors controlling a variety of physiological processes, exogenous opioid application results, therefore, in an imbalance in receptor activity and a potential plethora of side effects.

Sedation is a common short-term ADR because of the anticholinergic effect of opioids. Drowsiness, sedation, nausea and vomiting could all be seen after treatment with opioids, and usually occurs in dosage transition states. Sedation represents the best early clinical indicator of respiratory depression [18]. A number of blind studies confirm this effect which seems particularly evident for methylphenidate [19–21].

On the other side of the spectrum, opioids also appear to disturb the normal sleep cycles. This is likely due to the interference of this class of molecules with the action or binding of sleep-related neurotransmitters, such as noradrenaline, serotonin, acetyl choline, dopamine, histamine and gamma-aminobutyric acid [22]. Although this effect appears to be limited to the depth of sleep and duration of the REM (Rapid eye movement) phase rather than the quality of sleep itself [23, 24], this factor might be worth considering when opioid treatments worsen sleep disturbances derived from an underlying condition.

Constipation is also a common side effect reported in opioid users, due to the activation of mu receptors and the consequent modulation of gut motility [25]. Opioid-induced constipation is very diffused, with a single opioid treatment alone being able to induce constipation [26], this condition does not improve over time, and so its management should be planned in advance before the start of an opioid regimen. In recent studies, the naloxone-oxycodone combination has been shown to reduce constipation [25, 26], which favours an improved quality of life for patients.

Long-term use of opioids may also lead to additional complications, for example a hormonal imbalance [27, 28]. These ADRs are well known in the medical arena, to the point where the terms opioid endocrinopathy (OE) and opioid-induced androgen deficiency (OPIAD) both appear in the literature. Opioid users often display an imbalance in estrogen, testosterone, adrenocorticotropin, cortisol, and corticotropin-releasing hormone, luteinizing hormone, gonadotrophin-releasing hormone, dehydroepiandrosterone and dehydroepiandrosterone sulphates. This accounts for the increase reports of depression and sexual dysfunction among both sexes, while women are also at risk of a potential loss in bone mineral density [27, 28].

A well-known complication of opioid use is the potential development of physical addiction and opioid tolerance [29]. Both short- and long-term opioid use can induce these problems and due to the fact that they particularly affect chronic pain patients, incorrect use of opioids in this group of users could become both dangerous and ineffective.

Opioid tolerance is dependent on both the patient and the specific opioid employed [30]. This means that tolerance developed for a specific opioid does not automatically affect the efficacy of another opioid medication. However, in conjunction with the risk of hyperalgesia [31], which is, an increase in pain sensitivity also present in opioid users, this might still lead to an abuse of prescription medication, a particularly sensitive topic in opioid research.

Pruritus is another common adverse effect of opioids, more frequent with the parenteral route than oral. Opioid-induced pruritus is primarily mediated by mu-opioid receptors, serotonin receptors and to a lesser extent by histamine. The first-line treatment for pruritus should include low-dose nalbuphine, low-dose naloxone and ondansetron; antihistamines are less efficient. In addition to these common side effects, there are also ADRs for specific opioids. The most common ones are summarized in **Table 1**.

Gastrointestinal	Constipation Nausea Vomiting
Cutaneous	Pruritus Sweating
Neurologic	Sedation/fatigue Headache Delirium/confusion Clouded vision Dizziness
Autonomic	Xerostomia Bladder dysfunction (e.g. urinary retention) Postural hypotension

Table 1. Most commonly reported opioid-induced side effects [3].

To further reduce the ADRs caused by opioid administration, several measures have been suggested in the form of guidelines to ensure that an effort is being made on the part of the health care providers to reduce the amount of ADRs that occur with opioid drug administration.

The health care provider must ensure that before prescribing opioids to a patient, one has thoroughly documented the patient's diagnosis, medical well-being at the time and more importantly their psychological, psychiatric and social state, including whether or not the patient has abused any drugs in the past.

A patient who is now presenting with a pain condition should be asked questions regarding any previous medical or surgical treatments that may have been performed, along with clarifying and quantifying the present intensity of pain and how this may be affecting their daily activities of living.

Along with the patient's present physical state of health, a health care provider would also find it beneficial to inquire on the patient's living conditions, whether or not the patient has easy access to family and/or social support, and if the patient currently has a job or any domestic duties.

The psychiatric status of the patient is especially important. Knowing whether or not there has been a diagnosis of any psychiatric disorders in the past and how they were treated can greatly reduce the chances of the related ADRs or opioid addiction; some guidelines suggest to initiate with a low opioid dose and monitor the patient daily [32] when dealing with a patient who has a co-morbid psychiatric condition or a family history of psychiatric disorders.

Furthermore, substance use history is vital to formulate a comprehensive knowledge of the patient. A physician should inquire on the patient's history of substance use, abuse and addiction, namely marijuana, tobacco, benzodiazepines, opioids themselves, cocaine, amphetamines, barbiturates, hallucinogens and solvents.

After gathering all the information necessary to formulate a management plan, the physician should use this information to perform risk screening for the patient, assessing the potential for opioid drug misuse, overdose and addiction, looking at aberrant drug-related behaviours and if necessary, employing a urine drug screening.

Patients and their health care providers should then initiate goal setting in order to find out what the patient's goals are and how feasible the treatment could be, along with fully documenting what specific goals have been agreed on by the patient with the health care provider.

Additionally, documented informed consent for the use of opioids is suggesting, enabling the doctor and patient to explore the benefits, adverse effects. Medical complications and risks that may be encountered during the course of opioid treatment should also be determined and discussed with the patient, especially with high risk groups including the elderly, adolescent, pregnant, breastfeeding and those with co-morbid psychiatric conditions and those on long-term opioid treatment.

Moreover, one should verify and confirm that they have selected the most appropriate opioid for treatment of their patients, this should be done using peer-reviewed evidence which specifies which drug and what dose is used for first, second and third line treatment for the specific pain condition that the patient has.

After reviewing current data on the topic and starting a treatment regimen, one should continuously monitor the dose of opioid being given. If the patient is taking a dose on the higher end of the scale, the health care provider should re-asses the patient's pain condition to note if the medication is effective at reducing the pain (at least 30% reduction), and are there any non-opioid treatment options available.

Also, the doctor should clarify that all mental health disorders are adequately treated, that any ADRs are being managed and lastly if there is any sign of abnormal drug-related behaviours, the physician should then taper or switch the medication appropriately. After all these precautionary measures are taken, one should remember that arranging a consultation with an expert in pain or addiction management is always an option that could only benefit the patient greatly [33].

Health care providers should also consider alternative recommendations to replace long-term opioid treatment. Over the counter alternatives include acetaminophen and low dose NSAIDS. Although NSAIDs carry the well-known risk of organ failure and ulcer formation, NSAIDs at high doses are effective means of pain relief. Corticosteroids, serotonin inhibitors and norepinephrine inhibitors are all pharmacologic agents that can help alleviate pain.

Other measures which could be employed to reduce pain, with little to no risk to the patient, include the use of steroid injections for musculoskeletal pain, physical therapy, massage, exercise and chiropractic care [34].

3. NSAIDs

NSAIDs are generally considered non-specific analgesic medications and these are commonly prescribed for inflammation-derived acute pain. This class of drugs acts mainly through the inhibition COX (cyclooxygenase) synthesis, this then leads to a decreased in the synthesis of prostaglandin [35]. Being widely diffused, NSAIDs are often used in combination with further on-going treatments, leading to final effects dependent on drug-drug interactions [1]. However, prescribers should take into account the intrinsic risk of NSAIDs' ADRs (**Table 2**).

1. Gastrointestinal bleeding
2. Cardiovascular disease
3. Stroke
4. Thrombotic disease
5. Arrhythmia

Table 2. The intrinsic risk of ADRs associated with NSAIDs [7, 40].

Complications involving the gastrointestinal tract as a consequence of NSAID use are common, especially in combination with the presence of risk factors [36]. NSAIDs exert their effects through the inhibition of COX and the pharmacological inhibition of COX (both 1 and 2 isoenzymes) works to provide relief from the symptoms of inflammation and pain.

This NSAID-induced decrease in prostaglandin synthesis is responsible for side effects such as dyspepsia, abdominal pain, nausea, vomiting, heartburn, haemorrhage (NSAIDs could also lead to prolongation of bleeding time and a significantly increased risk of haemorrhage by altering vascular homeostasis), ulceration, perforation or obstruction [37].Therefore, COX-2 specific inhibitors, for example celecoxib, have a lower risk of causing gastrointestinal related ADRs [38].

NSAIDs are also a cause of renal complications. Acute renal failure is a possible consequence of NSAID use. While this is an intrinsic risk of NSAID medications, it is more likely to occur in geriatric patients and in patients using enzyme inhibitors (ACEIs) or angiotensin receptor II blockers [39]. NSAIDs are the class of medicines that are most commonly associated with hypersensitivity reactions. Because of this, it is generally not recommended to use NSAIDs even after having an unrelated hypersensitivity reaction or having positive allergy tests. NSAID-triggered hypersensitivity reactions can result in respiratory complications or in dermatological problems [40, 41].

Long-term NSAID use is often associated with cardiovascular complications such as strokes and myocardial infarctions, especially with COX-2 inhibitor therapy. This is an important factor to consider in patients with pre-existing cardiovascular diseases, where the use of NSAIDs could potentially worsen their condition, especially in combination with other drug treatments [42, 43]. Liver toxicity is also commonly associated with NSAID use, in particular nimesulide, making this medication particularly unsuitable for long-term applications in patients affected by chronic conditions [44].

Health care providers should also ensure that NSAIDs are prescribed properly and monitored closely considering the aforementioned ADRs; this can be done by precision treatment of patients.

Physicians should first consider prescribing the lowest effective dose of NSAIDs to those who have not found alleviation of pain after taking paracetamol. Patients who require NSAIDs have to be treated according to their gastrointestinal risk profile, because the use of NSAID is associated with increased ADRs of the entire GI tract, thus increasing mortality. Therefore, a gastro-protective pharmacologic agent such as misoprostol should be prescribed along with the NSAID even though it may not completely eradicate the risk of ADRs such as bleeding, the incidence of ulcer disease will be reduced [45].

Furthermore, physicians should be precise when evaluating patients for NSAID therapy especially in patients with existing cardiovascular conditions as the use of these medications could increase the risk of cardiovascular events occurring. Namely, celecoxib carries the highest risk of coronary artery events at high doses and thus one should consider an alternative like naproxen in place of its use [45].

4. Acetaminophen

Acetaminophen is often used as the first-line treatment for pain relief for many diagnoses across the fields of medicine, globally. As an over the counter medication, it is either prescribed by a doctor or bought by patients. The patients either complete the course as directed or they continue buying and self-treat with the medication, managing the doses on their own and subsequently increasing the dose with increasing pain. This behaviour, which is encouraged by some physicians, can be fatal and has been proven to be useless in most cases of long-term chronic pain management [46].

It is now known that acetaminophen is not effective in substantially reducing chronic pain conditions such as osteoarthritis, back pain or post-operative pain [47, 48]. A careful, systematic and thorough review of acetaminophen use becoming a public health and ethical concern must be gauged in depth across the globe. When one considers the ADRs associated with its use, acetaminophen as a first-line treatment for chronic pain seems to call for further evaluation; ADRs such as liver failure can occur in any patient demographic regardless of pre-existing conditions ranging from abnormal liver enzyme profiles to requiring liver transplantation.

Of note, hepatotoxicity is considered when more than 4 gm of acetaminophen have been administered in 1 day [49], but there have been cases of liver injury occurring even at lower doses [50]; geared with this information, physicians should begin to re-evaluate their stance on acetaminophen being completely safe for use with patients at home, regardless of their liver health status and especially in the setting of long-term chronic pain management.

5. Adjuvant therapy

Adjuvant analgesics are defined as drugs with a primary indication other than pain that have analgesic properties in some painful conditions. The group includes numerous drugs in diverse classes. Although the widespread use of these drugs as first-line agents, the term "adjuvant" is a misnomer, they usually are combined with a less-than-satisfactory opioid regimen, in particular when administered for cancer pain. Some adjuvant analgesics are useful in several painful conditions and are described as multipurpose adjuvant analgesics (antidepressants, corticosteroids, α_2-adrenergic agonists, neuroleptics), whereas others are specific for neuropathic pain (anticonvulsants, local anesthetics, N-methyl-D-aspartate receptor antagonists), bone pain (calcitonin, bisphosphonates, radiopharmaceuticals), musculoskeletal pain (muscle relaxants) or pain from bowel obstruction (octreotide, anticholinergics).

Antidepressants, namely triclyclics (TCAs), which are used as adjuvants for pain management, can sometimes cause lethal cardiotoxicity as an ADR. In order to reduce the likelihood of this, the prescribing physician is advised to order an electrocardiogram in those patients with a history of heart disease, or simply provide a better tolerated alternative, such as desipramine and nortripltyline. Orthostatic hypertension, acute glaucoma and cognitive impairment are also ADRs caused by TCAs which can be avoided by screening patients for pre-existing conditions and previous episodes of these diseases in order to reduce the likelihood of a reaction [51].

Corticosteroids, although well tolerated at moderated doses, can cause ADRs such as increasing the risk of peptic ulcer disease at a higher prolonged dose. One way to ameliorate this side effect is by prescribing a gastro-protective formulation, hence reducing the possible damage to the gastric lining [51].

Medications in the α_2-adrenergic drug class (clonidine and tizanidine) are only used as a last resort adjuvant, due to their serious side effects [51] which include somnolence and hypotension.

Olanzapine, along with other neuroleptics, are also used as an adjuvant only in cases where the patient is being treated for dementia or agitation. ADRs caused by olanzapine including tardive dyskinesia and neuroleptic malignant syndrome greatly reduce the quality of life of patients, which is undesirable [51].

Anticonvulsant drugs are now widely used to treat cancer-related neuropathic pain. Gabapentin and lamotrigine have both been proven to improve the condition of patients with neuropathic pain but these also cause side effects such as somnolence, dizziness and unsteadiness [51].

http://dx.doi.org/10.5772/67243

Calcitonin, another adjuvant, may cause a hypersensitivity reaction at the onset of administration when given subcutaneously, this requires skin testing, but has been identified, along with nausea as a minor side effect when used as an adjuvant in palliative care [51].

Radionuclide pharmaceutical agents have been used to treat metastatic bone disease, namely strontium and samarium, but using these medications can lead to myelosuppression, a severe unwanted ADR [51].

Therefore, it can be said that adjuvants also present with their own pertinent adverse drug reactions that could damper the overall effectiveness in improving the condition of a patient with long-term use, which does not improve the patient's quality of life.

6. Conclusions

Analgesics are essential pain relievers in modern medicine. However, analgesic misuse and their adverse effects can affect the efficiency of pain treatment and the eventual outcome could reduce the quality of life of patients. This review aims to highlight the most common adverse drug reactions of analgesic treatments and the possible safety risks involved with their use. Drug-drug interactions can be sometimes responsible for the adverse effects. However, a significant proportion of analgesic ADRs are preventable, which would reduce the patients' suffering. Acknowledging potential safety problems represents the first step for health professionals in assuring a safe and efficient analgesic treatment with minimum risks to patients. But being aware of the potential risks of the drugs should not be an impediment for health professionals to initiate analgesic therapy when necessary.

Author details

Silvia Ussai

Address all correspondence to: ussai.silvia@gmail.com

1 Bocconi University, MIHMEP, Milan, Italy

2 iRhythmia Research Centre, Bolzano, Italy

3 SIMED Medical Center, Gorizia, Italy

References

[1] Cazacu I, Mogosan C, Loghin F. Safety issues of current analgesics: an update. Clujul Med. 1957. 2015;88(2):128–36.

[2] IASP Taxonomy – IASP [Internet]. [cited 2016 May 30]. Available from: http://www.iasp-pain.org/Education/Content.aspx?ItemNumber=1698#Hyperalgesia

[3] Benyamin R, Trescot AM, Datta S, Buenaventura R, Adlaka R, Sehgal N, et al. Opioid complications and side effects. Pain Physician. 2008 Mar;11(2 Suppl):S105-120.

[4] Moore N, Pollack C, Butkerait P. Adverse drug reactions and drug-drug interactions with over-the-counter NSAIDs. Ther Clin Risk Manag. 2015;11:1061–75.

[5] Cabral DMC, Bracher ESB, Depintor JDP, Eluf-Neto J. Chronic pain prevalence and associated factors in a segment of the population of São Paulo City. J Pain Off J Am Pain Soc. 2014 Nov;15(11):1081–91.

[6] Patel KV, Guralnik JM, Dansie EJ, Turk DC. Prevalence and impact of pain among older adults in the United States: findings from the 2011 National Health and Aging Trends Study. Pain [Internet]. 2013 Dec [cited 2016 May 30];154(12). Available from: http://www.ncbi.nlm.nih.gov/pmc/articles/PMC3843850/

[7] Salomon L, Tcherny-Lessenot S, Collin E, Coutaux A, Levy-Soussan M, Legeron MC, et al. Pain prevalence in a French teaching hospital. J Pain Symptom Manage. 2002 Dec;24(6):586–92.

[8] Vallano A, Malouf J, Payrulet P, Baños JE, Catalan research group for studying pain in hospital. Prevalence of pain in adults admitted to Catalonian hospitals: a cross-sectional study. Eur J Pain Lond Engl. 2006 Nov;10(8):721–31.

[9] Tsang A, Von Korff M, Lee S, Alonso J, Karam E, Angermeyer MC, et al. Common chronic pain conditions in developed and developing countries: gender and age differences and comorbidity with depression-anxiety disorders. J Pain Off J Am Pain Soc. 2008 Oct;9 (10):883–91.

[10] Moore PN, Ganse EV, Parc J-ML, Wall R, Schneid H, Farhan M, et al. The PAIN study: paracetamol, aspirin and ibuprofen new tolerability study. Clin Drug Investig. 2012 Aug 29;18(2):89–98.

[11] Moore N, Charlesworth A, Van Ganse E, LeParc J-M, Jones JK, Wall R, et al. Risk factors for adverse events in analgesic drug users: results from the PAIN study. Pharmacoepidemiol Drug Saf. 2003 Oct 1;12(7):601–10.

[12] Zamora-Legoff JA, Achenbach SJ, Crowson CS, Krause ML, Davis JM, Matteson EL. Opioid use in patients with rheumatoid arthritis 2005-2014: a population-based comparative study. Clin Rheumatol. 2016 May;35(5):1137–44.

[13] Kongtharvonskul J, Anothaisintawee T, McEvoy M, Attia J, Woratanarat P, Thakkinstian A. Efficacy and safety of glucosamine, diacerein and nsaids in osteoarthritis knee: a systematic review and network meta-analysis. Bone Jt J. 2016 May 1;98–B(Suppl 8):120–120.

[14] Kongtharvonskul J, Anothaisintawee T, McEvoy M, Attia J, Woratanarat P, Thakkinstian A. Efficacy and safety of glucosamine, diacerein, and NSAIDs in osteoarthritis knee: a systematic review and network meta-analysis. Eur J Med Res. 2015;20:24.

[15] Furlan AD, Sandoval JA, Mailis-Gagnon A, Tunks E. Opioids for chronic noncancer pain: a meta-analysis of effectiveness and side effects. Can Med Assoc J. 2006 May 23;174 (11):1589–94.

[16] de Leon-Casasola OA. Opioids for chronic pain: new evidence, new strategies, safe prescribing. Am J Med. 2013 Mar;126(3, Supplement 1):S3–11.

[17] Trescot AM, Boswell MV, Atluri SL, Hansen HC, Deer TR, Abdi S, et al. Opioid guidelines in the management of chronic non-cancer pain. Pain Physician. 2006 Jan;9(1):1–39.

[18] Byas-Smith MG, Chapman SL, Reed B, Cotsonis G. The effect of opioids on driving and psychomotor performance in patients with chronic pain. Clin J Pain. 2005 Aug;21 (4):345–52.

[19] Bruera E, Miller MJ, Macmillan K, Kuehn N. Neuropsychological effects of methylphenidate in patients receiving a continuous infusion of narcotics for cancer pain. Pain. 1992 Feb;48(2):163–6.

[20] Wilwerding MB, Loprinzi CL, Mailliard JA, O'Fallon JR, Miser AW, van Haelst C, et al. A randomized, crossover evaluation of methylphenidate in cancer patients receiving strong narcotics. Support Care Cancer Off J Multinatl Assoc Support Care Cancer. 1995 Mar;3 (2):135–8.

[21] Bruera E, Chadwick S, Brenneis C, Hanson J, MacDonald RN. Methylphenidate associated with narcotics for the treatment of cancer pain. Cancer Treat Rep. 1987 Jan;71 (1):67–70.

[22] Moore P, Dimsdale JE. Opioids, sleep, and cancer-related fatigue. Med Hypotheses. 2002 Jan;58(1):77–82.

[23] Pickworth WB, Neidert GL, Kay DC. Morphinelike arousal by methadone during sleep. Clin Pharmacol Ther. 1981 Dec;30(6):796–804.

[24] Slatkin N, Rhiner M. Treatment of opioid-induced delirium with acetylcholinesterase inhibitors: a case report. J Pain Symptom Manage. 2004 Mar;27(3):268–73.

[25] DePriest AZ, Miller K. Oxycodone/naloxone: role in chronic pain management, opioid-induced constipation, and abuse deterrence. Pain Ther. 2014;3(1):1–15. doi:10.1007/s40122-014-0026-2.

[26] Mueller-Lissner S., "Fixed combination of oxycodone with naloxone: a new way to prevent and treat opioid-induced constipation"; Adv Therapy (2010) 27:581

[27] Li L, Setoguchi S, Cabral H, Jick S. Opioid use for noncancer pain and risk of myocardial infarction amongst adults. J Intern Med. 2013 May;273(5):511–26.

[28] Katz N, Mazer NA. The impact of opioids on the endocrine system. Clin J Pain. 2009 Feb;25(2):170–5.

[29] Warner EA. Opioids for the treatment of chronic noncancer pain. Am J Med. 2012 Dec;125 (12):1155–61.

[30] Eriksen J, Sjøgren P, Bruera E, Ekholm O, Rasmussen NK. Critical issues on opioids in chronic non-cancer pain: an epidemiological study. Pain. 2006 Nov;125(1–2):172–9.

[31] Lee M, Silverman SM, Hansen H, Patel VB, Manchikanti L. A comprehensive review of opioid-induced hyperalgesia. Pain Physician. 2011 Apr;14(2):145–61.

[32] Burian M, Geisslinger G. COX-dependent mechanisms involved in the antinociceptive action of NSAIDs at central and peripheral sites. Pharmacol Ther. 2005 Aug;107(2):139–54.

[33] Laine L. Gastrointestinal effects of NSAIDs and coxibs. J Pain Symptom Manage. 2003 Feb;25(2 Suppl):S32–40.

[34] Sostres C, Gargallo CJ, Arroyo MT, Lanas A. Adverse effects of non-steroidal anti-inflammatory drugs (NSAIDs, aspirin and coxibs) on upper gastrointestinal tract. Best Pract Res Clin Gastroenterol. 2010 Apr;24(2):121–32.

[35] Lazzaroni M, Battocchia A, Bianchi Porro G. COXIBs and non-selective NSAIDs in the gastroenterological setting: what should patients and physicians do? Dig Liver Dis Off J Ital Soc Gastroenterol Ital Assoc Study Liver. 2007 Jun;39(6):589–96.

[36] Lapi F, Azoulay L, Yin H, Nessim SJ, Suissa S. Concurrent use of diuretics, angiotensin converting enzyme inhibitors, and angiotensin receptor blockers with non-steroidal anti-inflammatory drugs and risk of acute kidney injury: nested case-control study. BMJ. 2013;346:e8525.

[37] Torres MJ, Barrionuevo E, Kowalski M, Blanca M. Hypersensitivity reactions to nonsteroidal anti-inflammatory drugs. Immunol Allergy Clin North Am. 2014 Aug;34(3):507–524, vii–viii.

[38] Sánchez-Borges M. Clinical management of nonsteroidal anti-inflammatory drug hypersensitivity. World Allergy Organ J. 2008 Feb;1(2):29–33.

[39] Coxib and traditional NSAID Trialists' (CNT) Collaboration, Bhala N, Emberson J, Merhi A, Abramson S, Arber N, et al. Vascular and upper gastrointestinal effects of non-steroidal anti-inflammatory drugs: meta-analyses of individual participant data from randomised trials. Lancet Lond Engl. 2013 Aug 31;382(9894):769–79.

[40] Gerstein NS, Gerstein WH, Carey MC, Kong Lam NC, Ram H, Spassil NR, et al. The thrombotic and arrhythmogenic risks of perioperative NSAIDs. J Cardiothorac Vasc Anesth. 2014 Apr;28(2):369–78.

[41] Suleyman H, Cadirci E, Albayrak A, Halici Z. Nimesulide is a selective COX-2 inhibitory, atypical non-steroidal anti-inflammatory drug. Curr Med Chem. 2008;15(3):278–83.

[42] Furlan AD, Reardon R. the National Opioid Use Guideline Group (NOUGG). Opioids for chronic noncancer pain: a new Canadian practice guideline. CMAJ : Can Med. Assoc J. 2010;182(9):923–30. doi:10.1503/cmaj.100187.

[43] National Opioid Use Guideline Group. Canadian guideline for safe and effective use of opioids for chronic non-cancer pain. Hamilton (ON): NOUGG; 2010. [(accessed 2010 May 3)].

[44] Hayden JA, van Tulder MW, Tomlinson G. Systematic review: strategies for using exercise therapy to improve outcomes in chronic low back pain. Ann Intern Med. 2005;142:776–785. doi:10.7326/0003-4819-142-9-200505030-00014.

[45] Scarpignato C, Lanas A, Blandizzi C, Lems WF, Hermann M, Hunt RH, International NSAID Consensus Group. Safe prescribing of non-steroidal anti-inflammatory drugs in patients with osteoarthritis – an expert consensus addressing benefits as well as gastrointestinal and cardiovascular risks. BMC Med. 2015;13:55.

[46] da Costa BR, Reichenbach S, Keller N, et al. Effectiveness of non-steroidal anti-inflammatory drugs for the treatment of osteoarthritis pain: a network meta-analysis. Lancet 2016;387:2093–105.

[47] Saragiotto BT, Machado GC, Ferreira ML, Pinheiro MB, Abdel Shaheed C, Maher CG. Paracetamol for low back pain. Cochrane Database Systematic Rev. 2016, Issue 6. Art. No.: CD012230. DOI: 10.1002/14651858.CD012230.

[48] Moore RA, Derry S, Aldington D, et al. Single dose oral analgesics for acute postoperative pain in adults: an overview of Cochrane reviews. Cochrane Database Syst Rev. 2015;9: CD008659.

[49] Fontana RJ. Acute liver failure including acetaminophen overdose. Med Clinics North Am. 2008;92(4):761–94. doi:10.1016/j.mcna.2008.03.005.

[50] Watkins PB, Kaplowitz N, Slattery JT, et al. Aminotransferase elevations in healthy adults receiving 4 grams of acetaminophen daily. JAMA. 2006;296:87–93.

[51] Lussier D, Huskey AG, Portenoy RK. Adjuvant analgesics in cancer pain management. The Oncologist. 2004;9(5):571–591. doi:10.1634/theoncologist.9-5-571. http://theoncologist.alphamedpress.org/content/9/5/571#cited-by. Accessed October 12, 2016.

Chapter 9

Pharmacologic Management of Low Back Pain

Dallas Schepers

Additional information is available at the end of the chapter

http://dx.doi.org/10.5772/66959

Abstract

Chronic back pain is a complex process and similar to how each patient has a very individualized disease process the treatment regimen should be similarly individualized. There are several different medication classes, each with a unique mechanism of action that can assist the practitioner in targeting a specific aspect of a patient's pain. The goal of this chapter will be to provide an adequate overview of the different medication classes while providing enough drug-specific information to guide the practitioner in selecting and developing an adequate multimodal analgesic regimen. When designing an analgesic regimen, an emphasis should be placed using a modified stepwise approach similar to the World Health Organization's analgesic ladder. There should be a focus on a multimodal analgesia utilizing nonopioid medications for chronic pain. Patient-specific factors should always be considered when choosing class, strength, dosage form and possible adjuvant medications. Just like patients, no analgesic regimen should be exactly the same.

Keywords: analgesics, paracetamol, nonsteroidal anti-inflammatories, neuropathic pain, opioids

1. Introduction

Chronic back pain is a complex process and similar to how each patient has a very individualized disease process the treatment regimen should be similarly individualized. There are several different medication classes, each with a unique mechanism of action that can assist the practitioner in targeting a specific aspect of a patient's pain. Additionally, patient-specific factors must be considered when developing a regimen to ensure adherence and improve outcomes. The goal of this chapter will be to provide an adequate overview of the steps a practitioner needs to take during the regimen development process and share enough drug-specific information to guide the practitioner in selecting the most efficacious and best suited agents for the individual patient.

Prior to initiating any pharmacologic treatment regimen for a patient, current consensus recommendations include discussing realistic expectations with the patient [1]. This should include patient's expectations of pain relief as well as functional goals that the patient should work toward. Additionally, the clinician should encourage self-care and education with evidence-based materials. It is important to emphasize to the patient that acute low back pain has very favorable improvement in the first month of recovery. Generally speaking, staying active and exercising should be highly encouraged for all patients. Bed rest should only be recommended if it improves severe pain symptoms and its duration should only be temporary. Patients should also be encouraged to resume activity as quickly as possible.

2. Multimodal and targeted treatment approaches

There are several important concepts that a clinician must understand before they can adequately start the treatment of low back pain. The first is that there is more data on the use of medication for acute low back pain than chronic low back pain [1]. This does not mean that specific pharmacologic agents are not effective in the setting of chronic low back pain, but simply that there is less evidence due to constraints in studying the long-term side effects [1]. When initiating the therapy, the clinician should focus on medications with the most known efficacy for the specific cause of pain and that have the least risk for serious side effects [1]. Specifically, the drug class and sometimes the even the individual drug chosen will be dictated by side effects (short and long term) and targeted mechanism of pain.

Treatment should include a targeted approach to the individual's cause of low back pain. The majority of low back pain is caused by a mechanical etiology [2]. These causes include degenerative disk or joint disease, vertebral fracture, and deformities and occur in up to 80–90% of patients. Neurogenic (e.g., herniated disks, spinal stenosis) inflammatory (e.g., rheumatoid arthritis, ankylosing spondylitis) and other less common causes (e.g., neoplasm, referred pain) make up the remainder of etiologies. The pharmacologic agents first selected should be completely dependent on the underlying etiology. However, as the pain progresses to a chronic state, a broader approach typically must be taken due to decreased efficacy of the targeted treatment.

The majority of this chapter will focus on the treatment of low back pain with an underlying mechanical etiology since it is by far the most common. However, if the cause of low back pain is inflammatory in nature, targeted therapy should also focus on treatment with anti-inflammatory agents. This may mean early use of nonsteroidal anti-inflammatories (NSAIDs) and treatment with corticosteroids or disease-modifying antirheumatic drugs (DMARDs) in patients with rheumatoid arthritis or ankylosing spondylitis [3]. Additionally, these disease states have a higher incidence of neuropathic pain and thus may require adjuvant medications that target this specific pain type. Some patients with mechanical low back pain also have increased pain due to spasticity and may benefit from treatment with antispasmodics. These agents will be discussed in much greater detail later, but to put it simply treatment should be tailored to the individual.

http://dx.doi.org/10.5772/66959

While the treatment of acute low back pain is normally fairly straight forward, its progression into chronic pain tends to complicate treatment. This is primarily due to the fact that chronic pain can often be associated with not only physical pain, but also deleterious cognitive and behavioral effects [4]. Because of this, a patient's rehabilitation program should emphasize a biopsychosocial model or one that involves a combination of physical, psychological and educational components [4, 5]. This also means that treatment (including medications) should be used to treat any psychological processes that may be worsening the perception of pain such as depression or anxiety.

Lastly, it is important to understand that medication alone will likely not completely alleviate a patient's pain, and it is even less likely to do so if the pain is chronic. Thus, treatment as a whole should be tailored to the individual and a holistic approach should be taken [4]. In addition to pharmacologic treatments, nonpharmacologic treatments including topical heat for acute pain or cognitive behavioral therapy, exercise therapy, spinal manipulation and interdisciplinary rehabilitation for subacute or chronic pain should be considered [6, 7]. However, for the purpose of this chapter, we will be focusing primarily on pharmacologic treatments and how they should be combined, implemented and optimized.

3. World Health Organization's stepwise approach to pain

In 1986, the World Health Organization (WHO) published an analgesic treatment model that described in detail the appropriate way to escalate therapy in chronic pain associated with cancer [8]. This stepwise model focused on the incremental escalation of treatment from non-opioid analgesics to low-strength opioids and eventually to medium- or high-strength opioids. Since its publication this model has been adapted into the treatment of all types of pain including acute, chronic and noncancer pain [9]. Many attribute this to the increased opioid utilization for the management of all types of pain [10]. Additionally, many argue that opioid medications are being over utilized and the stepwise approach, while simple, is not the most ideal method in treating chronic pain. Even if the stepwise model is not perfect in its original form, several key components should be considered when implementing or modifying an analgesic treatment regimen [9].

Whether the patient has acute or chronic pain, a couple of components of the WHO's stepwise approach are critical to follow no matter the circumstance [9]. These key aspects include that the prescriber should utilize oral medications whenever possible, prescribe analgesics at fixed intervals dictated by their duration of action, the specific analgesic chosen should be dependent on pain intensity and its effect should be evaluated by a validated pain intensity scale [8]. When looking at the complete analgesic regimen, it should be uniquely tailored to the individual and once a regimen is established, a written personal program should be given to the patient, so they can be held accountable to taking medications at their appropriate times and others (family, friends and medical professionals) know how they take their medications in case of emergency. While these components should be cemented in the care of any patient with low back pain, the ideal stepwise escalation, de-escalation or type of adjuvant medication depends upon the type of pain being treated and may not follow the originally proposed WHO's stepwise approach [9].

Several recommendations have been suggested for the alteration of the WHO's stepwise approach to pain [9]. The first is that when dealing with acute pain, it is sometimes necessary to start at a higher step than the first step of the ladder. This means that opposed to starting with a nonopioid agent alone, it may be necessary to start therapy with a weak, moderate or even strong opioid in addition to a nonopioid agent. However, because most acute pain resolves or markedly improves in a short period of time, there should be an emphasis on early alteration of the analgesic regimen. Rarely are opioids needed for longer than 7 days to treat acute pain [6]. The one major stipulation to treating acute pain in this way (skipping steps on the WHO's ladder) is that the provider is encouraged to rapidly step down the ladder or de-escalate therapy as pain diminishes or side effects are too severe. This requires a practitioner to have very close follow-up and may not be appropriate in all settings. This recommendation is not originally recommended by the WHO, but it is feasible when considering the acute pain process and the need to wean patients from regimens containing strong opioids [9].

As the patient transitions from an acute pain process to a chronic pain state (1–3 months), it is import to reassess the analgesic regimen. If de-escalation has not been performed, it should be done at this point to ensure that the patient is only prescribed the minimal amount of medications required to control their pain. When escalating in a stepwise manner, the cause and type of pain should be considered. The pain regimen should focus on nonopioid analgesics with nonsteroidal anti-inflammatories (NSAIDs) if the pain is caused or exacerbated by an inflammatory process. Adjuvant medications targeting neuropathic pain should be initiated and optimized at this time if there is a component of neuropathic pain [9]. Only when nonopioids and adjuvant medications have been fully optimized, an opioid should be scheduled at a fixed interval. Nonpharmacologic and nonopioid medications are preferred for chronic pain [6]. If the pain requires opioids, a weak opioid should be trialed first before escalating to a moderate or strong opioid [8, 9]. To appropriately escalate therapy, it is necessary to understand the specific attributes of each analgesic medication (nonopioids, opioids and adjuvants) so that the patient receives the maximum benefit while minimizing the potential for harm and side effects.

4. Paracetamol/acetaminophen

Paracetamol, also commonly referred to as acetaminophen, was first synthesized in 1878 by Morse, a researcher at Johns Hopkins Hospital [11]. It was not until 15 years later that paracetamol's antipyretic effects were first noted and a medical implication was suggested [11, 12]. The current consensus is that paracetamol is the first-line agent for both acute pain and chronic pain [1, 6, 11]. This is not because paracetamol is a more potent analgesic, but because it has a much better side effect profile than that of other nonopioid analgesics [1, 11].

Even though it has been well over a hundred years since its synthesis, not much is known about the mechanism of action of paracetamol and several have been proposed to explain

http://dx.doi.org/10.5772/66959

paracetamol's antipyretic and analgesics effects [11–13]. One in particular is that it indirectly inhibits the cyclooxygenase (COX) enzymes. The COX isoenzymes are responsible for converting arachidonic acid to prostaglandins, thromboxanes and prostacyclins. Prostaglandins are thought to be a primary mediator of pain, fever and inflammation both centrally and peripherally. Paracetamol is thought to only inhibit a certain isoenzyme of COX (COX-3) in the brain which is why many believe that it has minimal anti-inflammatory effects in peripheral tissues [11, 14]. While there are high concentrations of COX-1 and COX-2 in peripheral tissue, the proposed COX-3 enzyme is thought to have higher concentrations in the brain. It is through the inhibition of COX-3 that paracetamol may have its primary mechanism of action causing analgesic and antipyretic effects while exerting minimal anti-inflammatory effects [11, 12]. While this is a popular hypothesis, it does not explain the small amount of peripheral anti-inflammatory activity some researchers have found.

Another proposed hypothesis postulates that paracetamol inhibits COX isoenzymes in a unique manner and explains the mild anti-inflammatory effects it may have. Unlike NSAIDs, this hypothesis suggests paracetamol does not bind to the active site of COX to cause inhibition [11]. It instead reduces COX from its active form (Fe^{4+}) to its inactive form (Fe^{3+}) and in turn prevents the conversion of arachidonic acid to prostaglandins. Paracetamol's reducing effects are blocked by locally acting peroxides. This explains why paracetamol may be inactivated in the periphery where there are high levels of peroxides in the setting of cell damage, but not centrally where levels are significantly lower.

Side effects of paracetamol are relatively benign with the most worrisome being hepatotoxicity caused by toxic levels of its metabolite N-acetyl-p-benzoquinineimine (NAPQI) [11, 14]. Close to 40% of all acute liver failure cases in the United States and United Kingdom can be attributable to paracetamol intoxication. Approximately 90% of paracetamol is metabolized in the liver through glucuronidation or sulfation. The remainder of the drug's metabolism through the liver is through the cytochrome P450 (CYP450) system. The specific subfamily that has been implicated in the majority of this process is CYP2E1. As the glucuronidation and sulfation pathways are saturated, the metabolism through the CYP450 system proportionately increases and more NAPQI is produced. NAPQI then exerts its toxic effects by binding covalently to macromolecules of hepatocytes. Total daily doses of paracetamol alone or in combination with other analgesics should not be greater than 4 g a day with most regimens being 325–650 mg given every 4–6 h [1, 11, 15]. However, recent increases in the use of paracetamol-containing combination products have brought concern to overdose risk. Due to this, some clinicians recommend a maximum daily dose of 2.4–3.2 g a day, especially in the elderly [16–18]. Of note, paracetamol is commonly combined with opioid analgesics and is found to have additive analgesic effects when done so. The risk for overdose is increased in this setting due to patients taking paracetamol alone in addition to the combination product. In 2011, the Food and Drug Administration (FDA) of the United States limited the amount of paracetamol to 325 mg in combination products due to this increased risk.

Other patient populations at risk for toxicity include those that are malnourished, those taking CYP450 inducers (isoniazid, anticonvulsants) and those with heavy alcohol consumption

[11, 14]. Chronic alcoholism is especially worrisome for patients taking high doses of paracetamol on a daily basis. Chronic alcohol intake causes hepatotoxicity through a completely independent pathway as well as increasing CYP450 activity and depleting glutathione stores. Both of these increase the production of NAPQI. Therefore, in alcoholics, total daily doses should be limited to 2 g [18].

Other less common, but notable side effects of paracetamol therapy include hypersensitivity reactions and elevations in international normalized ration (INR) [11, 18, 19]. When patients were given 4 g of paracetamol a day for 14 days, there was a mild increase in INR as well as a mild decrease in vitamin K-dependent clotting factors. This supports closer monitoring when patients are being co-administered warfarin and paracetamol for long periods of time. Intravenous doses of 1 g have been shown to cause very minor decreases in platelet aggregation, but overall paracetamol should be considered safe to use in the setting of an elevated bleeding risk. It is because of the lack of side effects and relative tolerability of paracetamol that it is recommended as the first-line agent in treating acute and chronic pains.

5. Nonsteroidal anti-inflammatories

Similar to paracetamol, NSAIDs exert their analgesic, antipyretic and anti-inflammatory effects through the inhibition of COX isoenzymes [18, 20]. NSAIDs specifically target COX-1 and COX-2, and enzyme affinity varies among agents. It is this isoenzyme selectivity that determines the efficacy and safety profile of these agents. As a group, NSAIDs typically are used as second-line agents in the treatment of acute and chronic low back pains after paracetamol [1, 7]. NSAIDs are more potent analgesics when compared to paracetamol for the treatment acute pain, but they are also associated with gastrointestinal, renal and cardiovascular complications with chronic use [14, 21]. At high doses, NSAIDs can even have comparable analgesic effects to low-dose opioids without the respiratory depressant effects. When evaluating the clinical efficacy among NSAIDs, no study has shown that one agent is better than another [20]. Therefore, when selecting an agent, careful consideration of each agent's safety and pharmacokinetic profile should be considered.

There are several different classes of NSAIDs, and most classes have multiple agents as well. For the purposes of this chapter, we will be focusing on those agents commonly used to treat acute and chronic pains. In order to treat low back pain effectively, an NSAIDs must be available orally and have good bioavailability, a fast onset of action, convenient dosing interval and minimal drug-drug interactions (**Table 1**). Of note, several NSAIDs (diclofenac, ibuprofen and ketoprofen) have topical formulations that likely provide similar analgesic effects as their oral counter parts, but are associated with less systemic side effects [22]. Additionally, other dosage forms may be available to treat acute pain in patients unable to take oral medications. For example, there are intravenous formulations of ketorolac and ibuprofen that can be used in the hospitalized setting to treat acute pain. Similarly, rectal formulations are also available for several NSAIDs, but their long-term use for analgesia is inconvenient and comparative efficacy is unknown.

http://dx.doi.org/10.5772/66959

Drug name	Dosage forms	Typical dose (mg)	Dosing interval (h)	COX selectivity	Comments
Ketorolac	Oral; intravenous	10	4–6	COX-1	Potent analgesic
Ketoprofen	Oral (immediate release, extended release); Gel	Immediate release: 25–50; Extended release: 100	Immediate release: 6–8 Extended release: 24	COX-1	High incidence of GI side effects; maximum dose of 100 mg in patients with renal dysfunction
Indomethacin	Oral (immediate release, controlled release); Intravenous; Suppository	Immediate release: 25; Controlled release: 75	Immediate release: 8–12; Controlled release:	COX-1	High occurrence of headache as a side effect
Nabumetone	Oral	500–1000	12–24	COX-1	Long half-life (24 h) requires fixed interval dosing for best efficacy; well tolerated with less GI side effects; Variable dose reductions based on degree of renal dysfunction
Sulindac	Oral	150–200	12	Unselective	Undergoes enterohepatic recirculation
Naproxen	Oral (immediate release, extended release); Cream	Immediate release: 250–500; Extended release: 750	Immediate release: 12; Extended release: 24	Unselective	Long half-life (14 h) analgesic effect increases as it reaches steady-state (3 days)
Piroxicam	Oral	20	24	Unselective	Very long half-life (45–50 h) need to take on fixed interval for best efficacy
Ibuprofen	Oral; Cream; Intravenous; Suppository	200–600	6–8	Unselective	Very well tolerated at lower doses
Diflunisal	Oral	500–1000	8–12	Unselective	Weak antipyretic effects; excreted into breast milk
Meloxicam	Oral	7.5–15	24	COX-2	COX-2 selective at lower doses; long half-life (20 h) requires fixed interval dosing for best efficacy

Drug name	Dosage forms	Typical dose (mg)	Dosing interval (h)	COX selectivity	Comments
Diclofenac	Oral (immediate release, extended release); Suppository; Gel	Immediate release: 25–50; Extended release: 50–75	Immediate release: 6–8; Extended release: 24	COX-2	Edema is a common side effect (33% of patients)
Celecoxib	Oral	100–200	12	COX-2	Dose reduction is necessary in CYP2C9 poor metabolizers (*3/*3 allele) although not commonly known; May carry higher cardiovascular risk than other nonselective NSAIDs
Etodolac	Oral (immediate release, extended release)	Immediate release: 200–400; Extended release: 400–1000	Immediate release: 6–8; Extended release: 24	COX-2	Similar COX-2 selectivity as celecoxib

Table 1. Properties of common NSAIDs (ordered in increasing COX-2 selectivity).

The most common adverse reactions with chronic NSAID use are those associated with the upper GI tract [13, 19, 20]. These adverse reactions are dose dependent in nature, and patients are placed at increasing risk as doses are escalated for increased analgesia activity. For example, when ibuprofen is used at doses of 800–1200 mg a day, risk for GI bleed was not significantly different than placebo [13]. Additionally, as doses are escalated, the odds of a GI bleed nearly double when doses of ≤600 mg/day were compared to doses of >1200 mg/day [19]. Adverse reactions are uncommon with chronic NSAID use, with up to 20% of patients reporting dyspepsia during treatment [18, 20]. Other common adverse reactions include anorexia, nausea, abdominal pain and diarrhea.

GI adverse reactions are mediated through two possible mechanisms [18, 20]. Through inhibition of COX-1, NSAIDs decrease cytoprotective prostaglandin production in the gastric epithelial cells. This causes an increase in acid secretion, a decrease in mucosal blood flow and a decrease in the production of the protective mucous layer. The second proposed mechanism is through local irritation to mucosal cells. NSAIDs are week acids, and in the acidic environment of the stomach, they stay unionized and readily diffuse into mucosal epithelial cells. Once inside cells, these acids trap hydrogen ions and cause cell damage. Risk factors for NSAID-induced GI injury include age > 65 years, tobacco use, alcohol consumption, concurrent use of steroids, anticoagulation, prior history of GI ulceration and increasing dose or duration of NSAIDs. Of note, formulations whose goal is to decrease direct contact with gastric mucosa (e.g., enteric coating) have not shown to reduce the incidence of major GI adverse reactions. However, it is recommended to utilize acid suppression therapy (histamine blockers or proton pump inhibitors) in patients on chronic high doses of NSAIDs to aid in the prevention of gastric and duodenal ulcers [18, 19].

Due to these common side effects, a subset of NSAIDs was developed to selectively inhibit only the COX-2 isoenzyme. There are much lower concentrations of COX-2 in the upper GI tract, and by sparing inhibition to COX-1, the detrimental effects seen with nonselective NSAIDs on the GI mucosa are greatly diminished [19, 20]. Fortunately, this selective inhibition of COX-2 does not seem to decrease the analgesic effects of COX-2 selective NSAIDs when compared to nonselective NSAIDs [23]. However, because there are higher concentrations of COX-2 in cardiovascular (CV) tissue, COX-2 selective NSAIDs have been associated with increased CV risk. This has led to the majority of COX-2 selective agents to being pulled from the market [13]. With this consideration in mind, COX-2 selective NSAIDs may be advantages in patients with history of GI ulcers, dyspepsia, gastroesophageal reflux disease or other similar disorders and are otherwise good candidates for treatment with NSAIDs [20]. Similar to nonselective NSAIDs, use in the setting of acute pain is reasonable, but careful consideration must be made when used chronically as long-term risk likely outweighs benefit.

Another adverse effect of NSAIDs that goes hand in hand with the increased risk for GI adverse reactions is the risk of platelet inhibition. Through inhibition of the COX-1 isoenzyme, NSAIDs attenuate the production of thromboxane A2 [19]. By decreasing the production of thromboxane A2, NSAIDs reversibly inhibit platelet aggregation and clot formation and if combined with other drugs that carry a bleeding risk the effect is additive. One case-control study that looked at NSAID use combined with selective serotonin reuptake inhibitors found that the incidence of upper GI bleed or ulcer was three when the agents were used alone [24].

Other limiting factors shown with chronic therapy include an increased cardiovascular thrombotic risk, blood pressure and renal toxicity. While each of these adverse events occurs separately, they are intertwined through pathophysiology. CV risk is likely caused by decreased production of COX-2-dependent prostaglandins in the kidney. These prostaglandins normally blunt the effect that prothrombotic and atherogenic inputs have on the coronary vasculature [25]. Without this protection, the risk for CV-related events elevates. Blood pressure and renal toxicity are affected in a somewhat similar matter. In patients who have increased activation of the renin-angiotensin and elevated blood pressure, NSAIDs disrupt the tenuous balance that renal prostaglandins play a key role in maintaining homeostasis. When COX-2 is inhibited and these prostaglandins are reduced, antidiuretic hormone is blunted and chloride ions are reabsorbed to a greater degree. This causes sodium and water retention and an elevation in blood pressure [18]. A similar process is commonly described to explain the NSAID-induced renal injury. The same prostaglandins that regulate chloride reabsorption also maintain renal blood flow. Homeostasis normally occurs through reducing the effects of adrenergic or renin-angiotensin inputs. When removed, arterial constriction occurs, blood supply decreases and renal toxicity occurs [26].

Even with a large number of potential side effects, NSAIDs are a great option to treat low back pain, especially if it is only for a short duration. Caution should be advised when considering treating for longer durations and when a patient has co-morbid disease states or is at risk for adverse reactions. If it is used chronically, make sure the lowest efficacious dose is being used. Additionally, if a clinician commonly prescribes NSAIDs, they should be diligent in following new evidence on efficacy and safety of individual agents to assist them in selecting the most ideal one. When considering a patient's analgesic regimen, NSAIDs are a viable first- or second-line treatment choice if the risks for drug-related complications are low [1, 6]. In relation to the WHO's stepwise ladder, adding a NSAID is especially useful if a patient has an acute increase in pain (acute injury, worsening breakthrough pain, etc.) and even more so if the acute pain process has an inflammatory component. Ideally, when the acute pain event is resolved or mitigated, the clinician can shift back down the pain ladder and remove the NSAID from the regimen.

6. Adjuvant medications

Medications that fall into the adjuvant medication category have a unique place in therapy. These medications typically fall into two categories and can be added at any point in therapy (any step of the WHO's analgesic ladder). They should be used to tailor treatment and are a mainstay in the targeted treatment of the individual. The two categories are drugs that target neuropathic pain and drugs that target somatic pain through an indirect mechanism [8, 10]. When initiating an adjuvant medication, it should have a clear target and purpose to aid in decreasing pain. Adjuvants should not be used simply to lower opioid requirements, especially in patients, on lower doses, with minimal side effects as most adjuvants are not benign and many have severe side effects themselves [27].

Neuropathic pain is a type of pain that originates through a dysfunction in the peripheral or central nervous system [28, 29]. It is estimated to effect up to 7–8% of the general population in Europe and is often so severe that it is disabling to patients. It can be caused by several different disease processes including chronic radiculopathy and has a high incidence in low back pain caused by inflammatory causes.

Gabapentin and pregabalin exert their mechanism of action through binding to voltage-gated calcium channels and result in a decrease in release of the neurotransmitters glutamate and substance P [27, 28]. These agents are commonly considered first-line agents due to their high efficacy and a relatively benign side effect profile. Efficacy seems to increase as dose increases, but so do side effects. Most commonly, patients experience dizziness, sedation, peripheral edema and dry mouth [30]. Both agents can aid in sleep disturbances, and pregabalin has a mild anxiolytic effect as well. These agents have also been used in acute pain and are now recommended in the postoperative setting with more clinicians claiming these agents should be used as true analgesics and not as adjuncts [31].

Antidepressants can alter pain through several different mechanisms. These include modulation of monoamine activation, interacting with opioid pathways, inhibiting descending pain pathways and blocking ion channels that are important in pain transmission [27]. Tricyclic antidepressants (TCAs) have the most robust evidence to support their use in neuropathic pain. While the exact mechanism is unknown, it is likely mediated through blocking the reuptake of norepinephrine. These agents are antagonistic at N-methyl-D-aspartate (NMDA)

http://dx.doi.org/10.5772/66959

receptors and may have a roll at reducing hyperalgesia caused by central windup. Agents in this class include the secondary amines nortriptyline and desipramine and tertiary amines amitriptyline and imipramine. When compared to each other, no agent has been found to be superior to another. Despite this, nortriptyline and desipramine are typically considered the preferred agents due to better side effect profile. TCAs are associated with increased risk for sedation, orthostatic hypotension, dry mouth, constipation, urinary retention and cognitive impairment especially in the elderly [15, 23, 28].

TCAs are not the only antidepressants that have been looked at for the treatment of neuropathic pain. SSRIs and serotonin norepinephrine reuptake inhibitors (SNRIs) have also been evaluated. Even though the SSRIs citalopram and paroxetine have shown efficacy in treating neuropathic pain, they are typically not as preferred compared to TCAs and SNRIs because they are less efficacious [28]. Previously, TCAs had been preferred due to more evidence and lower costs. However, costs of both venlafaxine and duloxetine have decreased recently and use has increased. Some guidelines even support their use as first-line agents [29]. Of the two, duloxetine seems to be preferred because it is associated with less hypertension and is well tolerated in the elderly [16, 28, 29]. Patients should be counseled on the fact that treating pain with antidepressants can take up to 2.5 weeks to reach their full effect and this can decrease compliance.

Other common adjuvant medications commonly added to analgesic regimens include muscle relaxants, corticosteroids, local anesthetics and topical agents [27, 32]. Muscle relaxants as a group have varying mechanisms of action, some of which are not fully understood. These agents may be considered for acute pain relief, but have very limited data to support continued use. They should only be used in patients who have increased somatic pain due to spasticity. The primary side effect of this drug class is central nervous system adverse effects (sedation, fatigue, dizziness, etc.), but because these drugs are not related in mechanism, they each have their own safety profiles. Due to the lack of data and risk for severe side effects (e.g., hepatotoxicity of dantrolene) use of skeletal muscle relaxants for back pain not associated with severe spasticity is discouraged.

Topical lidocaine may be of an advantage for patients who complain of localized neuropathic pain [28]. Lidocaine decreases the frequency of Na+ channel opening, thereby decreasing pain transmission. When it is used topically, systemic absorption is decreased, which makes systemic adverse reactions very rare. Evidence for use in low back pain is lacking, but its use should be considered if a patient complains of localized neuropathic pain.

Patients who suffer from chronic low back pain are sometimes prescribed corticosteroids. Many different doses of prednisone and dexamethasone have been studied, but there is no general consensus on an effective dose or duration [27]. Many guidelines recommend the use of corticosteroids as no major study has shown long-term efficacy. If they are used, a single injection or short duration should highly be emphasized due to severe side effects of chronic use including immunosuppression, metabolic disorders and GI bleeding.

Addition of an adjuvant medication should directly target a cause of pain (neuropathy, muscle spasm, etc.), and efficacy should be evaluated after initiation and periodically throughout. If a medication is found to not be efficacious, it should be removed or replaced. For additional information, clinicians can refer to neuropathic pain guidelines that provide evidence-based recommendations for specific disease state-induced neuropathic pain [29]. If acute or chronic pain is completely neuropathic in nature, the WHO's stepwise ladder is not appropriate to follow and a medication regimen targeting neuropathy should be initiated.

7. Risk of opioids

After the addition of nonopioids and possible adjuvants, the WHO's analgesic ladder calls for low to strong opioids. However, if a patient is in severe acute pain, it is reasonable to start therapy with all three types of analgesics and then rapidly de-escalate to a lower step on the analgesic ladder [9]. When treating chronic pain, opioids should never be utilized as first-line agents outside of cancer or palliative care. Opioids have only been shown in the literature to have a short-term improvement in pain and carry a high risk for serious side effects and possibly even death [6]. Before initiating therapy, clinicians and patients should have a discussion regarding expected goals and potential risks. Goals should include how efficacy will be measured for both pain relief and functionality and what measures will indicate continued treatment. Patients should also be informed that opioids only show a short-term benefit in relieving pain and long-term efficacy is lacking. Expectations should be that opioids will likely never provide complete relief.

The addition of opioids to a chronic pain regimen should be considered carefully. Patients do not need to fail nonopioids or adjuvants prior to initiating opioids, benefits must simply outweigh the risks of starting opioid therapy [1, 8]. Another way to consider this is that opioids should be considered in patients with severe disabling pain that is likely not to be relieved from nonopioids and adjuvants alone. The worst risks are with overdose and potentially fatal respiratory depression. Overdose risk is dose dependent, and clinicians should be careful when doses are escalated. This is particularly important as there is technically no ceiling dose for opioids. Several other factors increase the risk for opioid-related overdose including methadone use, co-prescription with benzodiazepines, history of sleep-disordered breathing, reduced renal or hepatic function, increased age, pregnancy, history of substance abuse and psychiatric illness. Additionally, the risk of opioid-related overdose is elevated when starting patients on opioid therapy with long-acting or extended release formulations. For this reason, these dosage forms should only be utilized in opioid-tolerant patients. Risk mitigation strategies such as checking prescription refill history, urine drug screening and use of medications specifically for opioid use disorders (methadone, buprenorphine) increase retention in opioid treatment programs.

Prior to starting opioid therapy, the prescriber must fully understand the concepts of opioid abuse (opioid misuse disorders), tolerance and physical withdrawal [6]. Opioid abuse or opioid misuse disorders are described by patterned misuse of opioids that include unsuccessful attempts to curb use and results in social problems at home, work or school. Tolerance is simply a diminished response to a fixed dose of medication with repeated use. Physical dependence is when a medication causes the body to change in a way that when the medication is removed the body produces withdrawal symptoms. Both

http://dx.doi.org/10.5772/66959

physical dependence and tolerance can occur in the absence of opioid abuse. When treating a patient, it is necessary to keep these concepts separate and not to assume that because a patient is requiring higher doses of medication or is experiencing withdrawal symptoms that they are abusing opioids. Only after considering all of these things, a prescriber should initiate opioid therapy.

Opioid medications typically exert their analgesic effects through agonism at μ-, δ- and κ-opioid receptors [33, 34]. Opioid receptors are g-coupled protein receptors and are most commonly Gi/Go. Once these g-coupled protein receptors are activated, they decrease adenylyl cyclase activity, decrease calcium conductance and inhibit excitatory neurotransmission. This slows the transmission of pain that impulses both centrally and peripherally. Opioids activate centrally located receptors that play a key role in descending pain pathways and peripherally in the spinal cord. This spinal cord transmission regulates the relay of nociceptive pain inputs from the periphery to the brain. While all three opioid receptors mediate analgesia, activation of individual receptors will produce different effects [33]. μ-opioid receptors lower respiratory depression, sedation, euphoria, nausea, constipation and urinary retention. δ-opioid agonists have similar effects to those of μ-opioid agonists. These effects include respiratory depression, constipation and euphoria. While μ- and δ-opioid agonists have very similar effects, κ-opioid agonists have several unique effects. These agents can cause dysphoric, sedative, diuretic and sometimes aversive effects. An understanding of what receptor an individual opioid will activate will give the provider information in the common side effects that the medication will exhibit.

When acute or chronic low back pain necessitates the need to escalate to a weak opioid, the practitioner has several options to choose from. Drugs that are considered weak opioids are codeine, hydrocodone and oxycodone when used in combination with nonopioids (sometimes also tramadol), and all other full agonists (morphine, hydromorphone, oxycodone alone, oxymorphone and fentanyl) are considered moderate of strong opioids [15]. Weak opioids should be initiated with caution if the patient already is taking paracetamol at a fixed interval as it increases the risk of overdose. When starting opioid therapy with the intent to continue its long term, this initial phase should be considered a trial and should only be continued or escalated if pain relief occurs [6]. If a patient fails an initial trial of opioids, other agents should be considered for refractory pain. Once on opioid regimen is started, the practitioner should periodically assess the need to continue opioid therapy. If tolerance occurs or pain relief is reduced, the clinician should weight escalating therapy to a moderate or strong opioid versus the increase in risk. It is reasonable to abandon opioid therapy if, after an escalation in therapy, the patient does not experience an increase in analgesic effect.

8. Opioids

It is believed that opium was cultivated in Mesopotamia as early as 3400 BC [35]. Natural occurring opiates are the alkaloid compounds found in the poppy plant and include morphine and codeine while the term opioid refers to any compound that binds to opioid receptors. Narcotic originally was used to describe a medication that causes sleep, but the common misuse of drugs like quaaludes and barbiturates along with opioids caused this to become an umbrella term for drugs that are commonly abused. It is even used in a legal sense to describe the drugs of abuse. Even though opioids are grouped together, they have a wide range effects and each medication has unique properties (**Table 2**). There are four major opioid classes, and understanding each of the groups allows for easier prescribing as efficacy and side effects are similar within classes.

Drug name	pertinent dosage forms	Equianalgesic oral dose (mg)	Starting oral dose (mg)	Dosing interval (h)	Comments
Morphine	Immediate release extended release (Ms contin and kadian)	30	30–60	Immediate release: 4–6 Extended-release: 8–24	Several different extended-release formulations each with their own dosing interval recommendations Strong opioid
Codeine	Immediate release (combination with paracetamol)	200	30–60	4–6	Only available in combination with paracetamol Weak opioid
Hydromorphone	Immediate release Extended release	7.5	4–8	Immediate release: 4–6 Extended release: 12–24	Several different extended release formulations each with their own dosing interval recommendations Strong opioid
Hydrocodone	Immediate release (combination with paracetamol)	30	5–7.5	4–6	Only available in combination with paracetamol Weak opioid
Oxymorphone	Immediate release Extended release	10	5–10	Immediate release: 4–6 Extended release: 12	Strong opioid
Oxycodone	Immediate release (alone and combination with paracetamol) Extended release	20	15–30	Immediate release: 4–6 Extended release: 12	Can use lower starting doses if using combination product with paracetamol Weak opioid (combination product) Strong opioid (when used alone at higher doses)
Fentanyl	Transdermal; Submucosal	–	0.025	Transdermal: 24 Submucosal:	Use only in patients suffering from severe chronic pain

http://dx.doi.org/10.5772/66959

Drug name	pertinent dosage forms	Equianalgesic oral dose (mg)	Starting oral dose (mg)	Dosing interval (h)	Comments
Levorphanol	Immediate release	4	2–4	6–8	Half-life of 12–16 h; Good long-acting agent for those that cannot tolerate morphine or methadone
Methadone	Immediate release	Variable	2.5 (analgesic) 10–20 (withdrawal)	For analgesic effects: every 8 h To prevent withdrawal: every 24 h	Morphine (mg)/ methadone (mg) conversion changes as total daily doses of morphine increase 0–29 mg: 2/1 30–99 mg: 4/1 100–299 mg: 8/1 300–499 mg: 12/1 500–999 mg: 15/1 >1000 mg: 20/1

Table 2. Properties of common opioids.

The phenanthrenes are one of the larger classes of opioids and contain the prototypical opioid morphine. This class contains the most commonly used opioids including morphine, codeine, hydrocodone, hydromorphone, oxycodone, oxymorphone, levorphanol, buprenorphine, nalbuphine and butorphanol [35]. A majority of these agents are metabolized in the liver by the CYP450 isoenzyme CYP2D6. Some even require metabolism to exert analgesic effects. For example, codeine itself has no analgesic effect in its original state, and it is only through metabolism by CYPD6 to morphine that it can produce an analgesic effect [36]. A similar process happens to both hydrocodone and oxycodone to be converted to hydromorphone and oxymorphone. Similar to codeine, hydrocodone has been proposed to be a prodrug and its analgesic effect is dependent on activation by CYP2D6. Oxycodone, on the other hand, is a μ-opioid agonist and does not require activation by CYP2D6. A serious issue arises with the fact that CYP2D6 has a very dramatic range of activity from one person to the next. It has been reported in literature that through a mutation, some patients have no activity of CYP2D6 (codeine produces no analgesic effect) whatsoever while others may be classified as ultrarapid metabolizers. This may explain the wide range of reported efficacy in patients who are prescribed codeine- and hydrocodone-containing products.

Another common attribute of drugs in the phenanthrene class is that they are typically glucuronidated and eliminated via the kidneys. This is especially important for morphine whose glucuronidated metabolite, morphine-6-gucuronide, is responsible for its analgesic effects [37]. In young and healthy individuals, this is not of importance, but in elderly or those with markedly reduced renal function, morphine's analgesic effects are prolonged. Morphine prescribed at fixed intervals in this patient population should be closely monitored as the respiratory side effects may accumulate as the medication is cleared more and more slowly. Additionally, drugs in this class with a 6-hydroxyl group (morphine and codeine) are associated with a higher incidence of nausea than those in the class that do not [35].

Phenlyperidines include the agents' fentanyl, alfentanil, sufentanil and meperidine. Of these, fentanyl has the highest affinity for the μ-opioid receptor and is 80–100 times that of morphine [35, 37]. While incredibly potent fentanyl has a very short half-life leading to a short duration of action. Fentanyl's only advantage is that is highly lipophilic leading to its ability to be utilized nontraditional dosage forms. One of these dosage forms is the transdermal patch. Fentanyl transdermal patches should only be used in the most extreme cases of chronic low back pain. This dosage form possesses many nuances, and a complete understanding of them should be obtained before prescribing. When a fentanyl transdermal system is placed on a patient, it takes 6–12 h before taking effect [37]. Additionally, it will take 3–6 days to reach steady state and when removed a reservoir of drug will remain in effect up to 24 h. This makes initiating and weaning incredibly difficult and therefore should not be commonly done. Fentanyl also has a submucosal dosage form that may be beneficial in patients who suffer from acute breakthrough pain. The clinically applicability of this makes sense because of fentanyl's high potency and short duration of action. It is important to stress that this should not be prescribed on a regular basis and should only be utilized as a rescue medication in very rare cases. The majority of patients with chronic low back pain should not be prescribed fentanyl, but in rare circumstances, it may have clinical utility.

The other opioids in the phenlyperidine class should not be used in the treatment of low back pain. Meperidine is a relatively weak opioid agonist with poor oral absorption that fell out of favor due to its neurotoxic and anticholinergic side effects [23, 37]. Its metabolite normeperidine accumulates in patients with renal insufficiency and lowers seizure threshold. Additionally, it has significant drug-drug interactions with monoamine oxidase inhibitors that lead to severe respiratory depression. The other agents that are sufentanil and alfentanil in this drug class have little to no role in the treatment of low back pain due to their short duration and lack of specialized dosage forms.

The remaining classes of opioids consist of the benzomorphans and the diphenylheptanes. The only agent in the benzomorphan class is pentazocine, which is a mixed opioid agonist-antagonist. The diphenylheptaines include propoxyphene and methadone. While methadone has established itself in a highly specific role, propoxyphene has fallen out of favor dramatically [16]. Propoxyphene is thought to be no more efficacious than paracetamol, and it has a plethora of side effects. It has been associated with dizziness, weakness, paradoxical excitement, falls, visual disturbances and insomnia [35]. Propoxyphene itself is thought to act directly on the central nervous system and increase the risk for seizure activity which ultimately leads to the product being pulled off the market in the United States.

Several opioids have mixed agonist-antagonist activity and have only a limited role in the treatment of pain. These drugs provide small analgesic effects in patients with little or no prior opioid exposure and may exacerbate withdrawal symptoms in patients who have a physical dependence on opioid medications [35, 37]. Drugs in this group are pentazocine, butorphanol and nalbuphine. These agents have a ceiling effect on both analgesia and respiratory depression and have limited abuse potential. As doses escalate so do the antagonistic effects against other opioids. This places the patient at risk for withdrawal. Also, the risk for psychotomimetic side effects (delirium, delusions and hallucinations) increases in conjunction with the

http://dx.doi.org/10.5772/66959

dose [37]. Pentazocine has the highest incidence of these side effects. The role of these agents in pain is limited by their antagonistic effects and lack of convenient dosage forms. Only pentazocine is available in an oral dosage form and has fallen out of favor to treat acute or chronic pain. The partial agonist buprenorphine acts similarly to the agonist-antagonists with the one caveat that it is not associated with psychotomimetic side effects. Similar to the agonist-antagonists, it can produce withdrawal symptoms when administered to patients taking high doses of other opioid medications. It is also combined with naloxone to reduce the risk of abuse. Buprenorphine is available as a sublingual dosage form in the United States and a transdermal extended release system in Europe. The sublingual form is commonly used in the United States in addiction treatment programs.

Methadone is another opioid with a unique mechanism of action other than being a μ-opioid receptor agonist. This mechanism may be particularly advantageous for patients who have "opioid-resistant" pain states or have a neuropathic component to their pain [37]. Similar to some of the agents to treat neuropathy, the R-isomer of methadone is antagonistic at the NMDA receptor and may be beneficial in treating the effects of hyperalgesia and allodynia seen in chronic pain states [37]. Methadone should be used with caution as mentioned before its use increases the risk for overdose and a misunderstanding of its pharmacokinetics and pharmacodynamics perpetuates this effect. The terminal half-life of the drug is typically thought to be 15–60 h, but has been cited as up to 120 h [38]. Because of this, it may take a week or longer to reach steady state, and therefore, the drug should be titrated no more often than weekly. Additionally, the analgesic effect of methadone is roughly 4–8 h and should be dosed on an every 8-h interval. Due to this discrepancy, the drug has a high risk for accumulation and may put the patient at risk for sedation, confusion, respiratory depression, cardiac abnormalities and death. The general consensus is that a dose of 2.5 mg every 8 h is a safe starting dose for opioid-naive patients [38]. Careful monitoring should be performed on any patient starting on methadone. Another caveat to dosing methadone is that it has a nonlinear equianalgesic conversion. This means that patients on higher doses of opioids are more sensitive to the effects of methadone and when converting the ratio of morphine equivalents to methadone dose decreases. However, with caution, the practitioner can utilize this effect to their advantage in treating the most complicated of patients.

Lastly, there are two agents that are sometimes considered opioid analgesics, but have both opioid and nonopioid mechanisms. These two agents are tramadol and tapentadol. While both have activity at the μ-opioid receptor, this activity alone does not equate to the full analgesic effects seen with these agents [35, 39]. The remainder of their analgesic effects can be attributed to the inhibition of serotonin and norepinephrine reuptake. Similar to TCAs, this may be useful in treating neuropathic pain and caution should be used when combining therapy with other antidepressants or medications that increase the levels of serotonin as it increases the risk for serotonin syndrome [29]. Tramadol can be used for mild-to-moderate pain, but it should not be used as monotherapy when opioids are indicated based on the severity of pain. Tramadol's analgesic effect is at most equal to codeine and is probably less than that of hydrocodone [13, 16]. The maximum dose of tramadol is 100 mg every 6 h. Higher doses than 400 mg a day should not be used as it increases the risk for lethargy, nausea, tachycardia, agitation and hypertension. Additionally, tramadol has a neuroexcitatory effect so as doses increase so does the risk for seizures [13]. For these reasons, tramadol should be used either as an adjuvant medication or prior to stepping up to moderate or strong opioid-containing regimens and is often seen as adjunct medications.

9. Conclusion

By blending together all of the concepts in this chapter, a practitioner can provide the best treatment for their patients suffering from low back pain. Through an understanding of a modified WHO's stepwise approach and a thorough understanding of all of the drug class available to them, they should be able to escalate and de-escalate therapy in a safe and effective manner. The practitioner will need to set expectations, incorporate a multimodal treatment approach, analyze potential contraindications for specific drug therapy and provide the most ideal medication regimen. This regimen should be based on ease and appropriateness for the individual patient and should be executed with a complete understanding of every drug class mentioned in this chapter (paracetamol, NSAIDs, adjuvant and opioid medications). If this is done, the practitioner will truly be in expert in the pharmacologic management of low back pain.

Author details

Dallas Schepers

Address all correspondence to: dschep2@gmail.com

Mount Sinai Hospital, Chicago, IL, USA

References

[1] Chou R, Qaseem A, Snow V, et al. Diagnosis and treatment of low back pain: a joint clinical practice guideline from the American College of Physicians and the American Pain Society. Ann Intern Med. 2007;147(7):478–491.

[2] Karppinen J, Shen FH, Luk KDK, Andersson GBJ, Cheung KMC, Samartzis D. Management of degenerative disk disease and chronic low back pain. Orthop Clin North Am. 2011;42(4):513–528.

[3] Sarzi-Puttini P, Salaffi F, Di Franco M, et al. Pain in rheumatoid arthritis: a critical review. Reumatismo. 2014;66(1):18–27.

[4] Lee C, Crawford C, Swann S. Multimodal, integrative therapies for the self-management of chronic pain symptoms. Pain Med. 2014;15(S1):S76–S85.

http://dx.doi.org/10.5772/66959

[5] Kamper SJ, Apeldoorn AT, Chiarotto A, et al. Multidisciplinary biopsychosocial rehabilitation for chronic low back pain: Cochrane systematic review and meta-analysis. BMJ. 2015;350(Feb 18):h444.

[6] Dowell D, Haegerich TM, Chou R. CDC guideline for prescribing opioids for chronic pain—United States, 2016. JAMA. 2016;315(15):1624.

[7] Chou R, Huffman L. Nonpharmacologic therapies for acute and chronic low back pain: a review of the evidence for an American Pain Society/American College of Physicians clinical practice guideline. Ann Intern Med. 2007;147(7):492–504.

[8] World Health Organization. Cancer Pain Relief: With a Guide to Opioid Availability. 2nd ed. WHO; 1996.

[9] Vargas-Schaffer G. Is the WHO analgesic ladder still valid? Twenty-four years of experience. Can Fam Physician. 2010;56(6):514–517.

[10] Ballantyne JC, Kalso E, Stannard C. WHO analgesic ladder: a good concept gone astray. BMJ. January 2016;352:i20.

[11] Mattia C, Coluzzi F. What anesthesiologists should know about acetaminophen.pdf. Minerva Anestesiol. 2009;75(11):644–653.

[12] Botting RM. Mechanism of action of acetaminophen: is there a cyclooxygenase 3? Clin Infect Dis. 2000;31(Suppl 5):S202–S210.

[13] Sachs CJ. Oral analgesics for acute nonspecific pain. Am Fam Physician. 2005;71(5):913–918.

[14] Barkin RL. Acetaminophen, aspirin, or ibuprofen in combination analgesic products. Am J Ther. 2001;8(6):433–442.

[15] Kaye AD, Baluch A, Scott JT. Pain management in the elderly population: a review. Ochsner J. 2010;10(3):179–187.

[16] Cavalieri TA. Management of pain in older adults. J Am Osteopath Assoc. 2005;105 (3_suppl):12S–17S.

[17] Tracy B, Sean Morrison R. Pain management in older adults. Clin Ther. 2013;35(11): 1659–1668.

[18] Goser T, Smith E, FitzGerald G. Anti-inflammatory, antipyretic, and analgesic agents; pharmacotherapy of gout. In: Goodman & Gilman's: The Pharmacological Basis of Therapeutics. 12th ed. New York, NY: McGraw-Hill; 2011.

[19] Moore N, Pollack C, Butkerait P. Adverse drug reactions and drug-drug interactions with over-the-counter NSAIDs. Ther Clin Risk Manag. July 2015;11:1061-75.

[20] Green GA. Understanding NSAIDs: From aspirin to COX-2. Clin Cornerstone. 2001;3(5):50–59.

[21] Enthoven WT, Roelofs PD, Deyo RA, van Tulder MW, Koes BW. Non-steroidal anti-inflammatory drugs for chronic low back pain. In: The Cochrane Collaboration, ed. Cochrane Database of Systematic Reviews. Chichester, UK: John Wiley & Sons, Ltd; 2016.

[22] Derry S, Moore RA, Gaskell H, McIntyre M, Wiffen PJ. Topical NSAIDs for acute musculoskeletal pain in adults. In: The Cochrane Collaboration, ed. Cochrane Database of Systematic Reviews. Chichester, UK: John Wiley & Sons, Ltd; 2015.

[23] Gloth MF. Pain management in older adults: prevention and treatment. J Am Geriatr Soc. 2001;49(2):188–199.

[24] de Abajo FJ, Rodríguez LAG, Montero D. Association between selective serotonin reuptake inhibitors and upper gastrointestinal bleeding: Population based case-control study. Bmj. 1999;319(7217):1106–1109.

[25] Grosser T. Biological basis for the cardiovascular consequences of COX-2 inhibition: Therapeutic challenges and opportunities. J Clin Invest. 2005;116(1):4–15.

[26] Whelton A. Nephrotoxicity of nonsteroidal anti-inflammatory drugs: Physiologic foundations and clinical implications. Am J Med. 1999;106(5):13S–24S.

[27] Knotkova H, Pappagallo M. Adjuvant analgesics. Anesthesiol Clin. 2007;25(4):775–786.

[28] Moulin DE, Clark AJ, Gilron I, et al. Pharmacological management of chronic neuropathic pain–consensus statement and guidelines from the Canadian Pain Society. Pain Res Manag. 2007;12(1):13–21.

[29] Attal N, Cruccu G, Baron R, et al. EFNS guidelines on the pharmacological treatment of neuropathic pain: 2010 revision: Treatment of neuropathic pain. Eur J Neurol. 2010;17(9):1113–e88.

[30] Patel S. Neuropathic pain guidelines. SA Pharm J. 2015;82(5):23–26.

[31] Chou R, Gordon DB, de Leon-Casasola OA, et al. Management of Postoperative Pain: A clinical practice guideline from the American Pain Society, the American Society of Regional Anesthesia and Pain Medicine, and the American Society of Anesthesiologists' Committee on Regional Anesthesia, Executive Committee, and Administrative Council. J Pain. 2016;17(2):131–157.

[32] Hicks G, Duddleston D, Russel L, Shepherd J, Brown C. Low back pain. Am J Med Sci. 2002;324(4):207–211.

[33] Stein C. Opioids, sensory systems and chronic pain. Eur J Pharmacol. 2013;716(1–3): 179–187.

[34] Trang T, Al-Hasani R, Salvemini D, Salter MW, Gutstein H, Cahill CM. Pain and poppies: the good, the bad, and the ugly of opioid analgesics. J Neurosci. 2015;35(41):13879–13888.

[35] Trescot A, Datta S, Lee M, Hansen M. Opioid pharmacology. Pain Physician. 2008;11: S133–S153.

[36] Eichelbaum M, Evert B. Influence of pharmacogenetics on drug disposition and response. Clin Exp Pharmacol Physiol. 1996;23(10–11):983–985.

[37] Inturrisi CE. Clinical pharmacology of opioids for pain. Clin J Pain. 2002;18:S3–S13.

[38] Chou R, Fanciullo GJ, Fine PG, et al. Clinical guidelines for the use of chronic opioid therapy in chronic noncancer pain. J Pain. 2009;10(2):113–130.e22.

[39] Langford RM, Knaggs R, Farquhar-Smith P, Dickenson AH. Is tapentadol different from classical opioids? A review of the evidence. Br J Pain. 2016;101(4):217–221. doi:10.1177/2049463716657363

Section 2

Novel Research on Analgesics

Chapter 10

Paracetamol: Update on its Analgesic Mechanism of Action

Christophe Mallet, Alain Eschalier and
Laurence Daulhac

Additional information is available at the end of the chapter

http://dx.doi.org/10.5772/66649

Abstract

Paracetamol is the most widely used over-the-counter medication in the world. The mechanism of action of its analgesic effect was often considered as based on the mobilization of the cyclooxygenases and more recently on serotonergic pathways. A new metabolic pathway involving the generation of an active metabolite, AM404 (N-(4-Hydroxyphenyl)-5Z,8Z,11Z,14Z-eicosatetraenamide), in the brain by the fatty acid amide hydrolase (FAAH) enzyme, was recently identified. This chapter describes experimental data that have shown the involvement of this metabolic pathway in the analgesic action of paracetamol and its relationship with the cyclooxygenase and serotonergic systems. It also explains how new targets and systems, such as the cannabinoid and vanilloid systems and the calcium channel receptor Cav3.2, play a role in the action of paracetamol. Finally, it suggests how research on the mechanism of the clinically relevant effects of this long-established analgesic could lead to new therapeutic pain strategies.

Keywords: paracetamol, para-aminophenol, AM404, pain, FAAH, CB_1, TRPV1, Cav3.2, serotonin

1. Introduction

More than a century after its discovery, paracetamol (acetaminophen) is the most widely prescribed analgesic in the world. Although used as a treatment for moderate pain and fever for more than a century, the mechanisms of its analgesic action are poorly understood and are a topic of ongoing debate. This chapter presents and updates the preclinical data on the pharmacodynamics of the paracetamol. While the two main mechanisms are considered as based on the inhibition of cyclooxygenases and/or the activation of the serotonergic system [1], we show that the endocannabinoid and vanilloid systems and the T-type calcium-channel Cav3.2 are emerging as new targets of its action *via* complex metabolic and neuronal pathways.

2. Paracetamol, a prodrug of which AM404 is the active metabolite

In 2005, Högestätt et al. [2] showed that paracetamol, following its hepatic deacetylation to *p*-aminophenol, is metabolized in the brain by the fatty acid amide hydrolase (FAAH) enzyme to form AM404 (N-(4-Hydroxyphenyl)-5Z,8Z,11Z,14Z-eicosatetraenamide) (**Figure 1**).

After administration of deuterium-labeled paracetamol in rats, they detected deuterium-labeled AM404 and *p*-aminophenol in the brain. They further showed that formation of *p*-aminophenol was present in all tissues, with highest levels in the liver and that AM404 was mainly found in the brain. The latter results were confirmed in a recent study [3].

Incubation of brain homogenate with *p*-aminophenol *in vitro* but not with paracetamol (except at high doses) leads to the formation of AM404 [2]. This is not the case if brain

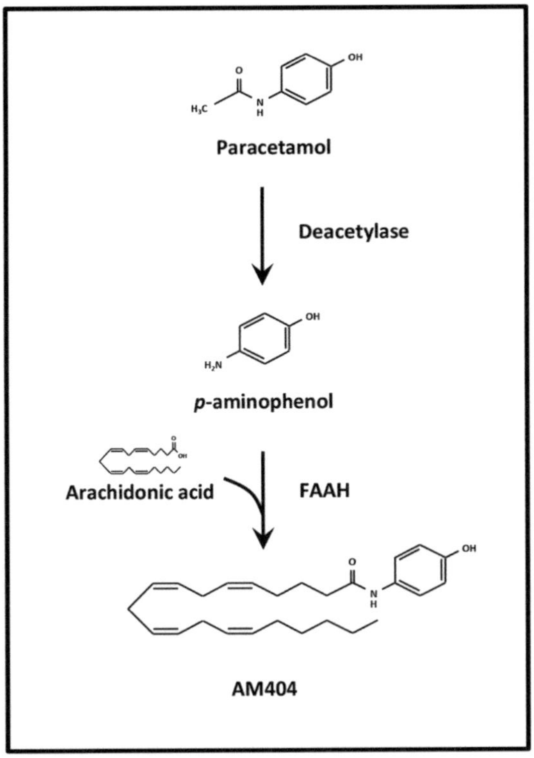

Figure 1. Metabolization of paracetamol into AM404. AM404: N-(4-hydroxyphenyl)-5Z,8Z,11Z,14Z-eicosatetraenamide. FAAH, fatty acid amide hydrolase.

http://dx.doi.org/10.5772/66649

homogenate is boiled, pretreated with PMSF (a broad-spectrum protease, esterase and amidase inhibitor [4]) or if brain homogenate comes from $FAAH^{-/-}$ mice. Incubation of isolated FAAH with *p*-aminophenol and arachidonic acid leads to the formation of AM404. *In vivo*, paracetamol does not produce AM404 in the brains of rats pretreated with PMSF or in $FAAH^{-/-}$ mice.

We speculated that this metabolic pathway was involved in its analgesic action and decided, therefore, to investigate the analgesic effect of paracetamol metabolites. Systemic administration of *p*-aminophenol or intracerebroventricular injection of AM404 produced an analgesic effect in animals.

We then investigated the involvement of FAAH in the action of paracetamol using mice deleted for the FAAH gene (genetic strategy) and systemic administration of PMSF or URB597, nonspecific and specific FAAH inhibitors, respectively, (pharmacological strategy) to inhibit the FAAH enzyme. Both strategies resulted in the abolition of paracetamol-induced (1) brain synthesis of AM404 and (2) analgesic action [5]. Likewise, the analgesic effect and brain formation of AM404 induced by *p*-aminophenol were decreased in $FAAH^{-/-}$ mice and in rats pretreated with PMSF [6].

The involvement of FAAH in the action of paracetamol was observed in different pain tests (paw pressure, von Frey, tail immersion and formalin tests) and modalities (thermal, mechanical and chemical *stimuli*) [5–7]. However, the experiments were conducted in naive animals, in a context far removed, therefore, from the clinical setting, in which paracetamol is used for pathological pain, notably nociceptive pain [8, 9]. Thus, the involvement of FAAH in the action of paracetamol was studied in a more relevant clinical context using an inflammatory mouse model submitted to thermal and mechanical *stimuli* to assess allodynia and hyperalgesia. The anti-allodynic and anti-hyperalgesic effects of paracetamol observed in this model were lost in $FAAH^{-/-}$ mice [10], which lend further weight to the involvement of the FAAH in inflammation.

Although it is now generally acknowledged that the action of paracetamol is central rather than peripheral, opinions still differ [11, 12]. FAAH is a ubiquitous enzyme [4]. Some authors detected AM404 in blood after paracetamol administration [13]. We investigated the peripheral versus central involvement of FAAH in the action of paracetamol studying its effect with an FAAH inhibitor that readily crosses the blood-brain barrier, URB597 and a peripherally restricted FAAH inhibitor, URB937 [14, 15] (**Figure 2A**).

The fact that the analgesic action of paracetamol is maintained after URB937 administration and lost after URB597 treatment [10] shows that only brain and not peripheral, FAAH is involved and thereby confirms the central action of paracetamol. As a counterproof, the peripherally restricted FAAH inhibitor URB937 was intracerebroventricularly injected and challenged with paracetamol (**Figure 2B**). A supra-spinal injection of URB937 in mice prior to paracetamol reversed its analgesic actions.

All these results show that supra-spinal FAAH is required for the desired effect of the paracetamol.

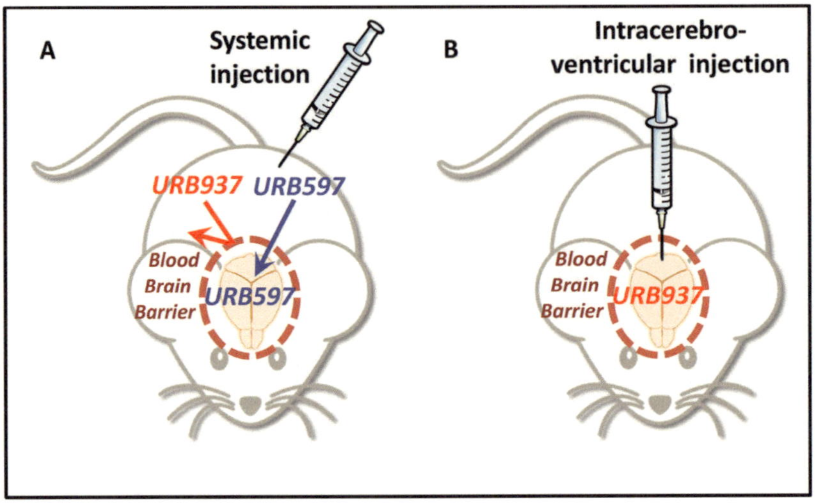

Figure 2. Pharmacological strategies to block central and/or peripheral FAAH. (A) Global or peripheral FAAH was inhibited by a systemic injection of URB597 (a brain permeant compound) or URB937 (a peripherally restricted FAAH inhibitor), respectively. (B) URB937 was supraspinally injected to specifically inhibit brain FAAH.

3. Different molecular targets of AM404

3.1. COX enzyme

The first historical hypothesis for the action of paracetamol, proposed by Flower and Vane, was the inhibition of COX [16]. In cell cultures, inhibition of COX by paracetamol was observed in different cell types, brain slices, or homogenates [16–18] with conflicting results [19]. Paracetamol seems to have only a weak inhibitory effect on prostaglandin production in cell culture, with IC_{50} values mostly around 100 μM [20]. In animals, paracetamol reduced prostaglandin in cerebrospinal fluid [21], the spinal cord [22] and the brain [23, 24]. Interestingly, AM404 was shown to be an inhibitor of COX on isolated COX-1 and COX-2 and in LPS-induced prostaglandin E_2 formation in RAW264.7 macrophages [2].

However, an orally administered analgesic dose of paracetamol (200 mg/kg) in mice did not affect brain prostaglandin E_2 (PGE_2) content, while a high intraperitoneal dose (300 mg/kg), which impairs mice locomotor activity, reduced the content of prostanoid levels in the brain (PGE_2), kidneys (PGE_2) and blood (thromboxane B_2) [7]. Paracetamol has a different pharmacological profile from that of the competitive COX inhibitor ibuprofen. In a context of noninflammatory pain, ibuprofen did not reduce pain, whereas paracetamol did, as observed in the first phase of formalin tests, tail immersion and von Frey tests in mice [7]. Altogether, these results indicate that the analgesic action of paracetamol cannot be attributed to inhibition of COX. Furthermore, the inhibitory effect of paracetamol on COX observed by some authors seems more closely related to its hypothermic/antipyretic effects than to its analgesic action [21, 23].

Further studies are needed before the involvement of COX can be fully ruled out. A study showing that PGs measured in mice after administration of 200 mg of paracetamol were not

http://dx.doi.org/10.5772/66649

decreased was performed with naive animals [7]. In a neuroinflammatory context such as chronic pain, in which PGs contribute to the maintenance of the process, it is possible that repeated administration of paracetamol could induce an inhibition of COX and that such a mechanism could be involved in the analgesic action of paracetamol.

3.2. CB_1 receptor

AM404 is able to indirectly activate the cannabinoid receptor CB_1 by inhibiting the degradation [25] and reuptake [26, 27] of anandamide. Involvement of this receptor in the action of paracetamol was confirmed by a study showing that CB_1 knockout mice and rats pretreated with a specific CB_1 antagonist (AM251) were insensitive to paracetamol [5, 28]. Corroborating these results, we showed that the analgesic effect of *p*-aminophenol was also suppressed by AM251 [6]. Interestingly, it was shown in a neuropathic rat pain model that the synergic or additive antinociception of paracetamol with gabapentin, memantine, or tramadol was attenuated by pretreatment with AM251 [29]. In the same study, the intrinsic analgesic effect of gabapentine, memantine, or tramadol was not affected by CB_1 receptor antagonist.

The involvement of CB_1 receptor seems independent of the potential inhibitory effect of AM404 on cannabinoid reuptake because the overall brain content of endocannabinoids (anandamide, 2-arachidonoylglycerol and palmitoylethanolamide) was not affected by an administration of paracetamol [7] or *p*-aminophenol [6] in mice or in rats. In addition, paracetamol does not bind directly CB_1 receptors [5]. Thus, the relationship between paracetamol and CB_1 remains to be elucidated.

3.3. TRPV1 receptor

Subsequent studies have shown that AM404 is also a potent activator of the capsaicin receptor TRPV1, as reported in patch-clamp experiments [30, 31]. Interestingly, local injection of AM404 in the paw of mice resulted in pain behavior (licking and lifting of the injected paw), a behavior not found in $TRPV1^{-/-}$ mice [7].

The contribution of TRPV1 to the action of paracetamol has been explored by both genetic and pharmacological approaches to inhibit it. Results showed that a genetic inactivation of TRPV1 abolished the antinociceptive effects of paracetamol in the mouse formalin, von Frey and tail immersion tests [7]. Pharmacological blockade of TRPV1 by capsazepine in rats also suppressed the analgesic effect of paracetamol [7]. Observations made on paracetamol can be extended to *p*-aminophenol, since pretreatment with capsazepine in rats or administration in $TRPV1^{-/-}$ mice prevented the antinociceptive effect of *p*-aminophenol [6]. Further, the analgesic effect of the intracerebroventricular injection of AM404 was lost in $TRPV1^{-/-}$ mice [7]. In a calcium imaging experiment, human embryonic kidney (HEK) cells, which constitutively expressed FAAH, were transfected with TRPV1. AM404 induced intracellular calcium mobilization [30]. This response was not observed in cells pretreated with capsazepine or in cells that were not transfected with TRPV1. In agreement with the previous results, bath application of *p*-aminophenol also induced an increase in intracellular calcium, smaller and slower than that of AM404. The calcium increase induced by *p*-aminophenol was abolished in cells either pretreated with capsazepine or not transfected with TRPV1 [30]. The effect of TRPV1 was due to metabolization of *p*-aminophenol into AM404 because *p*-aminophenol-induced calcium mobilization was lost in cells pretreated with an FAAH inhibitor.

To accurately establish the location of the involvement of TRPV1 in paracetamol action, systemic administration of paracetamol was challenged with the selective blockade of TRPV1 in the brain. Injection of capsazepine into the lateral ventricle of mice abolished the antinociceptive effects of paracetamol [7]. Similarly, the antinociceptive activity of *p*-aminophenol was also lost in mice intracerebroventricularly preinjected with capsazepine [6]. Collectively, these findings identify brain TRPV1 as an important effector of paracetamol.

3.4. Cav3.2 calcium channel

Arachidonic-related compounds such as anandamide and 2-arachidonylglycerol also interact with T-type calcium channels, especially the Cav3.2 subtype, an effect which mediates their analgesic property [32]. Silencing of Cav3.2 using oligonucleotide antisense [33], knockout mice [34], or pharmacological tools [35] resulted in impairment of pain in several pain tests, thereby confirming the strong role of this calcium channel in nociception. Because AM404 is the arachidonicrelated metabolite of paracetamol, the role of Cav3.2 in paracetamol action was investigated [30].

Mice with deletion of the Cav3.2$^{-/-}$ gene did not show any analgesic effect after paracetamol administration. In addition, the intracerebroventricular injection of AM404 did not induce an analgesic effect in these knockout mice.

To determine whether Cav3.2 in the brain is involved in the antinociceptive effect of paracetamol, we injected TTA-A2, a Cav3.2 blocker, intracerebroventricularly before administration of paracetamol. This treatment prevented the effect of paracetamol. Spinal involvement of Cav3.2 receptors was also studied by coadministering paracetamol with an intrathecal injection of TTA-A2. In contrast to the previous results, spinal blockade of Cav3.2 did not alter the analgesic effect of paracetamol, indicating that the antinociceptive effect of paracetamol is dependent on Cav3.2 located in the brain.

AM404 seems to have an indirect action because it only weakly inhibited Cav3.2 currents (IC_{50} = 13.7 μM) recorded in DRG neurons by a whole-cell patch clamp method [30]. By comparison, in the same assay, TTA-A2 had an IC_{50} of 9.0 nM. As expected, neither paracetamol nor *p*-aminophenol inhibited Cav3.2 currents.

We thus addressed the putative role of TRPV1, another calcium channel, in the mobilization of Cav3.2 in the analgesic action of paracetamol. To determine whether Cav3.2 was involved upstream or downstream of the action of TRPV1, we assessed the analgesic effect of intracerebroventricular injection of either TRPV1 agonist (capsaicin) or Cav3.2 antagonist (TTA-A2) in Cav3.2$^{-/-}$ and TRPV1$^{-/-}$ mice, respectively. Unlike the action of TTA-A2, which is maintained in TRPV1$^{-/-}$ mice, the analgesic effect of capsaicin is lost in Cav3.2$^{-/-}$ mice. These results show that brain TRPV1 activation needs Cav3.2 to mediate its action and suggest that the first target of AM404 is TRPV1.

To analyze more fully the relationship between TRPV1 and Cav3.2 channels, we performed electrophysiological recordings to study the Cav3.2 current in HEK cells stably expressing the human Cav3.2 sequence. In these cells, the Cav3.2 current induced by depolarization was not affected by the bath application of capsaicin. However, when the cells were transfected with TRPV1, application of capsaicin suppressed the Cav3.2 current.

Altogether, these behavioral and electrophysiological findings show that Cav3.2 and TRPV1 act sequentially in concert to support the analgesic action of paracetamol [30].

4. Involvement of the serotonergic system

The involvement of the serotonergic system in the action of paracetamol was first described by Tjolsen et al. [37] in 1991 and by Pini et al. [38] in 1996. They demonstrated that the analgesic effect of paracetamol was reduced after lesion of the serotonergic bulbospinal pathway by 5,6-dihydroxytryptamine or total depletion of the central serotonin (5-HT) synthesis by *p*-chlorophenylalanine. These results were confirmed by another team using 5,7-dihydroxytryptamine [39]. Studies showing that paracetamol did not bind serotonin receptors [38, 40] prompted investigation of the mobilization of the serotonin neurotransmitter. The results showed that paracetamol increased in a dose-dependent manner the tissue concentrations of 5-HT in the cortex, hypothalamus, striatum, hippocampus and brainstem [38, 41].

Later studies showed that the spinal role of 5-HT_{1A}, 5-HT_{2A}, 5-HT_{2C} and 5-HT_7 receptor subtypes of serotonin receptors was involved in the action of paracetamol [39, 42–48]. However, investigations of the involvement of 5-HT_3 receptors yielded conflicting results in both animals [36, 42, 43, 47, 49, 50] and humans [51–54]. Interestingly, some of these studies showed that tropisetron, a nonspecific 5-HT_3 receptor antagonist, blocked the analgesic effect of paracetamol. Libert et al. [36] reported that the inhibitory effect of tropisetron on the action of paracetamol was not mediated by 5-HT_3 receptor because (1) other 5-HT_3 antagonists (granisetron and ondansetron) or (2) antisense oligodeoxynucleotides directed against 5-HT_3 receptors did not reverse the paracetamol-induced antinociceptive effect, which suggests the involvement of a spinal tropisetron-sensitive receptor that is not the 5-HT_3 receptor. More work is needed to identify this spinal receptor.

These results should be treated with caution. Serotonin receptor subtypes are differently involved in paracetamol action, depending on the nature of the stimulus. For example, spinal 5-HT_{1A} is involved in the analgesic action of paracetamol assessed in the formalin test (chemical stimulus) [44] but not in the paw pressure test (mechanical stimulus) [47]. This discrepancy could be explained by the differential efficacy and power of serotonin itself relative to the noxious tests [55]. In addition, the analgesic action of spinal-administered serotonin, like that of paracetamol, is suppressed in the formalin test [44, 45] and conserved in the paw pressure test [45, 56] following the inhibition of spinal 5-HT_{1A} receptors.

Like paracetamol, *p*-aminophenol elicited antinociception through the serotonergic bulbospinal pathway because its effect was reversed after lesion of the pathway by 5,7-dihydroxytryptamine [6]. In addition, spinal pretreatment of rats with WAY-100,635, a 5-HT_{1A} receptor antagonist and tropisetron, a nonspecific 5-$HT_{3/4}$ receptor antagonist, reduced the analgesic effect of *p*-aminophenol in the formalin test and the paw pressure test, respectively [6].

In light of evidence showing that paracetamol and *p*-aminophenol involved CB_1 receptors [5], we investigated the serotonergic descending bulbospinal pathways and spinal 5-HT receptors in the antinociceptive effect of arachidonyl-2′-chloroethylamide (ACEA), a CB_1 receptor agonist. Our results showed that ACEA needed intact descending bulbospinal serotonergic pathways. Elsewhere, it was shown that the antinociceptive action of ACEA was suppressed by intrathecal injection of WAY-100,635 and tropisetron in the formalin test and the paw pressure test, respectively [5]. The similar serotonergic profiles of ACEA and paracetamol suggest that CB_1 receptor is an important link between paracetamol and serotonin in the production of antinociception.

5. New strategies to alleviate pain: pharmacological vectorization to target brain TRPV1 receptors

A high-concentration of capsaicin, an 8% patch (Qutenza®) is used clinically in Europe and the USA to alleviate neuropathic pain. It has been suggested that its action is due to defunctionalization of peripheral TRPV1 [57]. A systemic use of TRPV1 activators is to be avoided

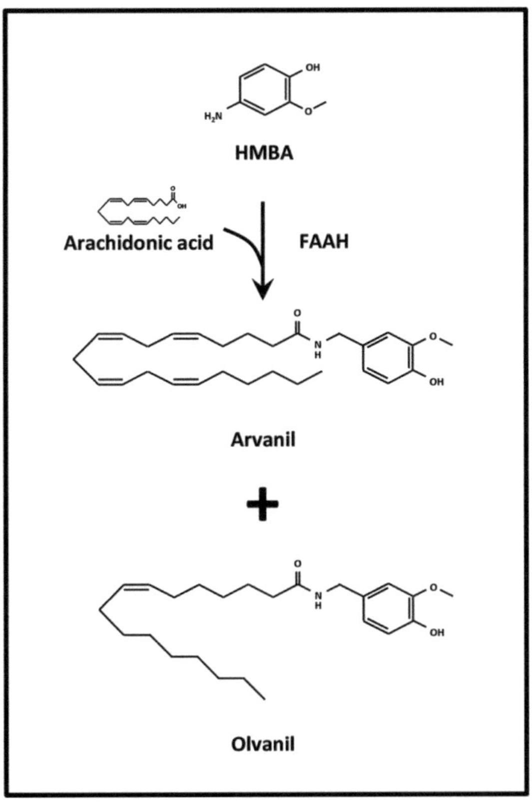

Figure 3. FAAH-dependent formation of arvanil and olvanil from HMBA.

because of their high toxicity, which entails the risk of, notably, pulmonary and cardiovascular adverse effects [58–60]. Metabolites of capsaicin could be mutagenic at very high doses as well [61]. On the basis of the study of the mechanism of action of paracetamol, we propose that brain TRPV1 should be specifically targeted for the pharmacological management of pain. New substrates of FAAH, analogs of paracetamol or *p*-aminophenol, can be synthesized with the idea that the arachidonic acid-conjugated metabolites would be a potent TRPV1 activators.

To validate this strategy, we studied, with E.D. Högestätt and P.M. Zygmunt, 4-hydroxy-3-methoxybenzylamine (HMBA), a primary amine analog of *p*-aminophenol. HMBA produced arvanil and olvanil *in vitro* in brain homogenates and *in vivo* in mouse brain [6] (**Figure 3**).

Administered in mice or in rats, it had an analgesic effect. Both the formation of arvanil and olvanil and the analgesic effect induced by HMBA were FAAH-dependent. These two effects were lower in $FAAH^{-/-}$ mice than in their $FAAH^{+/+}$ littermates. Arvanil and olvanil are potent TRPV1 activators [6, 62]. This mechanism of action contributed to the action of HMBA because, like that of paracetamol and *p*-aminophenol, its analgesic effect was suppressed after a genetic ($TRPV1^{-/-}$ mice) or pharmacological (rats pretreated with capsazepine) blockade of TRPV1. Finally, as with paracetamol or *p*-aminophenol, intracerebroventricular injection of the TRPV1 blocker capsazepine prevented the antinociceptive effect of HMBA [6].

Taken together, these data provide evidence of concept for the use of a pharmacological vectorization strategy aimed specifically at activating supraspinal TRPV1 to alleviate pain.

6. Conclusion

All these recent findings prompt us to propose a novel view of paracetamol as a prodrug that needs to overcome a two-step metabolism to form AM404, its active metabolite, which mediates the analgesic effect via different supra-spinal targets to activate the bulbospinal serotonergic pathways (**Figure 4**).

Interestingly, the involvement of the FAAH metabolic pathway and cannabinoid system is specifically related to their antinociceptive action and not to their hypothermic/antipyretic action [63, 64].

Several other concepts of the mechanism of action of paracetamol have been forwarded, including the involvement of the opioid [13, 65–68], adrenergic [69–71] and cholinergic [72, 73] systems and that of nitric oxide synthetase [74–77], adenosine receptors [48, 78, 79] and calcium channel TRPA1 [80]. However, other studies have yielded conflicting findings notably concerning the opioid [40, 81, 82], adrenergic [37, 71, 83] and cholinergic [84] systems.

The huge number of putative targets for the action of paracetamol and the complex relationship between all the different neurological systems complicate the study of the molecular mechanism of its analgesic action. The relationship between the putative targets needs further investigation to provide an overall view of the action of paracetamol. The understanding of the neurological and molecular actions of clinically used analgesics such as paracetamol could pave the way for the discovery of new analgesic compounds.

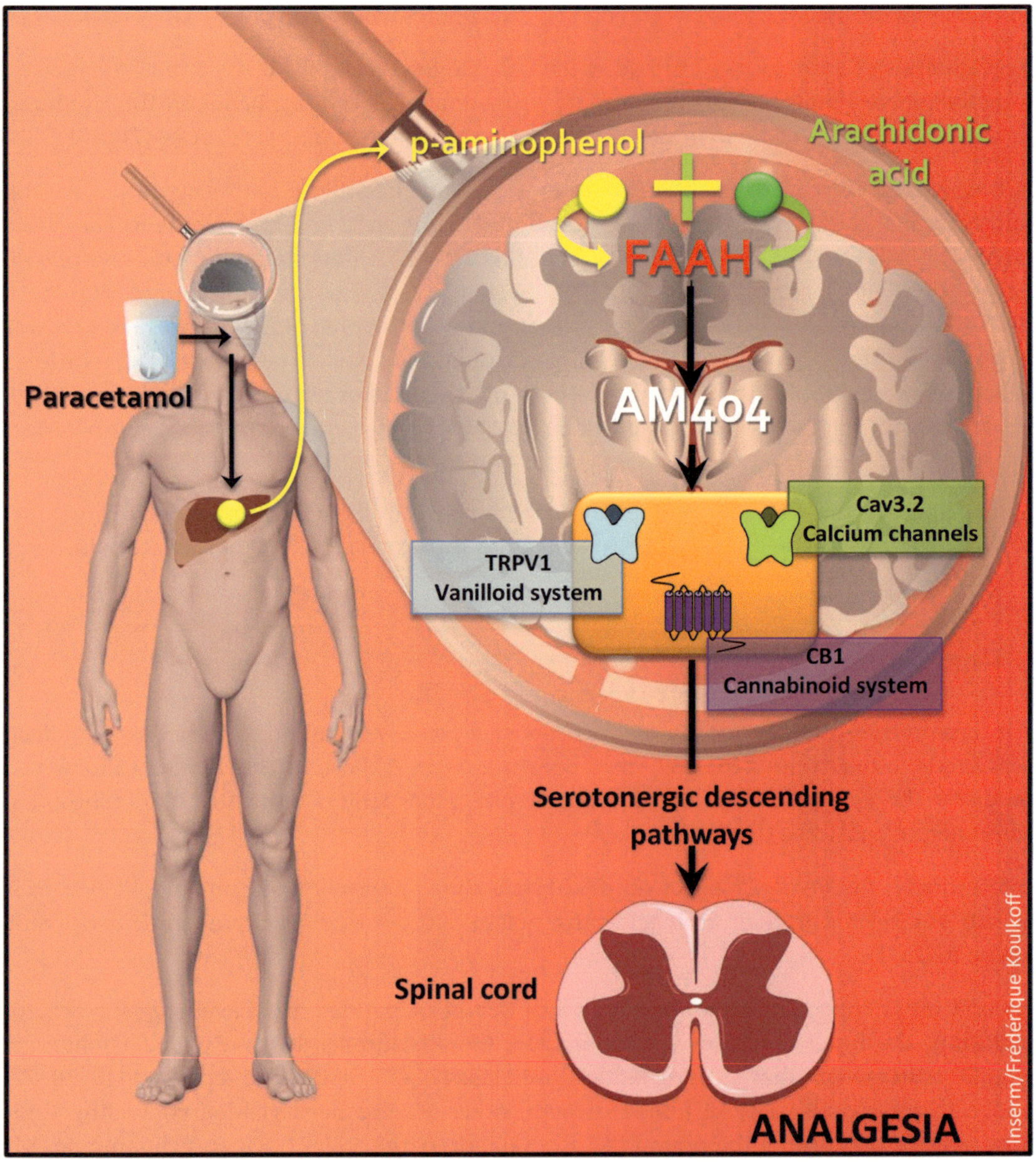

Figure 4. Proposed sequential mechanisms for the antinociceptive effect of paracetamol. (1) Deacetylation of paracetamol in *p*-aminophenol in the liver. (2) FAAH-dependent metabolism of *p*-aminophenol into AM404 in the brain. (3) Direct and/or indirect involvement of supra-spinal CB_1 receptors by this metabolite. (4) Reinforcement of the serotonergic bulbospinal pathways and (5) Involvement of spinal pain-suppressing serotonergic receptors. © Frédérique Koulkoff/ Inserm from Mallet/UMR 1107/Neuro-Dol Inserm.

Author details

Christophe Mallet[1,2*], Alain Eschalier[1,2,3] and Laurence Daulhac[1,2]

*Address all correspondence to: christophe.mallet@udamail.fr

1 University of Clermont Auvergne, Fundamental and Clinical Pharmacology of Pain, Clermont-Ferrand, France

2 Inserm U 1107, Neuro-Dol, Clermont-Ferrand, France

3 CHU Clermont-Ferrand, Department of Pharmacology, Clermont-Ferrand, France

References

[1] C. Mallet, A. Eschalier, Pharmacology and mechanism of action of acetaminophen, in: Pharmacology of Pain, International Association for the Study of Pain, Seattle, (2010). pp. 65–86.

[2] E.D. Högestätt, B.A. Jonsson, A. Ermund, D.A. Andersson, H. Bjork, J.P. Alexander, B.F. Cravatt, A.I. Basbaum, P.M. Zygmunt, Conversion of acetaminophen to the bioactive N-acylphenolamine AM404 via fatty acid amide hydrolase-dependent arachidonic acid conjugation in the nervous system, J Biol Chem. 280 (2005) 31405–31412.

[3] S. Muramatsu, S. Shiraishi, K. Miyano, Y. Sudo, A. Toda, M. Mogi, M. Hara, A. Yokoyama, Y. Kawasaki, M. Taniguchi, Y. Uezono, Metabolism of AM404 from acetaminophen at human therapeutic dosages in the rat brain, Anesth Pain Med. 6 (2016) e32873. doi:10.5812/aapm.32873.

[4] D.G. Deutsch, N. Ueda, S. Yamamoto, The fatty acid amide hydrolase (FAAH), Prostaglandins Leukot Essent Fatty Acids. 66 (2002) 201–210.

[5] C. Mallet, L. Daulhac, J. Bonnefont, C. Ledent, M. Etienne, E. Chapuy, F. Libert, A. Eschalier, Endocannabinoid and serotonergic systems are needed for acetaminophen-induced analgesia, Pain. 139 (2008) 190–200.

[6] D.A. Barrière, C. Mallet, A. Blomgren, C. Simonsen, L. Daulhac, F. Libert, E. Chapuy, M. Etienne, E.D. Högestätt, P.M. Zygmunt, A. Eschalier, Fatty acid amide hydrolase-dependent generation of antinociceptive drug metabolites acting on TRPV1 in the brain, PLoS One. 8 (2013) e70690. doi:10.1371/journal.pone.0070690.

[7] C. Mallet, D.A. Barriere, A. Ermund, B.A. Jonsson, A. Eschalier, P.M. Zygmunt, E.D. Hogestatt, TRPV1 in brain is involved in acetaminophen-induced antinociception, PLoS One. 5 (2010). http://www.ncbi.nlm.nih.gov/entrez/query.fcgi?cmd=Retrieve&db=PubMed&dopt=Citation&list_uids=20862299.

[8] R.D. Altman, J.R. Zinsenheim, A.R. Temple, J.E. Schweinle, Three-month efficacy and safety of acetaminophen extended-release for osteoarthritis pain of the hip or knee:

a randomized, double-blind, placebo-controlled study, Osteoarthr Cartil. 15 (2007) 454–461. doi:10.1016/j.joca.2006.10.008.

[9] A. Wegman, D. van der Windt, M. van Tulder, W. Stalman, T. de Vries, Nonsteroidal antiinflammatory drugs or acetaminophen for osteoarthritis of the hip or knee? A systematic review of evidence and guidelines, J Rheumatol. 31 (2004) 344–354.

[10] R. Dalmann, L. Daulhac, M. Antri, A. Eschalier, C. Mallet, Supra-spinal FAAH is required for the analgesic action of paracetamol in an inflammatory context, Neuropharmacology. 91 (2015) 63–70. doi:10.1016/j.neuropharm.2014.11.006.

[11] M. Dani, J. Guindon, C. Lambert, P. Beaulieu, The local antinociceptive effects of paracetamol in neuropathic pain are mediated by cannabinoid receptors, Eur J Pharmacol. (2007). http://www.ncbi.nlm.nih.gov/entrez/query.fcgi?cmd=Retrieve&db=PubMed&dopt=Citation&list_uids=17651722.

[12] S.H. Ferreira, B.B. Lorenzetti, F.M. Correa, Blockade of central and peripheral generation of prostaglandins explains the antialgic effect of aspirin like drugs, Pol J Pharmacol Pharm. 30 (1978) 133–140.

[13] V. Ruggieri, G. Vitale, L.A. Pini, M. Sandrini, Differential involvement of opioidergic and serotonergic systems in the antinociceptive activity of N-arachidonoyl-phenolamine (AM404) in the rat: comparison with paracetamol, Naunyn Schmiedebergs Arch Pharmacol. 377 (2008) 219–229.

[14] J.R. Clapper, G. Moreno-Sanz, R. Russo, A. Guijarro, F. Vacondio, A. Duranti, A. Tontini, S. Sanchini, N.R. Sciolino, J.M. Spradley, A.G. Hohmann, A. Calignano, M. Mor, G. Tarzia, D. Piomelli, Anandamide suppresses pain initiation through a peripheral endocannabinoid mechanism, Nat Neurosci. 13 (2010) 1265–1270. doi:10.1038/nn.2632.

[15] G. Moreno-Sanz, B. Barrera, A. Guijarro, I. d'Elia, J.A. Otero, A.I. Alvarez, T. Bandiera, G. Merino, D. Piomelli, The ABC membrane transporter ABCG2 prevents access of FAAH inhibitor URB937 to the central nervous system, Pharmacol Res. 64 (2011) 359–363. doi:10.1016/j.phrs.2011.07.001.

[16] R.J. Flower, J.R. Vane, Inhibition of prostaglandin synthetase in brain explains the antipyretic activity of paracetamol (4-acetamidophenol), Nature. 240 (1972) 410–411.

[17] A. Greco, M.A. Ajmone-Cat, A. Nicolini, M.G. Sciulli, L. Minghetti, Paracetamol effectively reduces prostaglandin E2 synthesis in brain macrophages by inhibiting enzymatic activity of cyclooxygenase but not phospholipase and prostaglandin E synthase, J Neurosci Res. 71 (2003) 844–852.

[18] M.G. Sciulli, F. Seta, S. Tacconelli, M.L. Capone, E. Ricciotti, G. Pistritto, P. Patrignani, Effects of acetaminophen on constitutive and inducible prostanoid biosynthesis in human blood cells, Br J Pharmacol. 138 (2003) 634–641.

[19] T.A. Swierkosz, L. Jordan, M. McBride, K. McGough, J. Devlin, R.M. Botting, Actions of paracetamol on cyclooxygenases in tissue and cell homogenates of mouse and rabbit, Med Sci Monit. 8 (2002) BR496–BR503.

[20] G.G. Graham, R.O. Day, M.K. Milligan, J.B. Ziegler, A.J. Kettle, Current concepts of the actions of paracetamol (acetaminophen) and NSAIDs, Inflammopharmacology. 7 (1999) 255–263. doi:10.1007/s10787-999-0008-x.

[21] W. Feldberg, K.P. Gupta, Pyrogen fever and prostaglandin-like activity in cerebrospinal fluid, J Physiol. 228 (1973) 41–53.

[22] U.S. Muth-Selbach, I. Tegeder, K. Brune, G. Geisslinger, Acetaminophen inhibits spinal prostaglandin E2 release after peripheral noxious stimulation, Anesthesiology. 91 (1999) 231–239.

[23] S.S. Ayoub, R.M. Botting, S. Goorha, P.R. Colville-Nash, D.A. Willoughby, L.R. Ballou, Acetaminophen-induced hypothermia in mice is mediated by a prostaglandin endoperoxide synthase 1 gene-derived protein, Proc Natl Acad Sci USA. 101 (2004) 11165–11169.

[24] S.S. Ayoub, P.R. Colville-Nash, D.A. Willoughby, R.M. Botting, The involvement of a cyclooxygenase 1 gene-derived protein in the antinociceptive action of paracetamol in mice, Eur J Pharmacol. 538 (2006) 57–65.

[25] S.T. Glaser, N.A. Abumrad, F. Fatade, M. Kaczocha, K.M. Studholme, D.G. Deutsch, Evidence against the presence of an anandamide transporter, Proc Natl Acad Sci USA. 100 (2003) 4269–4274.

[26] M. Beltramo, N. Stella, A. Calignano, S.Y. Lin, A. Makriyannis, D. Piomelli, Functional role of high-affinity anandamide transport, as revealed by selective inhibition, Science. 277 (1997) 1094–1097.

[27] A. Giuffrida, M. Beltramo, D. Piomelli, Mechanisms of endocannabinoid inactivation: biochemistry and pharmacology, J Pharmacol Exp Ther. 298 (2001) 7–14.

[28] A. Ottani, S. Leone, M. Sandrini, A. Ferrari, A. Bertolini, The analgesic activity of paracetamol is prevented by the blockade of cannabinoid CB1 receptors, Eur J Pharmacol. 531 (2006) 280–281.

[29] A.T. Hama, J. Sagen, Cannabinoid receptor-mediated antinociception with acetaminophen drug combinations in rats with neuropathic spinal cord injury pain, Neuropharmacology. 58 (2010) 758–766. doi:10.1016/j.neuropharm.2009.12.010.

[30] N. Kerckhove, C. Mallet, A. François, M. Boudes, J. Chemin, T. Voets, E. Bourinet, A. Alloui, A. Eschalier, Ca(v)3.2 calcium channels: the key protagonist in the supraspinal effect of paracetamol, Pain. 155 (2014) 764–772. doi:10.1016/j.pain.2014.01.015.

[31] P.M. Zygmunt, H. Chuang, P. Movahed, D. Julius, E.D. Hogestatt, The anandamide transport inhibitor AM404 activates vanilloid receptors, Eur J Pharmacol. 396 (2000) 39–42.

[32] G. Barbara, A. Alloui, J. Nargeot, P. Lory, A. Eschalier, E. Bourinet, J. Chemin, T-type calcium channel inhibition underlies the analgesic effects of the endogenous lipoamino acids, J Neurosci. 29 (2009) 13106–13114.

[33] E. Bourinet, A. Alloui, A. Monteil, C. Barrere, B. Couette, O. Poirot, A. Pages, J. McRory, T.P. Snutch, A. Eschalier, J. Nargeot, Silencing of the Cav3.2 T-type calcium channel gene in sensory neurons demonstrates its major role in nociception, Embo J. 24 (2005) 315–324.

[34] S. Choi, H.S. Na, J. Kim, J. Lee, S. Lee, D. Kim, J. Park, C.C. Chen, K.P. Campbell, H.S. Shin, Attenuated pain responses in mice lacking Ca(V)3.2 T-type channels, Genes Brain Behav. 6 (2007) 425–431. doi:10.1111/j.1601-183X.2006.00268.x.

[35] A. Francois, N. Kerckhove, M. Meleine, A. Alloui, C. Barrere, A. Gelot, V.N. Uebele, J.J. Renger, A. Eschalier, D. Ardid, E. Bourinet, State-dependent properties of a new T-type calcium channel blocker enhance Ca(V)3.2 selectivity and support analgesic effects, Pain. 154 (2013) 283–293. doi:10.1016/j.pain.2012.10.023.

[36] F. Libert, J. Bonnefont, E. Bourinet, E. Doucet, A. Alloui, M. Hamon, J. Nargeot, A. Eschalier, Acetaminophen: a central analgesic drug that involves a spinal tropisetron-sensitive, non-5-HT(3) receptor-mediated effect, Mol Pharmacol. 66 (2004) 728–734.

[37] A. Tjolsen, A. Lund, K. Hole, Antinociceptive effect of paracetamol in rats is partly dependent on spinal serotonergic systems, Eur J Pharmacol. 193 (1991) 193–201.

[38] L.A. Pini, M. Sandrini, G. Vitale, The antinociceptive action of paracetamol is associated with changes in the serotonergic system in the rat brain, Eur J Pharmacol. 308 (1996) 31–40.

[39] A. Dogrul, M. Seyrek, E.O. Akgul, T. Cayci, S. Kahraman, H. Bolay, Systemic paracetamol-induced analgesic and antihyperalgesic effects through activation of descending serotonergic pathways involving spinal 5-HT(7) receptors, Eur J Pharmacol. (2011). doi:10.1016/j.ejphar.2011.12.016.

[40] T. Pelissier, A. Alloui, F. Caussade, C. Dubray, A. Cloarec, J. Lavarenne, A. Eschalier, Paracetamol exerts a spinal antinociceptive effect involving an indirect interaction with 5-hydroxytryptamine3 receptors: *in vivo* and *in vitro* evidence, J Pharmacol Exp Ther. 278 (1996) 8–14.

[41] J.P. Courade, F. Caussade, K. Martin, D. Besse, C. Delchambre, N. Hanoun, M. Hamon, A. Eschalier, A. Cloarec, Effects of acetaminophen on monoaminergic systems in the rat central nervous system, Naunyn Schmiedebergs Arch Pharmacol. 364 (2001) 534–537.

[42] A. Alloui, T. Pelissier, C. Dubray, J. Lavarenne, A. Eschalier, Tropisetron inhibits the antinociceptive effect of intrathecally administered paracetamol and serotonin, Fundam Clin Pharmacol. 10 (1996) 406–407.

[43] A. Alloui, C. Chassaing, J. Schmidt, D. Ardid, C. Dubray, A. Cloarec, A. Eschalier, Paracetamol exerts a spinal, tropisetron-reversible, antinociceptive effect in an inflammatory pain model in rats, Eur J Pharmacol. 443 (2002) 71–77.

[44] J. Bonnefont, A. Alloui, E. Chapuy, E. Clottes, A. Eschalier, Orally administered paracetamol does not act locally in the rat formalin test: evidence for a supraspinal, serotonin-dependent antinociceptive mechanism, Anesthesiology. 99 (2003) 976–981.

[45] J. Bonnefont, E. Chapuy, E. Clottes, A. Alloui, A. Eschalier, Spinal 5-HT1A receptors differentially influence nociceptive processing according to the nature of the noxious stimulus in rats: effect of WAY-100635 on the antinociceptive activities of paracetamol, venlafaxine and 5-HT, Pain. 114 (2005) 482–490.

[46] J. Bonnefont, L. Daulhac, M. Etienne, E. Chapuy, C. Mallet, L. Ouchchane, C. Deval, J.P. Courade, M. Ferrara, A. Eschalier, E. Clottes, Acetaminophen recruits spinal p42/p44 MAPKs and GH/IGF-1 receptors to produce analgesia via the serotonergic system, Mol Pharmacol. 71 (2007) 407–415.

[47] J.P. Courade, C. Chassaing, L. Bardin, A. Alloui, A. Eschalier, 5-HT receptor subtypes involved in the spinal antinociceptive effect of acetaminophen in rats, Eur J Pharmacol. 432 (2001) 1–7.

[48] J. Liu, A.R. Reid, J. Sawynok, Antinociception by systemically-administered acetaminophen (paracetamol) involves spinal serotonin 5-HT7 and adenosine A1 receptors, as well as peripheral adenosine A1 receptors, Neurosci Lett. 536 (2013) 64–68. doi:10.1016/j.neulet.2012.12.052.

[49] P. Girard, Y. Pansart, M.C. Coppe, B. Niedergang, J.M. Gillardin, Modulation of paracetamol and nefopam antinociception by serotonin 5-HT(3) receptor antagonists in mice, Pharmacology. 83 (2009) 243–246.

[50] V. Minville, O. Fourcade, J.X. Mazoit, J.P. Girolami, I. Tack, Ondansetron does not block paracetamol-induced analgesia in a mouse model of fracture pain, Br J Anaesth. 106 (2011) 112–118.

[51] R. Jokela, J. Ahonen, E. Seitsonen, P. Marjakangas, K. Korttila, The influence of ondansetron on the analgesic effect of acetaminophen after laparoscopic hysterectomy, Clin Pharmacol Ther. 87 (2010) 672–678. doi:10.1038/clpt.2009.281.

[52] G. Pickering, M.A. Loriot, F. Libert, A. Eschalier, P. Beaune, C. Dubray, Analgesic effect of acetaminophen in humans: first evidence of a central serotonergic mechanism, Clin Pharmacol Ther. 79 (2006) 371–378.

[53] L. Ramirez, J. Cros, B. Marin, P. Boulogne, A. Bergeron, G.E. de Lafont, F. Renon-Carron, M.A. de Vinzelles, V. Guigonis, N. Nathan, P. Beaulieu, Analgesic interaction between ondansetron and acetaminophen after tonsillectomy in children: the Paratron randomized, controlled trial, Eur J Pain. 19 (2015) 661–668. doi:10.1002/ejp.587.

[54] E. Tiippana, K. Hamunen, V. Kontinen, E. Kalso, The effect of paracetamol and tropisetron on pain: experimental studies and a review of published data, Basic Clin Pharmacol Toxicol. 112 (2013) 124–131. doi:10.1111/j.1742-7843.2012.00935.x.

[55] L. Bardin, M. Bardin, J. Lavarenne, A. Eschalier, Effect of intrathecal serotonin on nociception in rats: influence of the pain test used, Exp Brain Res. 113 (1997) 81–87.

[56] L. Bardin, J. Lavarenne, A. Eschalier, Serotonin receptor subtypes involved in the spinal antinociceptive effect of 5-HT in rats, Pain. 86 (2000) 11–18.

[57] P. Anand, K. Bley, Topical capsaicin for pain management: therapeutic potential and mechanisms of action of the new high-concentration capsaicin 8% patch, Br J Anaesth. 107 (2011) 490–502. doi:10.1093/bja/aer260.

[58] W. Johnson, Final report on the safety assessment of capsicum annuum extract, capsicum annuum fruit extract, capsicum annuum resin, capsicum annuum fruit powder, *Capsicum frutescens* fruit, capsicum frutescens fruit extract, capsicum frutescens resin and capsaicin, Int J Toxicol. 26 Suppl 1 (2007) 3–106. doi:10.1080/10915810601163939.

[59] H. Knotkova, M. Pappagallo, A. Szallasi, Capsaicin (TRPV1 Agonist) therapy for pain relief: farewell or revival?, Clin J Pain. 24 (2008) 142–154.

[60] A. Patapoutian, S. Tate, C.J. Woolf, Transient receptor potential channels: targeting pain at the source, Nat Rev Drug Discov. 8 (2009) 55–68.

[61] Y.J. Surh, S.S. Lee, Capsaicin in hot chili pepper: carcinogen, co-carcinogen or anticarcinogen? Food Chem Toxicol. 34 (1996) 313–316.

[62] L. De Petrocellis, T. Bisogno, J.B. Davis, R.G. Pertwee, V. Di Marzo, Overlap between the ligand recognition properties of the anandamide transporter and the VR1 vanilloid receptor: inhibitors of anandamide uptake with negligible capsaicin-like activity, FEBS Lett. 483 (2000) 52–56.

[63] S.S. Ayoub, G. Pryce, M.P. Seed, C. Bolton, R.J. Flower, D. Baker, Paracetamol-induced hypothermia is independent of cannabinoids and transient receptor potential vanilloid-1 and is not mediated by AM404, Drug Metab Dispos. 39 (2011) 1689–1695. doi:10.1124/dmd.111.038638.

[64] G. Corley, S.M. Rawls, Opioid, cannabinoid CB1 and NOP receptors do not mediate APAP-induced hypothermia in rats, Pharmacol Biochem Behav. 92 (2009) 503–507. doi:10.1016/j.pbb.2009.01.020.

[65] M. Bujalska, Effect of nonselective and selective opioid receptors antagonists on antinociceptive action of acetaminophen [part III], Pol J Pharmacol. 56 (2004) 539–545.

[66] L.A. Pini, G. Vitale, A. Ottani, M. Sandrini, Naloxone-reversible antinociception by paracetamol in the rat, J Pharmacol Exp Ther. 280 (1997) 934–940.

[67] R.B. Raffa, D.J. Stone, R.J. Tallarida, Discovery of "self-synergistic" spinal/supraspinal antinociception produced by acetaminophen (paracetamol), J Pharmacol Exp Ther. 295 (2000) 291–294.

[68] M. Sandrini, G. Vitale, L.A. Pini, G. Lopetuso, P. Romualdi, S. Candeletti, Nociceptin/orphanin FQ prevents the antinociceptive action of paracetamol on the rat hot plate test, Eur J Pharmacol. 507 (2005) 43–48.

[69] H.F. Miranda, G. Pinardi, Isobolographic analysis of the antinociceptive interactions of clonidine with nonsteroidal anti-inflammatory drugs, Pharmacol Res. 50 (2004) 273–278. doi:10.1016/j.phrs.2004.02.008.

[70] G. Pinardi, F. Sierralta, H.F. Miranda, Adrenergic mechanisms in antinociceptive effects of nonsteroidal anti-inflammatory drugs in acute thermal nociception in mice, Inflamm Res. 51 (2002) 219–222.

[71] R.B. Raffa, D.J. Stone, R.J. Tallarida, Unexpected and pronounced antinociceptive synergy between spinal acetaminophen (paracetamol) and phentolamine, Eur J Pharmacol. 412 (2001) R1–R2.

[72] H.F. Miranda, F. Sierralta, G. Pinardi, Neostigmine interactions with nonsteroidal anti-inflammatory drugs, Br J Pharmacol. 135 (2002) 1591–1597.

[73] G. Pinardi, F. Sierralta, H.F. Miranda, Atropine reverses the antinociception of nonsteroidal anti-inflammatory drugs in the tail-flick test of mice, Pharmacol Biochem Behav. 74 (2003) 603–608.

[74] R. Bjorkman, K.M. Hallman, J. Hedner, T. Hedner, M. Henning, Acetaminophen blocks spinal hyperalgesia induced by NMDA and substance P, Pain. 57 (1994) 259–264.

[75] M. Bujalska, Effect of nitric oxide synthase inhibition on antinociceptive action of different doses of acetaminophen, Pol J Pharmacol. 56 (2004) 605–610.

[76] M. Bujalska, W.S. Gumulka, Effect of cyclooxygenase and NO synthase inhibitors on antinociceptive action of acetaminophen, Pol J Pharmacol. 53 (2001) 341–350.

[77] L. Godfrey, I. Bailey, N.J. Toms, G.D. Clarke, I. Kitchen, S.M. Hourani, Paracetamol inhibits nitric oxide synthesis in murine spinal cord slices, Eur J Pharmacol. 562 (2007) 68–71.

[78] L. Godfrey, L. Yan, G.D. Clarke, C. Ledent, I. Kitchen, S.M. Hourani, Modulation of paracetamol antinociception by caffeine and by selective adenosine A2 receptor antagonists in mice, Eur J Pharmacol. 531 (2006) 80–86.

[79] J. Sawynok, A.R. Reid, Caffeine inhibits antinociception by acetaminophen in the formalin test by inhibiting spinal adenosine A_1 receptors, Eur J Pharmacol. 674 (2012) 248–254. doi:10.1016/j.ejphar.2011.10.036.

[80] D.A. Andersson, C. Gentry, L. Alenmyr, D. Killander, S.E. Lewis, A. Andersson, B. Bucher, J.L. Galzi, O. Sterner, S. Bevan, E.D. Högestätt, P.M. Zygmunt, TRPA1 mediates spinal antinociception induced by acetaminophen and the cannabinoid Δ(9)-tetrahydrocannabiorcol, Nat Commun. 2 (2011) 551. doi:10.1038/ncomms1559.

[81] H. Madenoğlu, M. Kaçmaz, R. Aksu, C. Bicer, G. Yaba, K. Yildiz, K. Doğru, A. Boyaci, Effects of naloxone and flumazenil on antinociceptive action of acetaminophen in rats, Curr Ther Res Clin Exp. 71 (2010) 111–117. doi:10.1016/j.curtheres.2010.03.001.

[82] G. Pickering, F. Moustafa, S. Desbrandes, J.M. Cardot, D. Roux, C. Dubray, Paracetamol and opioid pathways: a pilot randomized clinical trial, Fundam Clin Pharmacol. 27 (2013) 339–345. doi:10.1111/j.1472-8206.2011.01010.x.

[83] M. Bujalska, Effect of cyclooxygenase and NO synthase inhibitors administered centrally on antinociceptive action of acetaminophen (Part II), Pol J Pharmacol. 55 (2003) 1001–1011.

[84] K.S. Abelson, M. Kommalage, A.U. Hoglund, Spinal cholinergic involvement after treatment with aspirin and paracetamol in rats, Neurosci Lett. 368 (2004) 116–120.

Chapter 11

Voltage-Gated Calcium Channel Antagonists: Potential Analgesics for Jejunal Pains

Kania Bogdan Feliks and Danuta Wrońska

Additional information is available at the end of the chapter

http://dx.doi.org/10.5772/66597

Abstract

The significant role of voltage-gated calcium channel (VGCC) L-type antagonists used concomitantly with opioids in attenuation of clinical pain has been confirmed. The aim of this study is to evaluate the comparable effect of intracerebroventricularly (*i.c.v.)* administered diltiazem, nifedipine and/or verapamil – specific antagonists of VGCCs – in the dose of 1.0 and 2.0 mg *in toto* on behavioral signs, clinical symptoms, rumen motor activity and biochemical (plasma cortisol and catecholamine—CA) parameters in sheep that have undergone experimental duodenal distension (DD) and to determine whether voltage-gated calcium channel inhibitors (VGCCIs) exert any anti-nociceptive effects under these conditions. The study was carried out using 24 mature, behind reproductive season crossbred ewes, each weighing 32–42 kg. DD was managed by inclusion and the distension of stretching balloon (having 40 mL of water 39°C temperature—DD40). After 5 min of DD40, the signs were observed: an important augmentation of behavioral nociceptive signs, particularly looking around, defecation, head movement, stretching, grinding, lying down, tachycardia, hyperventilation, inhibition of ruminal contractions (70% approximately, during 15 min) and an increase in plasma catecholamine concentration (over sevenfold increase of epinephrine (E): from 0.24 ± 0.12 in control to 2.98 ± 0.21 mM L^{-1} during 2 h following DD, 2-times norepinephrine (NE): from 1.29 ± 0.23 in control to 2.51 ± 0.30 mM L^{-1} and 124% increase of dopamine (DA): from 0.94 ± 0.02 in control to 2.10 ± 0.35 mM L^{-1}). VGCCI infusion administered 10 min before duodenal distension diminished severity of jejunal nociceptive reactions, for instance, behavioral symptoms, cardiac acceleration, increase in the number of respiration, inhibition of the reticulum and rumen hypomotility, and effortlessly abolished the increasing presence of plasma cortisol and biogenic amines (CA) release. We suggest that the increase and insistence of visceral hyperalgesia stimulate the flow of Ca^{2+} ion flow, provoking neurohormones/neuromediators liberatione and cytoplasmic membrane responsiveness modulation. This result confirmed analgesic effects of VGCCIs L- and/or R-type (nimodipine, lercanidipine, SNX-482) obtained by other authors and also suggests that these channels play a crucial role in the modulation of acute visceral hyperalgesia in sheep and may be a therapeutic target for new drugs.

Keywords: duodenal distension, diltiazem, nifedipine, verapamil, behavioral signs, clinical symptoms, rumen motility, blood plasma cortisol, catecholamine concentration, sheep

1. Introduction

A calcium channel is an ion channel which displays selective permeability to calcium ion (Ca^{2+}). It is sometimes synonymous as voltage-dependent calcium channel (VDCC) [1], although there are also ligand-gated calcium channels (LGCCs) [2]. Voltage-gated calcium channels (VGCCs) are found in excitable cells (e.g., glial cells, muscle, neurons, etc.) [3–6]. There are at least six classes of VGCCs (L-, N-, P/Q-, R- and the T-type channels) that are distributed according to cell type and location, and that may be distinguished by electrophysiological, pharmacological, and structural characteristics. No small organic ligands are clinically available for other than the L-type channels, although there are a number of experimental compounds for the T- and N-type channels [7].

It is known that VGCCs exert a regulatory control of CNS, cardiac, and muscularly activities and that their activity disorders can provide raise to physiopathological cases extending from cardiac and vascular disorders to central nervous system pathologies. Voltage-gated calcium channels inhibitors (VGCCIs) have been applied profitably to treat epilepsy and are arising as probable curative pathways as long as pathology, such as algesia, Parkinson's disease, anxiety, and addiction [8]. Therefore, calcium channels can be drug targets for nervous system diseases, and potential challenges and opportunities for the development of new clinically effective calcium channel inhibitors [8].

L-type VGCCs are located in neuronal cells, dendrites, spinal cord, adrenal gland, skeletal cardiac and smooth muscles, and many other locations [9–14]. L-type calcium currents typically require strong depolarization for their activation and are blocked by different antagonists (VGCCIs) including dihydropyridines (nifedipine), benzothiazepines (diltiazem), and phenylalkylamines (e.g., verapamil). VGCCIs are a class of drugs that disrupts the movement of calcium ions through calcium channels. These substances, by relaxing the smooth muscle tone, are commonly used to treat high blood pressure (hypertension), migraines, *angina pectoris*, Raynaud's disease, and also cluster headaches [9, 14]. In palliative medicine, they are used as analgesic drugs and in veterinary, they are used to treat experimental duodenal acute pain (colic) in sheep [15, 16]. Since high density of these channels are found in sinoatrial and atrioventricular nodes, VGCCIs decrease impulse conduction through these nodes and are used as antiarrhythmic agents.

The mode of action of verapamil similarly to diltiazem and nifedipine, is based on binding with the largest subunit α_1 of Ca^{2+} channels. This subunit incorporates the conduction pore, voltage sensor, gating apparatus, and several regulation sites, e.g., by second messengers, drugs, and toxins. VGCCIs inhibit Ca^{2+} ions influx to the cells, which are the main Ca^{2+} currents in muscle and endocrine cells initiating many activities, such as gene expression, muscle contraction (excitation-contraction coupling), hormone secretion, neurotransmitter release, cell growth and regulation, neurons migration, cell damage, and death or finally cell survival [17].

Acute intestinal distension ("colic"), similarly as functional gastrointestinal disorders, inflammatory bowel disease or irritable bowel syndrome causes visceral hypersensitivity and may produce persistent pain [17, 18]. Visceral pain is described as pressure-like, intermittently squeezing or cramp, not well localized, vague in character, and difficult for patients to describe [19]. Visceral pain is frequently accompanied by nausea, sweating, defecation, vocalization, grinding, head movement, hyperventilation, hypertension, tachycardia, hypercortisolemia, and hypercatecholaminemia (**Table 1**).

Accompanying symptoms	**0–5**			**5–10**		**10–15**		**25–30**	**55–60**	**120 min**	
	DD	**1 2**	**3**	**DD**	**1**	**2 3 DD**	**1 2**	**3 DD**	**1 2 3 DD**	**1 2 3 DD**	**1 2 3**
Inhibition ruminal activity	4+	− +	−	4+	−	± − 3+	2 +	+ −	− − − −	− ± − −	− − −
Looking around	3+	± ±	±	2+	±	± ± +	+ +	+ −	− − + −	− − − −	− − −
Defecation	3+	− −	−	+	−	± − −	± −	± −	− ± + −	− − − −	− − −
Head movements	3+	− −	−	2+	±	± ± −	− −	− −	− ± + −	− − − −	− ± −
Stretching	2+	− −	−	−	+	− − −	− +	± −	− − − −	− − − −	− − −
Grinding	2+	± ±	±	±	−	+ + −	± ±	± −	− − − −	− − − −	− − −
Lying down	2+	− −	−	−	+	− − −	± ±	− −	− − − −	− − − −	− − −
Bleating	+	− −	−	−	+	− − −	− −	− −	+ + + +	− − − −	− − −
Tachycardia	4+	± 3+	3+	±	4+	− ± 4+	− 3+	± 3+	− ± ± 3+	− ± ± 3+	− − −
Hyperventilation	4+	± −	±	3+	−	− ± 4+	− −	± 3+	− − − 3+	− − − 3+	− − −

1, Diltiazem + DD40; 2, Nifedipine + DD40; 3, Verapamil + DD40.

Table 1. The effect of duodenal distension (DD40) on the ruminal motility (inhibition in % 5 min^{-1} in comparison to the control values) [10] and behavioral symptoms (number·5 min^{-1}) in sheep before and after voltage-gated calcium channels inhibitor pretreatment at a dose of 1 or 2 mg *in toto* (i.e. 25 or 50 $\mu g{\cdot}kg^{-1}$ B.W.; n = 6).

Gastrointestinal sensory system consist intrinsic (enteric) sensory afferents and extrinsic (vagus, spinal cord, pelvic) afferents. Intrinsic sensory system functions independently of the CNS. Enterochromaffin cells within mucosa and enteroendocrine cells release 5-HT, CCK, orexin, and leptin which modulates and regulates motor activity of intestine [20, 21]. The submucosal enteric plexus and myenteric plexus have a high degree of synaptic interactions (enteric nervous system or a "gut brain"), which can be either inhibitory or stimulatory for the purpose of regulating gastrointestinal motility and peristalsis [22, 23].

Mechanisms of the reception, transduction, transformation and modulation of nociceptive stimulus, and reaction diminishing response on nociception are regulated by afferent systems to CNS and efferent systems from CNS "stimulating" reaction, but quenching (pain-gated).

Several data show antinociceptive/antistressoric effects of organic Ca^{2+} inhibitors of L-VGCCs in acute duodenal pain of sheep [16, 20]. These inhibitors potentiate the analgesic action of κ-opioidergic receptor agonists [15], as well as morphine by decreasing opioids' tolerance [24]. It was also shown by Bongianni et al. [25] that VGCCIs suppress not only metabolic but also behavioral expression of the morphine withdrawal syndrome. In experiments performed on mice, it was shown that verapamil blocked amphetamine and also physostigmine induced footshock-induced aggression [26]. It was postulated by Michaluk et al. [27] that VGCCIs show antinociceptive properties; but they also change the territorial behavior of animals [28] and conspecific aggression in fish [29]. Such effects were probably caused by the inhibition of Ca^{2+} entry into neurons, preventing the appearance of synaptic vesicles in axon terminal, and release of neurotransmitter into the synaptic cleft. Davis and Bauer [14] have shown in experiments performed on rats, that activation of L-VGCCs are necessary for the long-term retention of fear excitation.

A duodenal and/or colonic distension method, provoking jejunal pain, stimulates hypothalamic-pituitary-adrenal-cortical (HPA) and sympatico-adrenal system (SAS), pathways that revealed as an increase in cortisol and CA in blood plasma [18, 20]. A different role of L-type antagonists for VGCC has been previously identified in different types of experimental and clinical pain in man and animals. Present study examined comparative role of VGCC blockers from different chemical groups—diltiazem, nifedipine, and verapamil administered *i.c.v.* in the same four different doses (0.25, 0.5, 1.0 and/or 2.0 mg *in toto*)—to estimate the comparable effect on the development of pain-related symptoms, clinical signs, plasma cortisol and catecholamine level, and the inhibition of ruminal motor activity caused by 5 min lasting mechanical duodenal distension (DD) in the sheep.

2. Material and methods

2.1. Preparation of animals

Experiment was carried out on 24 mature crossbred ewes, Polish merino sheep weighing 32–42 kg B.W., being *in anoestrus* period accordingly to the earlier described methods [16, 18, 20]. Food was removed 24 hours prior to the experiment. Analgesia was initiated by *i.m.* ketamine (Calypsovet, 20 mg kg^{-1} B.W., Gedeon Richter, Budapest, Hungary) administration, and 15 min later, *i.v.* infusion of pentobarbital anaesthesia in the dose of 20 mg kg^{-1} B.W. (Vetbutal, BIOWET, Pulawy, Poland) was performed. During unconsciousness, a T-shaped silicon cannula (inside diameter of 21 mm) was inserted into the duodenum (12–15 cm from pylorus). Secondly, an identical cannula was inserted into the dorsal sac of the rumen, using techniques described previously [30] on all animals. Simultaneously, under the same general anaesthesia/analgesia, a permanent stainless steel cannula, 29 mm length and 2 mm in diameter (guide cannula), was inserted into the lateral cerebral ventricle (on the left and/or the right side) of the brain, 10 mm above the bregma and 5 mm laterally from the midline suture using stereotaxic method described by Sorraing et al [31]. After recovery from surgery, the animals were

http://dx.doi.org/10.5772/66597

placed in metabolic cages at constant temperature (18–20°C) for at least 14 days prior to beginning of the experiment [20].

Investigations were performed in four steps (groups, each of six animals for every drug). Every exercise was carried together on two unfed animals, placed in separate boxes at seven days interruption. Blood collection was performed 30 min prior to investigation, in 0 time and 5, 10, 15, 30, 60, and 120 min (**Figure 1**).

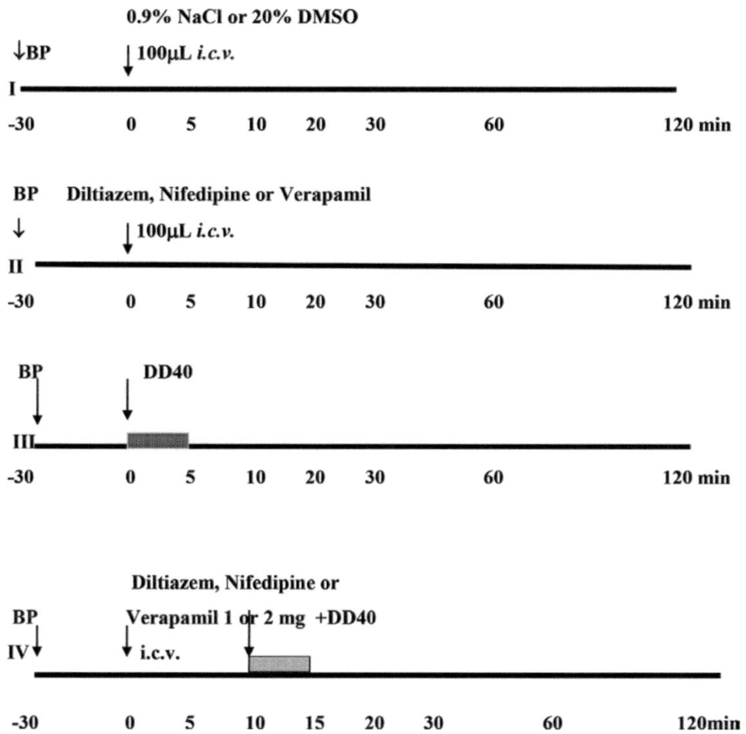

Figure 1. Experimental timelines for the four test group and blood sampling: Control: 0.9% solution NaCl or 20% DMSO—100 μL *i.c.v.* Diltiazem, nifedipine, or verapamil—1.0 or 2.0 mg *in toto* in 100 μL of 0.9% NaCl or 20% DMSO *i.c.v.* DD40—duodenal distension—40 mL water (temp. = 39°C) placed into rubber balloon. Duodenal distension + drug treatment. The time at which the intraduodenal balloon was inserted is marked with the letters: BP.

In the first experimental group, a 60 min recording of the ruminal motility was performed in each animals (n = 6) receiving 100 μL of 20% DMSO (control for nifedipine) or 0.9% NaCl (control for diltiazem and/or verapamil), during 1 min infusion (20 min after the 1st venous blood collection) into the lateral ventricle of the brain (*i.c.v.*); the rumen contraction was registered for 90 min (schema of the blood collection, it was respectively to **Figure 1**).

The second group of sheep (n = 6) were subjected to VGCCIs treatment alone, after 60 min control recording of rumen motility. Every animal received each dose of the substance (with 7 days interval). After the second collection of the venous blood, the sheep were *i.c.v.* given a 1 min lasting infusion of 100 μL of nifedipine in 20% DMSO solution (diltiazem or verapamil in 0.9% NaCl solution) in a dose of 0.25 mg in the first, 0.5 in the second, 1.0 mg in the third or 2.0 mg *in toto* (6.25, 12.5, 25.0 or 50.0 μg kg^{-1} B.W.) in 4 weeks and then the registration was maintained for the next 90 min.

In the third group of sheep (n = 6), after 30 min of control registration of the rumen motility, a rubber balloon (10 cm long) was inserted into the duodenum *via* the duodenal fistula. After placing the balloon in the jejunum, soon after the 2nd blood collection (0 time), the balloon was filled with 40 mL of warm water (DD40) and the distension was maintained for 5 min [28]. Then, the recording of ruminal contractions was continued for 60–90 min. Ten minutes before DD40, each animal received *i.c.v.* infusion of 100 μL of solvents for the drugs tested (**Figure 1**).

In the fourth group of sheep (n = 6), after 30 min of control registration of the rumen motility, a rubber balloon (10 cm long) was inserted into the duodenum and 30 min after the animals received the 100 μL *i.c.v.* infusion of diltiazem, nifedipine (in 20% DMSO solution) or verapamil at a dose of 0.25 mg in the first, 0.5 mg in the second, 1.0 in the third or 2.0 mg *in toto* in the 4th week (the same mode it was used for diltiazem, nifedipine and verapamil experimentation). After 10 min of the diltiazem, nifedipine or verapamil, 1-minute infusion duodenum was distended for 5 min with the balloon containing 40 mL of water (DD40) at body temperature. After the 5 min distension was over, the recording was continued for 60–90 min.

Experimental procedure lasted for 10 months. The doses of 1.0 and 2.0 mg diltiazem, nifedipine or verapamil *in toto* were effective in premedication contra DD40 only.

2.2. Mechanography

The ruminal contractions were analyzed using the electronic tensometric recorder PIT 212 (COMT, Bialystok, Poland). The analysis of mechanograms and calculations of results were performed similarly as in a case of electromyographic recording [32]. The number of the rumen motor activity was determined by the frequency on mechanograms, with 5 min intervals before and after the DD40.

2.3. The estimation of blood cortisol and catecholamine (CA) levels

Blood samples for the analysis of CA estimation were collected from the jugular external vein (according to a scheme described above—**Figure 1**). Blood samples were placed in 10 mL test tubes containing reduced glutathione (0.05 mM). The plastic tubes were maintained on ice, and after the centrifugation, plasma was stored at −80°C, until the beginning of the analytical process. The detection of CA levels was performed by radioimmunoassay using REA kits (CATECHOLA, Czech Republic). The sensitivity of this method was for E, 0.37, for NE, 0.53, and for DA, 0.85 nM L^{-1}. The intra serial error for E was of 3%, for NE 4.2%, and for DA 6.1%, whereas the error among the series was of 4.2, 7.4, and 6.6%, respectively.

Cortisol levels were detected by radioimmunoassay (RIA), according to previous experiments [18]. The mean intra and inter assay of the method was of 9.5 pg, for a sample of 10 μL (ORION DIAGNOSTICA, Espoo). Δ_{max} concentration for each hormone was the difference between the basal concentration and the highest concentration measured.

2.4. The determination of cardiac and ventilation rates

The heart and respiratory rates were measured by determining the number of heart frequencies, as well as by observing the respiratory thoracic movements, using the stethoscope for 1 min. These estimations were detected out by the same person prior to blood test for analysis, according to earlier article [20].

The lack of effect of solvents was determined in preliminary experiments [29, 32].

2.5. Statistical analysis

Statistical significance of the results was carried out through the comparison of control values with those obtained after mechanical distension (duodenal distension—DD40), as well as after VGCCIs premedication and concurrent DD40, using a multifactorial analysis of variance (ANOVA). The statistical significance of the results was detected with a post hoc Tukey-Kramer test; the results are shown as a mean ± SEM. A p value, less than 0.05 was considered statistically significant in all tests.

The researches were performed according to the rules of the Principles of Laboratory Animal Care (NIH publication no. 86-23, revised 1985), as well as the specific national laws on protection of animal (National Law for Animals Protection – 1997, Dz. U.23 XI; Permission of 3rd Local Ethical Commission No. 9/2001 issued 11.01.2001).

3. Results

The influence of DD on behavioral signs, clinical symptoms, reticulo-ruminal contraction and blood plasma cortisol, and CA level was investigated. Before the physiological experimentation, no alteration was observed neither in the physiological behavior of two animals, simultaneously tested in individual cages, nor in the motoric and behavioral response to environmental factors. The mean cardiac frequency was 75.2 (±5.11) and the number of breathing was 35.6·min^{-1} (±4.21), and the reticulo-ruminal frequency was 6.45 ± 0.75 c × 5 min^{-1} in 30 min, before DD. After the implantation of an empty rubber balloon into the duodenum, the observed changes were NS in animal behavior or in the heart beat (70.5 beats·min^{-1} (±8.2)), respiration frequency (42.1 ± 6.35·min^{-1}, **Table 1**) and reticulo-ruminal contractions (6.12 ± 0.28 c·5 min^{-1}). Five-minute duodenal distension induced highly statistically significant alterations in the behavioral signs of animals [10].

3.1. The effect of DD on the behavioral and clinical symptoms, blood plasma cortisol, and/or catecholamine level

Duodenal distension by 40 mL of warm water resulted in a significant increase in the behavioral pain responses: motility, bleating, teeth grinding, prostration, wetting, defecation, tachycardia (from 60 ± 3 beats·min^{-1} to 86 ± 6.2 beats·min^{-1}), hyperventilation (from 36.3 ± 3.6 number·min^{-1} to 50.3 ± 4.5 number·min^{-1}), inhibition of reticulo-rumen contractions rate (from 6.15 ± 0.54 c × 5 min^{-1} in control to 1.09 ± 0.33 c × 5 min^{-1} during DD and to 1.35 ± 0.52

c × 5 min^{-1} 10 min after DD (**Figure 2**; p = 0.001), from −82.2% to −78.0% during 15–20 min; a significant increase in plasma cortisol concentration from 10.51 ± 2.66 ng·mL^{-1} in control to 24.72 ± 8.25 ng·mL-1 during DD and to 34.44 ± 5.46 ng·mL^{-1} ($p \leq 0.01$) 10 min after DD (**Figure 3**); a statistically significant increase of plasma catecholamine concentration (over seven-fold increase of E from 0.34 ± 0.12 nM·L^{-1} in control to 2.87 ± 0.65 nM L^{-1}, during 2 hours following the DD (**Figure 4**); 100% NE—from 1.29 ± 0.23 nM·L^{-1} in control to 2.32 ± 0.24 nM·L^{-1}—120 min after DD (**Figure 4**) and 126% increase of DA from 0.93 ± 0.02 nM L^{-1} in the control to 2.33 ± 1.16 nM L^{-1}, 120 min after DD) (**Figure 4**).

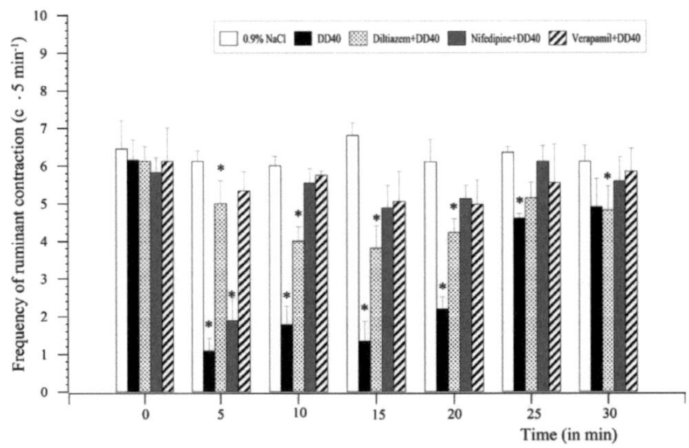

Figure 2. Influence of *i.c.v.* 1 min infusion after 10 min pretreatment of different voltage-gated calcium channels inhibitor (diltiazem, nifedipine or verapamil) in different doses (1.0 or 2.0 mg/animal) per number of reticulo-ruminal contractions (c × 5 min^{-1}) in sheep in comparison with the group with duodenal distension, DD40 (x ± SEM, n = 6). Mean values of results obtained from the same blood collection (time point) with different superscript sign $p \leq 0.001$–0.05 level in comparison to DD40 value.

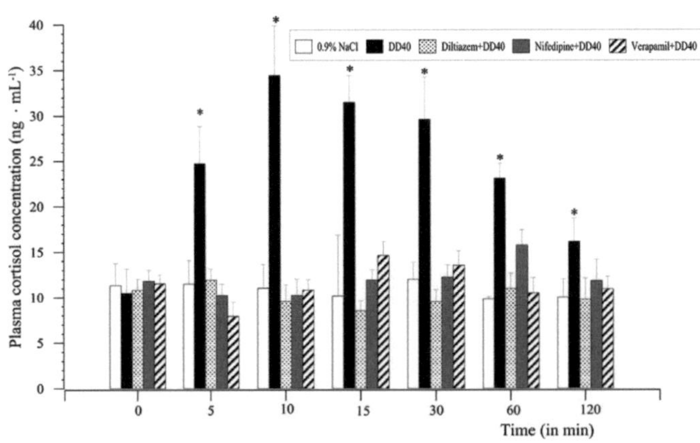

Figure 3. Comparative analysis of 10 min premedication influence with *i.c.v.* diltiazem, nifedipine, and/or verapamil (in doses 1.0 and/or 2.0 mg/animal) and DD40 on plasma cortisol concentration in sheep, in comparison to DD40 value at $p \leq 0.001$–0.05 (x ± SEM, n = 6).

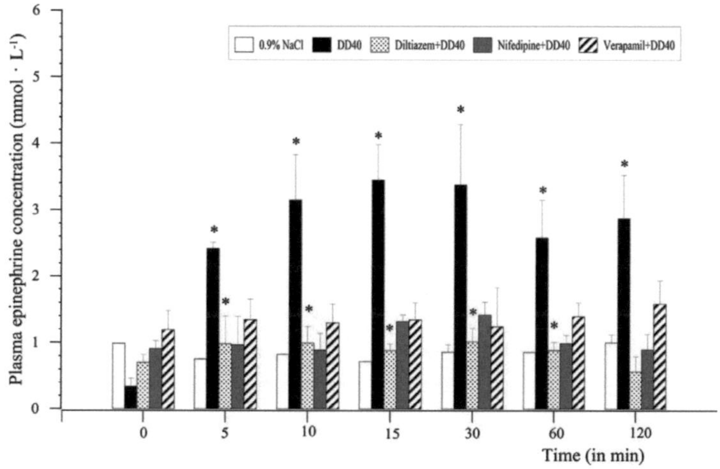

Figure 4. Comparative analysis of duodenal distension and premedication with different diltiazem, nifedipine and verapamil doses (1.0 or 2.0 mg/animal) on plasma epinephrine concentration in comparison with DD40 (x ± SEM, n = 6, p ≤ 0.001–0.05). Mean values of results obtained from the same blood collection (time point).

3.2. The influence of VGCCIs premedication on the behavioral changes, clinical symptoms, rumen motility, plasma cortisol, and catecholamine level in animals with/without DD

I.C.V. infusion of 1 min diltiazem, nifedipine or verapamil in doses of 0.25, 0.50, 1.0 or 2.0 mg *in toto*, did not have any significant influence on the behavioral and clinical symptoms (**Table 1**), rumen contractions count (**Figure 2**), cortisol (**Figure 3**), and CA's level in blood plasma (**Figures 4–6**).

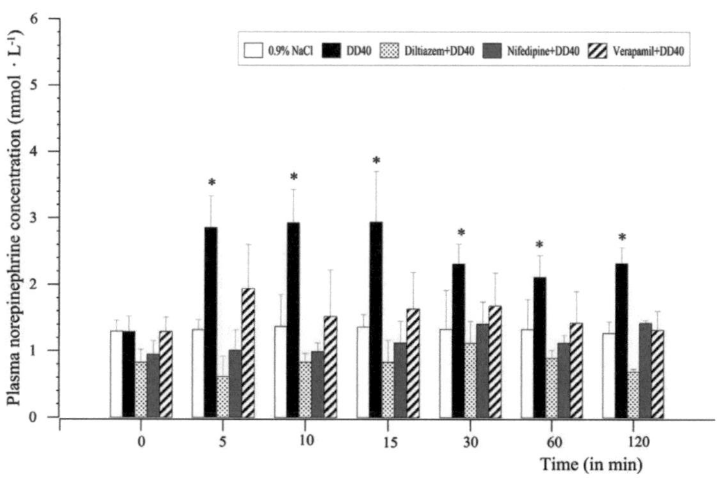

Figure 5. Comparative analysis of duodenal distension and premedication with different diltiazem, nifedipine and verapamil doses (1.0 or 2.0 mg/animal) on plasma norepinephrine concentration in comparison with DD40 (x ± SEM, n = 6, p ≤ 0.001–0.05). Mean values of results obtained from the same blood collection (time point).

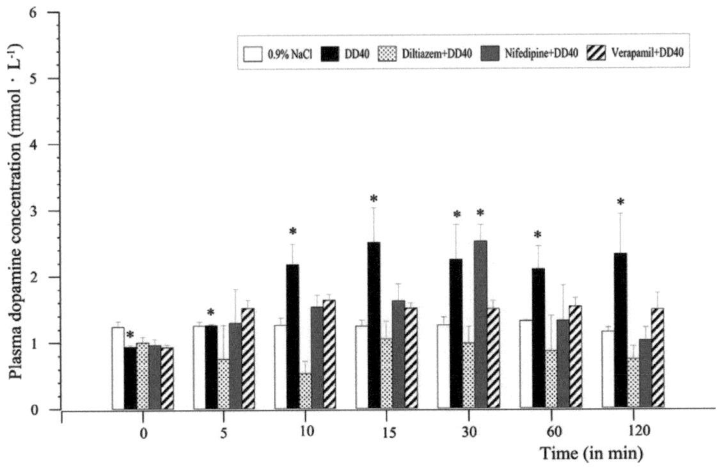

Figure 6. Comparative analysis of duodenal distension and premedication with different diltiazem, nifedipine and verapamil doses (1.0 or 2.0 mg/animal) on plasma dopamine concentration in comparison with DD40 (x ± SEM, n = 6, $p \leq 0.001$–0.05). Mean values of results obtained from the same blood collection (time point).

I.C.V. infusion of diltiazem, nifedipine, and verapamil (1.0 or 2.0 mg *in toto*), 10 min before the DD inhibited and/or completely attenuated the beginning of clinical symptoms of jejunal nociception, provoked by duodenal distension (**Table 1**). In control animals before premedication, intense acceleration of cardiac beats was observed (mean from 70 to 102 beats·min^{-1}) and in the animals treated with diltiazem or verapamil, it was decreased to 63–86 beats·min^{-1}; after nifedipine premedication, the DD caused an increased cardiac frequency from 68 to 90 beats·min^{-1}. Respiration frequency was 50 and 34·min^{-1}, respectively.

Drugs	Control	5 min	10 min	15 min	20 min	25 min	30 min
0.9% NaCl	6.45 ± 0.75	6.12 ± 0.28	6.00 ± 0.25	6.80 ± 0.33	6.10 ± 0.60	6.35 ± 0.15	6.11 ± 0.43
DD40	6.15 ± 0.54	1.09 ± 0.33*	1.78 ± 0.49*	1.35 ± 0.52*	2.20 ± 0.31*	0.61 ± 0.12*	4.91 ± 0.75
Diltiazem + DD40	5.00 ± 0.61*	4.00 ± 0.38*	3.80 ± 0.60*	4.23 ± 0.36*	5.14 ± 0.42	4.82 ± 0.64	6.12 ± 0.40
Nifedipine + DD40	5.82 ± 0.45	1.89 ± 0.81*	5.54 ± 0.23	4.88 ± 0.62	5.12 ± 0.74	6.11 ± 1.11	5.59 ± 1.22
Verapamil + DD40	6.12 ± 0.89	5.33 ± 0.51	5.75 ± 0.11	5.05 ± 0.80	4.97 ± 0.65	5.55 ± 1.02	5.85 ± 0.61

Value are mean ± SEM of 6 sheep, and indicate significant difference corresponding from control group.
ẍ ± SEM, n = 6.
*$p \leq 0.001$–0.05.

Table 2. Frequency of ruminal contraction of the five groups (control, DD40, diltiazem + DD40, nifedipine + DD40, verapamil + DD40) during the course of the experiments.

VGCCIs premedication caused that inhibition of rumen frequency after 5 min DD, decreasing from average 6.12 ± 0.40 to 5.00 ± 0.61, in 5 min, and 4.00 ± 0.38 c × 5min^{-1}, in 10 min, after DD,

http://dx.doi.org/10.5772/66597

but not from 6.15 ± 0.54 in control to 1.09 ± 0.33 c × 5 min^{-1} after DD (**Table 2**, **Figure 2**). Plasma cortisol concentration changed from 10.83 ± 1.19 in control to 11.95 ± 1.25, during (NS), and 9.53 ± 1.36 (NS) 30 min, after DD, but not increased from 10.51 ± 2.66 in control to 24.72 ± 8.25, during DD, and 34.44 ± 5.46 (+227.7%) 10 min, after DD (p<0.001, **Figure 3**). Diltiazem premedication caused that increase of plasma CA concentration after 5 min DD, decreased E from average +606.41% in control to +23.02%, during 120 min after DD (**Figure 4**); NE from +120.95% in control to −21%, during 120 min after DD (**Figure 5**) and DA from +124.2% in control to −24,8%, during 120 min after diltiazem premedication (**Figure 6**).

Nifedipine *i.c.v.* premedication caused that inhibition of rumen frequency after 5 min DD, decreased from average 5.82 ± 0.45 to 1.89 ± 0.81 (−69%) in 5 min only, during DD, and 5.54 ± 0.23 (−5.2%) 10 min, after DD, but not from 6.15 in control to 1.78 c × 5 min^{-1} (−71.%), after DD (**Figure 2**). Nifedipine premedication diminished the increase in plasma cortisol concentration from 11.81 ± 1.13 ng L^{-1} (NS) in control to 10.25 ± 1.65 ng · L^{-1} (NS) in 10.00 and to 11.85 ng L^{-1} 120 min after DD (**Figure 3**). Premedication by 1 min *i.c.v.* nifedipine infusion caused that increase of plasma catecholamine concentration, after 5 min DD, statistically significantly decreased from average 0.34 to 2.98 nM L^{-1} (+767.8%) in DD and from 0.91 in control to 1.08 nM L^{-1} (+23%) to E, from +98.5 to +23.7%, to NE, and from +124.2 in control to 61.3% to DA, during 120 min after DD (**Figures 4–6**).

Verapamil *i.c.v.* premedication by 1 min infusion caused that inhibition rumen frequency after 5 min DD, decreased from 6.12 ± 0.89 to 5.38 ± 0.53 (−12.1%) during 30 min after DD and by average 44.7% in comparison to DD only (**Table 2**). In the same time, verapamil premedication caused that increase of plasma cortisol concentration after 5 min DD, decreased from average 11.53 ± 0.98 in control to 7.91 ± 1.58 (−36.1%; p<0.05) during DD and 11.39 ± 1.48 ng·L^{-1} (NS) during 120 min after DD and by −153% (p<0.001) in comparison to DD group (**Table 3**).

	Control	5 min	10 min	20 min	30 min	60 min	120 min
0.9% NaCl	11.35 ± 2.40	11.50 ± 2.61	11.05 ± 2.58	10.17 ± 6.71	12.01 ± 1.86	9.87 ± 0.25	10.02 ± 2.02
DD40	10.51 ± 2.66	24.72 ± 8.25*	34.44 ± 5.46*	31.52 ± 2.91*	29.65 ± 4.61*	23.10 ± 1.61*	16.16 ± 2.56*
Diltiazem + DD40	10.83 ± 1.19	11.95 ± 1.25	9.58 ± 1.81	8.52 ± 1.13	9.53 ± 1.36	10.99 ± 1.68	9.8 ± 2.31
Nifedipine + DD40	11.81 ± 1.13	10.25 ± 1.51	10.25 ± 1.17	11.94 ± 1.65	12.25 ± 1.39	15.75 ± 1.69	11.85 ± 1.35
Verapamil + DD40	11.53 ± 0.98	7.91 ± 1.58*	10.83 ± 1.17	14.63 ± 1.53	13.53 ± 1.58	10.49 ± 1.69	10.96 ± 1.36

*p ≤ 0.001–0.05.

Table 3. Comparative analysis *i.c.v.* diltiazem, nifedipine, or verapamil (in the doses 2 mg *in toto*) premedication influence and DD40 on plasma cortisol concentration changes in sheep.

Verapamil *i.c.v.* premedication caused that plasma epinephrine after 5 min DD increased, but nonsignificantly from average 1.19 ± 0.29 in control to 1.36 ± 0.59 (+14.7%), during 120 min after DD, but not from 0.34 ± 0.12 in control to 2.99 ± 0.81 nM L^{-1}, e.g., +767.8% (p<0.001), during

120 min after DD (**Table 4**). Decrease of epinephrine plasma concentration by verapamil premedication was 753.08%.

Verapamil *i.c.v.* premedication caused that increase of plasma norepinephrine concentration after 5 min DD, increased from average 1.29 ± 0.22 in control to 1.58 ± 0.84 nM L^{-1}, during 120 min after DD, but not from 1.29 ± 0.23 in control to 2.50 ± 0.42 nM L^{-1} (+98.56%), during 120 min after DD. Decrease in norepinephrine concentration by verapamil premedication was 75.71%.

Catecholamine	**Time (in min)**						
	0	**5**	**10**	**15**	**30**	**60**	**120**
Epinephrine							
0.9% NaCl (100 μL)	0.98 ± 0.00	0.75 ± 0.00	0.82 ± 0.00	0.71 ± 0.00	0.85 ± 0.11	0.85 ± 0.00	0.99 ± 0.12
DD40	0.34 ± 0.12	2.42 ± 0.09	3.15 ± 0.68	3.45 ± 0.53	3.38 ± 1.82	2.58 ± 1.13	2.87 ± 0.65
Diltiazem + DD40	0.70 ± 0.12	0.98 ± 0.42	0.99 ± 0.25	0.88 ± 0.10	1.01 ± 0.20	0.88 ± 0.12	0.56 ± 0.23
Nifedipine + DD40	0.90 ± 0.12	0.97 ± 0.14	0.89 ± 0.25	1.31 ± 0.58	1.41 ± 0.38	0.99 ± 0.18	0.90 ± 0.41
Verapamil + DD40	1.19 ± 0.29	1.34 ± 0.31	1.30 ± 0.28	1.34 ± 0.26	1.24 ± 0.59	1.39 ± 0.21	1.58 ± 0.35
Norepinephrine							
0.9% NaCl (100 μL)	1.30 ± 0.16	1.32 ± 0.15	1.37 ± 0.48	1.36 ± 0.19	1.33 ± 0.58	1.33 ± 0.44	1.28 ± 0.17
DD40	1.29 ± 0.23	2.85 ± 0.48	2.93 ± 0.51	2.94 ± 0.76	2.31 ± 0.30	2.11 ± 0.32	2.32 ± 0.24
Diltiazem + DD40	0.82 ± 0.20	0.61 ± 0.31	0.83 ± 0.13	0.83 ± 0.33	1.12 ± 0.33	0.89 ± 0.12	0.69 ± 0.04
Nifedipine + DD40	0.95 ± 0.06	1.01 ± 0.14	0.99 ± 0.28	1.12 ± 0.38	1.41 ± 1.22	1.12 ± 0.72	1.43 ± 1.23
Verapamil + DD40	1.29 ± 0.22	1.94 ± 0.66	1.52 ± 0.42	1.63 ± 1.12	1.68 ± 1.10	1.42 ± 0.48	1.32 ± 0.24
Dopamine							
0.9% NaCl (100 μL)	1.23 ± 0.08	1.24 ± 0.06	1.26 ± 0.10	1.24 ± 0.09	1.25 ± 0.12	1.31 ± 0.01	1.15 ± 0.07
DD40	0.93 ± 0.02	1.26 ± 0.01	2.18 ± 0.30	2.51 ± 0.52	2.25 ± 0.52	2.10 ± 0.35	2.33 ± 1.16
Diltiazem + DD40	0.99 ± 0.09	0.75 ± 0.51	0.53 ± 0.18	1.05 ± 0.26	0.98 ± 0.25	0.86 ± 0.53	0.74 ± 0.19
Nifedipine + DD40	0.96 ± 0.02	1.29 ± 0.12	1.53 ± 0.42	1.62 ± 0.28	2.52 ± 1.41	1.32 ± 0.19	1.02 ± 0.32
Verapamil + DD40	0.92 ± 0.04	1.51 ± 0.12	1.63 ± 0.09	1.51 ± 0.08	1.50 ± 0.12	1.53 ± 0.13	1.48 ± 0.25

Table 4. Comparative analysis *i.c.v.* diltiazem, nifedipine, and verapamil (in the dose of 1.0 or 2.0 mg *in toto*) premedication influence and DD40 on concentration epinephrine, norepinephrine and dopamine plasma level changes in sheep in comparison to the control values (x̄ ± SEM; n = 6).

I.C.V. verapamil premedication caused that plasma dopamine concentration after 5 min DD increased from 0.92 ± 0.04 in control to 1.52 ± 0.13 nM L^{-1}, during 120 min after DD (+65.04%),

http://dx.doi.org/10.5772/66597

but not from 0.93 ± 0.02 in control to 2.33 ± 1.16, during 120 min after DD (+126.3%; $p<0.001$, **Table 4**). Decrease in dopamine concentration by verapamil premedication was 61.26% ($p<0.01$).

4. Discussion

The results of this experiment showed that 1 min diltiazem, nifedipine, and/or verapamil (VGCCIs) *i.c.v.* infusion in doses 0.25, 0.5, 1.0, or 2.0 mg *in toto*, given 10 min before DD, decreased the intensity of visceral nocifensive responses, such as behavioral changes, tachycardia, hyperventilation, reticulo-ruminal motility inhibition, and efficiently prevented the appearance of cortisol and catecholamine concentration in the blood plasma, after two higher doses. It was established that these results revealed that the development and persistence of acute duodenal pain depends on the activation of Ca^{2+} ion flux, leading to neurohormones release and modulation of membrane excitability. It seems that VGCCIs given *i.c.v.* 10 min prior to DD, which was evoked by the darting pain, blocked specific receptors $\alpha(1)$ subunits of voltage-gated calcium channels in effector tissues, attenuate depolarization of cellular membranes, and liberation of neurotransducers important for pain perception in small ruminants. The confirmed analgesic effect of L-type VGCCIs proposes that these L-type VGCCs play a crucial role in the modulation of acute experimental visceral pain in sheep. The important significance of VGCC L-type inhibitors, applied together with opioids in weakness of clinical nociception, have been revealed by Gullapalli and Ramarao [33], that L-type channel modulation by 1,4-dihydropyridines (nimodipine and lercanidipine) potentiates kappa-opioid receptor agonist induced acute analgesia and inhibits the development of tolerance in rats using the tail-flick test. Nimodipine (1 $mg{\cdot}kg^{-1}$; *i.p.*) and lercanidipine (0.3 $mg{\cdot}kg^{-1}$; *i.p.*) used in this study produced no tail-flick analgesia, but administered that in these doses, 15 min prior analgesic doses of selective kappa-opioid agonists (U 50,488, PD 117,302 and U 69,593) significantly potentiated the analgesia produced by three kappa-opioid receptor agonists. These results strongly suggested a functional role of L-type Ca^{2+} channels in the regulation of pain sensitivity and mechanism of kappa-opioid analgesia. Last results by Qian et al. [17] suggest also, an important role of VGCCs in rat visceral hypersensitivity by 2,4,6-trinitrobenzenesulfonic acid provoked car nimodipine and SNX-482 prevented it.

In our study, saline and 20% DMSO *i.c.v.* infused during 1 min in volume of 100 μL did not change the ruminal motor activity during 30 min before DD40 and after introduced empty balloon, it was 1.38 ± 0.14 $c{\cdot}min^{-1}$. The results obtained were nonsignificant in comparison with the results obtained after the intraduodenal balloon placed and no influencing on the interpretation of the results obtained. Mechanical duodenal distension by balloon 10 cm in length with 40 mL of warm water (DD40) provoked during and after 5 min total inhibition of spiking activity [30, 32] or contraction of the rumen and duodenum during 8–12 min ($p \leq 0.01$, **Figure 2**), approximately 85%. These effects, lasting 20 min after DD termination (average 47.3%) were statistically significant ($p \leq 0.05$) in comparison to the control values (**Figure 2**). During 5 min episode of DD40, only one to two ruminal contractions were registered in six animals tested. Singular contraction recurred after terminations of DD40 immediately, but their number did not exceed the values of control contractions.

It is known that DD40 provoked stimulation of behavioral signs, clinical symptoms, and statistically significant increase in plasma cortisol and catecholamine concentrations (**Table 1**, **Figures 3–6**). *I.C.V.* premedication, by VGCCIs attenuated ruminal motor inhibition by 5 min episode DD, provoked during 30 min average 39.4%, e.g., from 56.8% after DD to 24.2, 18.1 and 9.6% after diltiazem, nifedipine, and verapamil premedication, respectively. The most preventing for the 5 min DD inhibitory influence on ruminal motility was verapamil in comparison to the control values. All the VGCCIs in premedication use inhibited statistically significant behavioral signs, such as looking around, defecation and/or urination, head movements, lying down, and clinical symptoms, such as tachycardia and hyperventilation by 120 min after DD persistent (**Table 1**).

Five-minute DD episode increased the plasma cortisol concentration average for 153% during 120 min after DD, in comparison to the control values. Ten-minute VGCCIs premedication diminished the plasma cortisol release by an average of 139.5 % (diltiazem), and 141% (nifedipine and verapamil) ($p \leq 0.001$; **Table 3**, **Figure 3**) respectively.

Five-minute DD episode increased the plasma catecholamine concentration average: E 768%, NE 98.5%, and DA 124% during 120 min after DD. Diltiazem, nifedipine, and verapamil minimized the increase of plasma catecholamine concentration, which was caused by visceral pain, provoked by duodenal distension. Average of catecholamine release inhibition by VGCCIs were for E—773.3%, NA—90%, and DA—90.2%, during 120 after 5 min DD episode ($p \leq 0.001$; **Table 4**, **Figures 4–6**). The most anticatecholaminergic activity was detected for diltiazem. In our study, we found that all the VGCCIs—whatever their chemical origin—in premedication attenuated vegetative signs and clinical symptoms, HPA and SAS stimulation axes caused by acute 5 min duration nocifensive factor (duodenal distension) in sheep.

This confirms the results obtained by Qian et al. [17] that $Ca_v1.2$ and $Ca_v2.3$ channels in colonic primary sensory neurons play an important role in visceral inflammatory hyperalgesia, which may be a potential therapeutic target, because L-type and R-type selective colonic channel blockers may block calcium currents which are importantly increased in colonic dorsal root ganglion (DRG) neurons of 2,4,6-trinitrobenzenesulfonic acid-treated rats in comparison with control animals. The author cited above concluded that L-type channel antagonist (nimodipine) and R-type channel antagonist (SNX-482) attenuates visceral pain in 2,4,6-trinitrobenzenesulfonic acid intrathecal injected. The results obtained confirm the hypothesis that L-type and/or R-type calcium channels play a more crucial role in pathology of visceral pain in animals.

A moderate degree of mechanical duodenal distension (DD20 and DD30) in sheep reduced the frequency of forestomach and abomasum motor activity by 45 and 52%, respectively [30], whereas, strong distension (DD40 and DD80) provoked the total contraction inhibition in conscious animals accompanied by the acute visceral pain [21, 33]. There is a direct relationship between the viscero-visceral reflex and visceral pain [34]. Visceral pain is a general sign involved in many gastro-duodenal and gastro-colonic disorders, such as colic, inflammatory

http://dx.doi.org/10.5772/66597

processes, and other diseases. These symptoms are accompanied by stimulation of the HPA (neuropeptides, hormones, e.g., cortisol) and SAS (catecholamine, 5-HT, neuropeptides) axes and the exacerbation of motivational and motor CNS structures (limbic system) involved in many quinine, neuropeptides, and necrohormones release useful in alarm reactions and defense of animals.

I.C.V. application of VGCCIs in 10 min premedication prevented nocifensive signs of behavior, clinical symptoms, increase plasma cortisol and catecholamine concentration in periphery, and perhaps in CNS structures, as well. The molecular mechanisms of these processes are the result of the L-type voltage-gated calcium channel inhibitors blockage of specific Ca^{2+} receptors by the drugs tested. Calcium channels receptor blockage by VGCC inhibitors attenuates visceral pain by inhibiting nocifensive neurohormone/neurotransmitters release in CNS and in peripheral nervous system, due to the fact that Ca^{2+} ions cannot bind to their specific receptor for depolarization of presynaptic neuronal membrane and promote the release of nocifensive substances.

4.1. Other types of calcium channel blockers used in the treatment of pain

Voltage-gated calcium channels are made with subunit α_1 which forms a channel pore and subunit $\alpha_{2\delta}$, which facilitates movement to the membrane surface [35]. There are ten different $\alpha_{1\delta}$ subtypes and four $\alpha_{2\delta}$. $\alpha_{2\delta1}$ and $\alpha_{2\delta2}$ subtypes bind gabapentin and pregabalin. Subtype 1 exists principally in the intermediate matrix (dentate gyrus, insula, cortex, and amygdala) [36].

Subtypes $\alpha_{2\delta1}$ exhibit expression also in dorsal root ganglia, spinal cord and in the small intestine smooth muscle, together with N-type calcium channels [36]. Subtype 2 is found in the periaqueductal gray matter, spinal cord and as diffused all over CNS, but not in the colon or duodenal smooth muscle [37]. Pregabalin and gabapentin bind with subtypes $\alpha_{2\delta}$ in the cytoplasm and prevent calcium channels expression on the plasmatic membranes [38]. Preventing the binding and expression blocks calcium conductance and in consequence substance P (SP), calcitonin gene related peptide (CGRP) and glutamate cannot be released from primary afferent neurons [35, 39]. Prevention of nocifensive neurotrasmitters release by gabapentine and pregabaline occurs only during pathological processes, in which calcium channels are up-regulated and activated [40]. Both pregabaline and gabapentine are central analgesics [39]. Gabapentinoids inhibited visceral hypersensitivity in the experimental animals, as well as irritable bowel syndrome in humans [41]. Smalls doses of gabapentine administered with morphine inhibit *i.p.* acid injection induced writhing syndrome in rats, which were ineffective when the drugs were applied separately.

Gabapentenoids not only inhibit central nociceptive transmission, but also enhance the intestine susceptibility to distension, possibly by blockage of $\alpha_{2\delta}$ subtypes in the smooth muscle [42, 43].

Other calcium channels can be also involved in the development of visceral hypersensitivity. Stimulation of T-type calcium channels, subtype $Ca_v3.2$ on the primary signaling visceral afferents was associated with symptoms similar to the irritable bowel syndrome in the animal model. Behavioral symptoms resolved after the application of T-type calcium channels inhibitor [44]. Afferent transduction from mesentery in the experimental intestinal ischaemia was blocked by nifedipine, an L-type calcium channels inhibitor [45].

5. Conclusion

The results of this investigation indicates, that VGCCIs can be applied effectively in visceral pain modulation of animals and could be paid to the use of this kind of medicine, perhaps in human pain treatment as well.

Author details

Kania Bogdan Feliks[1*] and Danuta Wrońska[2]

*Address all correspondence to: bkania@ur.krakow.pl

1 Veterinary Institute, University Center for Veterinary Medicine Jagiellonian University& Agricultural University, Hugon Kołłątaj Agricultural University in Cracow, Al Mickiewicza Cracow, Poland

2 Department of Physiology and Endocrinology of Animals, Faculty of Animal Science, Hugon Kołłątaj Agricultural University in Cracow, Al. Mickiewicza Cracow, Poland

References

[1] Dorland's M Dictionary. Calcium Channels. 32nd Edition, Elsevier, USA, 2016.

[2] Striggow F, Ehrlich BE. Ligand gated calcium channels inside an aut. Curr. Opin. Cell. Biol. 1996; 8: 490–495.

[3] Catteral WA, Perez-Reyes E, Snutch TP, Striessing J. International Union of Pharmacology. XLVIII. Nomenclature and structure-function relationships of voltage-gated calcium channels. Pharmacol. Rev. 2005; 57: 411–425.

[4] Yamagake M, Namiki A. Calcium channels – basic aspects of their structure, function and gene encoding; anesthetic action on the channels – a review. Can. J. Anaesth. 2002; 49: 151–164.

[5] Rang H, Ritter JM, Flower RJ, Henderson G. How drugs act: cellular aspects – excitation, contraction and secretion. In: Rang & Dale's Pharmacology. 8th Edition, Elsevier Churchill Livingstone, 2016; pp. 50–65.

http://dx.doi.org/10.5772/66597

[6] Morgan AJ, Platt FM, Lloyd-Evans E, Galione A. Molecular mechanisms of endolysosomal Ca^{2+} signaling in health and disease. Biochem. J. 2011; 439: 349–374.

[7] McDonough SI. Calcium Channel Pharmacology. Kluwer Academic/Plenum, New York, 2004.

[8] Zamponi GW. Targeting voltage-gated calcium channels in neurological and psychiatric diseases. Nat. Rev. Drug Discov. 2016; 15: 19–34.

[9] Leone M, Franzini A, Proietti Cecchini A, Mea E, Brogi G, Bussone G. Management of chronic cluster headache. Curr. Treat. Options Neurol. 2011; 13: 56–70.

[10] Guttierez-Martin Y, Martin-Romero FJ, Henao F. Store-operated calcium entry in differentiated C2C12 skeletal muscle cells. Biochem. Biophys. Acta. 2005; 1711: 33–40

[11] Sicca D. Calcium channel blockers and the kidney. Clin. Cornerstone. 2004; 6: 39–52.

[12] Long W, Zhao Y, Zhang L, Longo LD. Role of Ca^{2+} channels in NE induced increase in $[Ca^{2+}](i)$ and tension in fetal and adult cerebral arteries. Am. J. Physiol. 1999; 277: R286–R294.

[13] Yamagishi S, Takeuchi M. Nifedipine inhibits tumor necrosis factor-alpha-induced upregulation of monocyte chemoattractant protein-1 mRNA levels by suppressing CD40 expression in endothelial cells. Drug. Exp. Clin. Res. 2005; 31: 13–17.

[14] Davis SE, Bauer EP. L-type voltage-gated calcium channels in basolateral amygdala are necessary for fear extinction. J. Neurosci. 2012; 32: 13582–13586.

[15] Leblondel G, Allain P. Ca^{2+} uptake and energy supply of sheep heart mitochondria in presence of some calcium antagonists. Res. Commun. Chem. Pathol. Pharmacol. 1984; 44: 499–502.

[16] Kania BF, Ŝutiak V. Influence of centrally administered diltiazem on behavioral response, clinical symptoms, reticulo-ruminal contraction and plasma catecholamine level after experimentally induced duodenal distension in sheep. Res. Vet. Sci. 2011; 90: 291–297.

[17] Qian A, Song D, Li Y, Liu X, Tang D, Yao W, Yuan Y. Role of voltage gated Ca^{2+} channels in rat visceral hypersensitivity change induced by 2,4,6-trinitrobenzene sulfonic acid. Mol. Pain. 2013; 9: 15 DOI: 10.1186/1744-8069-9-15

[18] Kania BF, Wrońska D. Supraspinal basis of analgesic and clinical effects of the metabotropic glutamate $mGluR_1$ antagonist during colonic distension in sheep. Small Rum. Res. 2014; 117: 84–93.

[19] Bielefeldt K, Christianson JA, Davis RM. Basic and clinical aspects of visceral sensation: transmission in the CNS. . Neurogastroenterol. Motil. 2005; 17: 488–499.

[20] Kania BF, Brytan M, Tomaszewska D. Centrally administered verapamil prevents the autonomic reaction to visceral pain in sheep. Res. Vet. Sci. 2009; 86: 121–128.

[21] Brikas P, Kania BF, Fioramonti J, Buéno L. Central and peripheral serotonergic influences on viscerovisceral inhibitory reflex during duodenal distension in sheep. Dig. Dis. Sci. 1993; 38: 1079–1086.

[22] Blackshaw LA, Brookes SJ, Grundy D, Scheman M. Sensory transmission in the gastrointestinal tract. Neurogastroenterol. Motil. 2007; 19: 1–3.

[23] Ossipov MH, Morimura K, Porreca F. Descending pain modulation and chronification of pain. Curr. Opin. 2014; 8: 143–151.

[24] Shimizu N, Kishioka S, Maeda T, Fukazawa Y, Yamamoto C, Ozaki M, Yamamoto H. Role of pharmacokinetic effects in the potentiation of morphine analgesia by L-type calcium channel blockers in mice. J. Pharmacol. Sci. 2004; 94: 240–245.

[25] Bongianni F, Carla V, Moroni F, Pellegrini-Giampietro DE. Calcium channel inhibitors suppress the morphine-withdrawal syndrome in rats. Br. J. Pharmacol. 1986; 88: 561–567.

[26] Srivastava SK, Nath C. The differential effects of calcium channel blockers in the behavioral despair test in mice. Pharmacol. Res. 2000; 42: 293–297.

[27] Michaluk J, Karolewicz B, Antkiewicz-Michaluk L, Vetulani J. Effects of various Ca^{2+} channel antagonists on blond pressure in the rat. Eur. J. Pharmacol. 1998; 352: 189–197.

[28] Kavaliers M. Aggression and defeat-induced opioid analgesia displayed by mice are modified by calcium channel antagonists and agonists. Neurosci. Lett. 1987; 74: 107–111.

[29] Kania BF, Dębski B, Wrońska D, Zawadzka E. Verapamil – L-type voltage-gated calcium channel inhibitor diminishes aggressive behavior in male Siamese fighting fish. Pol. J. Vet. Sci. 2015; 18: 401–406.

[30] Kania BF, Zaremba-Rutkowska M, Romanowicz K. Experimental intestinal stress induced by duodenal distension in sheep. J. Anim. Feed Sci. 1999; 8: 233–245.

[31] Sorraing JM, Fioramonti J, Buéno L. Central and peripheral serotonergic control of forestomach motility in sheep. J. Vet. Pharmacol. Ther. 1985; 8: 312–319.

[32] Kania BF, Brikas P, Buéno L, Fioramonti J, Zaremba–Rutkowska M. The evaluation of the role of CCK in the opioid modulation of the motility of the gastrointestinal tract in sheep. J. Vet. Pharmacol. Ther. 1999; 22: 153–160.

[33] Gullapalli S, Ramarao P. L-type Ca^{2+} channel modulation by dihydropyridines potentiates kappa-opioid receptor agonist induced acute analgesia and inhibits development of tolerance in rats. Neuropharmacology. 2002; 42: 467–475.

[34] De Ponti F, Azpiroz F, Malagelada JR. Reflex gastric relaxation in response to distension of the duodenum. Am. J. Physiol. 1987; 252: G595–G601.

[35] Gale JD, Houghton LA. Alpha 2 delta (α(2)δ) ligands, gabapentin and pregabalin: what is the evidence for potential use of these ligands in irritable bowel syndrome. Front. Pharmacol. 2011; 2: 28.

[36] Taylor CP, Garrido R. Immunostaining of rat brain, spinal cord, sensory neurons and skeletal muscle for calcium channel alpha2-delta ($\alpha2\delta$) type 1 protein. Neuroscience. 2008; 155: 510–521.

[37] Cole RI., Lechnaer SM, Williams LE. Differential distribution of voltage-gated calcium channel alpha-2 delta ($\alpha2\delta$) subunit mRNA-containing cells in the rat central nervous system and the dorsal root ganglia. J. Comp. Neurol. 2005; 491: 246–269.

[38] Mich PM, Horne WA. Alternative splicing of the Ca^{2+} channel β4 subunit confers specificity for gabapentin inhibition of $Ca_v2.1$ trafficking. Mol. Pharmacol. 2008; 74: 904–912.

[39] Field MJ, Cox PJ, Stott E. Identification of the α2-δ-1 subunit of voltage-calcium calcium channels as a molecular target for pain mediating the analgesic actions of pregabalin. Proc. Nat. Acad. Sci. USA. 2006; 103: 17537–17542.

[40] Dooley DJ, Donovan CM, Pugsley TA. Stimulus-dependent modulation of ^3H norepinephrine release from rat neocortical slices by gabapentin and pregabalin. J. Pharm. Exp. Ther. 2000; 295: 1086–1093.

[41] Stepanovic-Petrovic RM, Tomic MA, Vuckovic SM. The antinociceptive effects of anticonvulsants in a mouse visceral pain model. Anesth. Analg. 2008; 106: 1897–1903.

[42] Lee KJ, Kim JH, Cho SW. Gabapentin reduces rectal mechanosensitivity and increases rectal compliance in patients with diarrhoea-predominant irritable bowel syndrome. Aliment. Pharmacol. Ther. 2005; 22: 981–988.

[43] Ravnefjord A, Brusberg M, Larsson H, Lindström E, Martinez V. Effects of pregabalin on visceral pain responses and colonic compliance in rats. Brit. J. Pharmacol. 2008; 155: 407–416.

[44] Marger F, Gelot A, Alloui A. T-type calcium channels contribute to colonic hypersensitivity in a rat model of irritable bowel syndrome. Proc. Natl. Acad. Sci. USA. 2011; 108: 11268–11273.

[45] Jiang W, Kirkup AJ, Grundy D. Mast cells drive mesenteric afferent signaling during acute intestinal ischemia. J. Physiol. 2011; 589: 3867–3882.

Chapter 12

Interaction of Non-Steroidal Anti-Inflammatory Drugs (NSAIDs) with Reactive Oxygen Species (ROS): Possible Biomedical Implications

Norman A. García, Mabel Bregliani and Adriana Pajares

Additional information is available at the end of the chapter

http://dx.doi.org/10.5772/66478

Abstract

The present chapter deals on the interaction of nonsteroidal anti-inflammatory drugs (NSAIDs), diflunisal, indomethacin, meloxicam, tenoxicam and piroxicam with reactive oxygen species (ROS) photogenerated in aqueous solution by the vitamin riboflavin employed as a dye sensitizer. Simple techniques as substrate and oxygen consumption and more sophisticated time-resolved spectroscopic methods were employed for the kinetic and mechanistic evaluation of the deactivation of the *in situ* generated ROS singlet molecular oxygen ($O_2(^1\Delta_g)$), superoxide radical anion ($O_2^{\bullet-}$) and hydrogen peroxide (H_2O_2) by the mentioned NSAIDs. Results could be prudently extrapolated to a possible action of NSAIDs in the retardation or inhibition of neuroinflammatory disorders, in which oxidative agents such as ROS were found to be upregulated. Despite the potential benefit, some adverse effects in humans reported in relation with high doses of NSAIDs alert about the cares that have to be taken about their use.

Keywords: antioxidants, NSAIDs, photosensitization, riboflavin, ROS

1. Introduction

In the last decades, it has been a widespread use of an increasing number of chemical compounds with analgesic, antipyretic, and anti-inflammatory properties. In order to remark their differences with other group of medicines which presents known bad side effects, they were labeled as nonsteroidal anti-inflammatory drugs with the acronym NSAIDs [1–3].

At the same time, many neuroinflammatory mediators, including oxidative agents such as reactive oxygen species (ROS), were found to be upregulated in neurodegenerative disorders (ND) that affect human brain areas [4, 5]. This fact immediately allows the proposal of some kind of cause-effect link between the presence of ROS, oxidation processes, neuroinflammation, and ND pathogenesis [4, 5].

Oxidative stress is a process that occurs in early stages of ND and is considered an identifier mark for their detection as could be evaluated by DNA, RNA, lipids, and protein oxidation levels [6–8]. Simultaneously, several studies have observed an inverse correspondence between prolonged NSAID administration and the development of some ND in humans, (for review, see Ref. [9]). So, it is now accepted that NSAIDs could play a protective role on many ND and one of the reasons of the great interest for getting more insight into the elucidation of the pathways and mechanisms of the oxidative processes in which several NSAIDs and different ROS take part.

The present chapter will analyze the results presented in two relatively recent papers that have been dedicated to evaluate the possible action of some NSAIDs as protectors against ROS-mediated oxidation/deterioration of biological targets [10, 11]. Those research works are focused on NSAIDs from different chemical structure classes, one salicylic acid derivative, diflunisal (DFN), an indolic acid derivative, indomethacin (IMT) (**Figure 1**) and the enolic acid derivatives, oxicams, represented by meloxicam (MEL), tenoxicam (TEN) and piroxicam (PIR) (**Figure 2**).

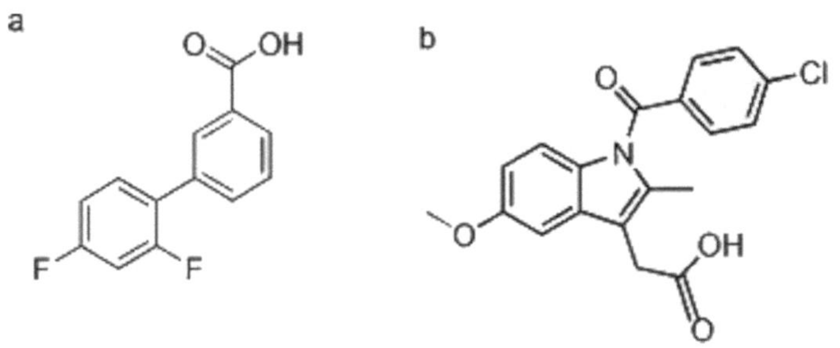

Figure 1. Chemical structures of **a:** 2′,4′-difluoro-4-hydroxyphenyl-3-carboxylic acid, diflunisal (DFN) and **b:** 2-{1′-[(4-chlorophenyl)carbonyl]-5-methoxy-2-methyl-1H-indol-3-yl} acetic acid, indomethacin (IMT).

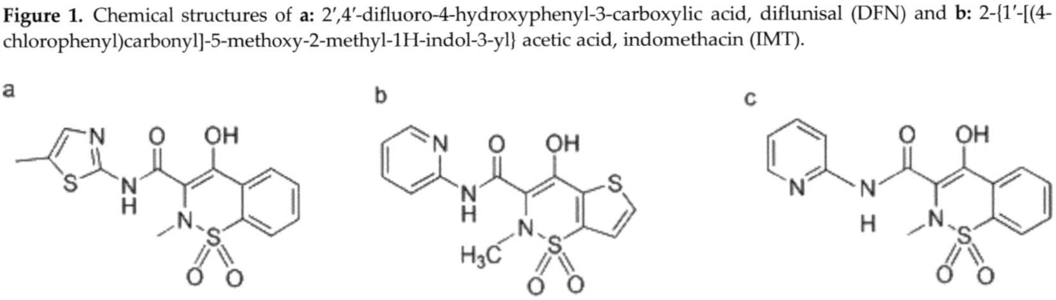

Figure 2. Chemical structures of **a:** [4-hydroxy-2-methyl-N-(5-methyl-2-thiazolyl)-2H-1,2-benzothiazine-3-carboxamide 1,1 dioxide], meloxicam (MEL), **b:** [4-hydroxy-2-methyl-N-(pyridin-2-yl)-2H-thieno(2,3-e)-1,2 thiazine-3-carboxamide 1,1-dioxide], tenoxicam (TEN) and **c:** [4-hydroxy-2-methyl-N-(pyridin-2-yl)-2H-1,2-benzothiazine-3-carboxamide 1,1-dioxide], piroxicam (PIR).

2. Oxidation processes

Many compounds in the presence of oxygen and any electron donor can generate different ROS—by energy and/or electron transfer processes—like singlet molecular oxygen, $O_2(^1\Delta_g)$, superoxide radical anion ($O_2^{\bullet-}$) or hydrogen peroxide (H_2O_2) among others. An interesting example of those compounds is vitamin B2, riboflavin (Rf), a naturally occurring endogenous compound of singular importance, present in practically all living organisms. Rf absorbs energy in the wavelength range of visible light, being a well-known photosensitizer for oxidative processes [12, 13]. Upon selective absorption of energy, Rf is promoted from its ground state to electronically excited singlet state ($^1Rf^*$) (Eq. (1)).

$$Rf + h\upsilon \rightarrow {}^1Rf^* \quad (1)$$

The generated $^1Rf^*$ can decay to the original ground state or produce the electronically excited triplet state ($^3Rf^*$) (Eq. (2)).

$$^1Rf^* \rightarrow {}^3Rf^* \quad (2)$$

The $^3Rf^*$ may react with the ground state oxygen ($O_2(^3\Sigma_g^-)$) (Eq. (3)) to form superoxide radical anion ($O_2^{\bullet-}$), with a very low quantum yield (0.009) (Krishna, 1991).

$$^3Rf^*(^3\Sigma_g^-) \rightarrow Rf^{\bullet+} + O_2^{\bullet-} \quad (3)$$

In living organisms, a great number of biomolecules essential to life such as DNA, RNA, lipids, and proteins, can be oxidized by the generated ROS producing oxidative stress [6–8, 14]. Among other substrates, NSAIDs are compounds that can be oxidized in the presence of Rf-generated ROS and as shown can act as quenchers of electronically excited states of Rf (Eqs. (4) and (5)).

$$^1Rf^* + NSAIDs \rightarrow Rf + NSAIDs \text{ or } P(4) \;\; \text{rate constant } {}^1k_q \quad (4)$$

$$^3Rf^* + NSAIDs \rightarrow Rf^{\bullet-} + NSAIDs^{\bullet+} \;\; \text{rate constant } {}^3k_q \quad (5)$$

The protonation of $Rf^{\bullet-}$ at neutral pH can generate the species $RfH^{\bullet}$ ($pK_a = 8.3$), (Eq. (6)).

$$Rf^{\bullet-} + H^+ \rightleftarrows RfH^{\bullet} \quad (6)$$

Its bimolecular decay through a disproportionation reaction can yield the ground state of the vitamin and fully reduced Rf (Eq. (7)).

$$2RfH^{\bullet} \rightarrow Rf + RfH_2 \quad (7)$$

The last product, in the presence of ground state oxygen, is reoxidized to Rf radical and superoxide radical anion ($O_2^{\bullet-}$) (Eq. (8)).

$$RfH_2 + O_2(^3\Sigma_g^-) \rightarrow RfH_2^{\bullet+} + O_2^{\bullet-} \quad \text{rate constant } k_8 \tag{8}$$

The electron transfer process, in Eq. (8) is relevant as a source of H_2O_2 (Eq. (9)), another important already-mentioned ROS.

$$RfH_2^{\bullet+} + O_2^{\bullet-} \rightarrow Rf + H_2O_2 \tag{9}$$

In parallel, the generated $O_2^{\bullet-}$ can chemically react with a substrate, according to Eqs. (10) and (11), respectively, illustrates the processes that occur with NSAIDs.

$$O_2^{\bullet-}\ \text{NSAIDs} \rightarrow P(10) \quad \text{rate constant } k_{10} \tag{10}$$

$$H_2O_2 + \text{NSAIDs} \rightarrow P(11) \tag{11}$$

Another possible pathway for $^3Rf^*$ is the energy transfer reaction with $O_2(^3\Sigma_g^-)$ which generates $O_2(^1\Delta_g)$, with reported quantum yield of 0.49 in water [15] (Eq. (12)).

$$^3Rf^* + O_2(^3\Sigma_g^-) \rightarrow Rf + O_2(^1\Delta_g) \text{ rate constant } k_{ET} \tag{12}$$

The $O_2(^1\Delta_g)$ formed may be physically quenched either by the solvent (Eq. (13)).

$$O_2(^1\Delta_g) \rightarrow O_2(^3\Sigma_g^-) \tag{13}$$

or by a substrate, as happens in the presence of NSAIDs (Eq. (14)).

$$O_2(^1\Delta_g) + \text{NSAIDs} \rightarrow O_2(^3\Sigma_g^-) + \text{NSAIDs} \quad \text{rate constant } k_q \tag{14}$$

Finally, Eq. (15) represents the main pathway of substrate disappearance in $O_2(^1\Delta_g)$ mediated processes.

$$O_2(^1\Delta_g) + \text{NSAIDs} \rightarrow P(15) \text{ rate constant } k_r \tag{15}$$

k_t being the overall rate constant for physical plus chemical quenching processes (Eq. (16)).

$$k_t = k_r + k_q \tag{16}$$

In order to get more insight into the behavior of NSAIDs toward Rf-generated ROS several *in vitro* experiments were performed.

2.1. Stationary photolysis: riboflavin-photosensitization

In complex biological structures, Rf and NSAIDs may occupy the same locations. Kinetic and mechanistic aspects of their mutual interaction constitute the crucial information for understanding the behavior of NSAIDs toward Rf-generated ROS and the potential *in vivo* consequences.

Using a home-made photolyzer, aerated neutral aqueous solutions of each of the following NSAIDs DFN, IMT, MEL, TEN, and PIR, were irradiated with the light of a 150W quartz-halogen lamp, in the presence of Rf as a sensitizer. All the NSAIDs used as substrates are transparent to visible light. Nevertheless, in order to assure that they do not absorb any incident radiation, a cut-off filter at 400 nm was employed. The processes were followed by the absorption spectra using a diode array spectrophotometer (Hewlett Packard 8452A). The light irradiation induced changes in the absorption spectra of the mixtures 0.05 mM DFN + 0.04 Rf (**Figure 3**), 0.05 mM IMT + 0.04 mM Rf (**Figure 3**, inset A) and 0.05 mM MEL + 0.04 mM Rf (**Figure 4**). The processes could be monitored from the absorbance decay at the respective absorption maxima for each substrate. In this way, the rates of sensitized photoxygenation for each NSAID were determined.

In parallel experiments, using a specific oxygen electrode (Orion 97-08) the oxygen concentration was measured during irradiation of the same mixtures in aqueous solutions in a closed Pyrex cell [10]. Under these conditions, all the NSAIDs under study showed oxygen consumption. Regarding the oxicams family, TEN and PIR presented the lowest rate of oxygen consumption. It was a little bit higher for MEL (**Figure 4**, inset B). In the corresponding set for DFN and IMT, the rate of oxygen uptake was significantly higher for the latter (**Figure 3**, inset B).

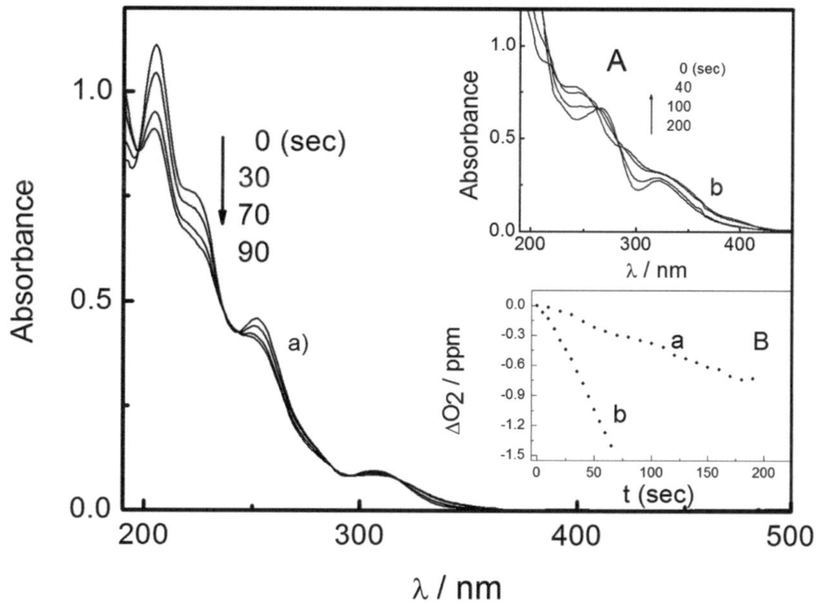

Figure 3. Changes in UV-vis absorption spectra of a pH 7 aqueous solution of 0.05 mM DFN plus 0.04 mM Rf upon photoirradiation taken vs. a 0.04 mM Rf aqueous solution (spectrum **a**). Cut-off 400 nm interference filter, under air-saturated conditions. Numbers on the spectra represent photoirradiation time in seconds. (**Inset A**) Changes in UV-vis absorption spectrum of a pH 7 aqueous solution of 0.05 mM IMT plus 0.04 mM Rf upon photoirradiation taken vs. a 0.04 mM Rf aqueous solution (spectrum **b**). Cut-off 400 nm interference filter, under air-saturated conditions. Numbers on the spectra represent photoirradiation time in seconds. (**Inset B**) Oxygen consumption vs. photoirradiation time in pH 7 aerated aqueous solutions for the systems: a: Rf (A_{446} = 0.46) plus DFN (0.4 mM); b: Rf (A_{446} = 0.46) plus ITM (0.4 mM). Reprinted from Purpora et al. [10], © (2013), with permission from The American Society of Photobiology, a Wiley Company, John Wiley & Sons, Inc.

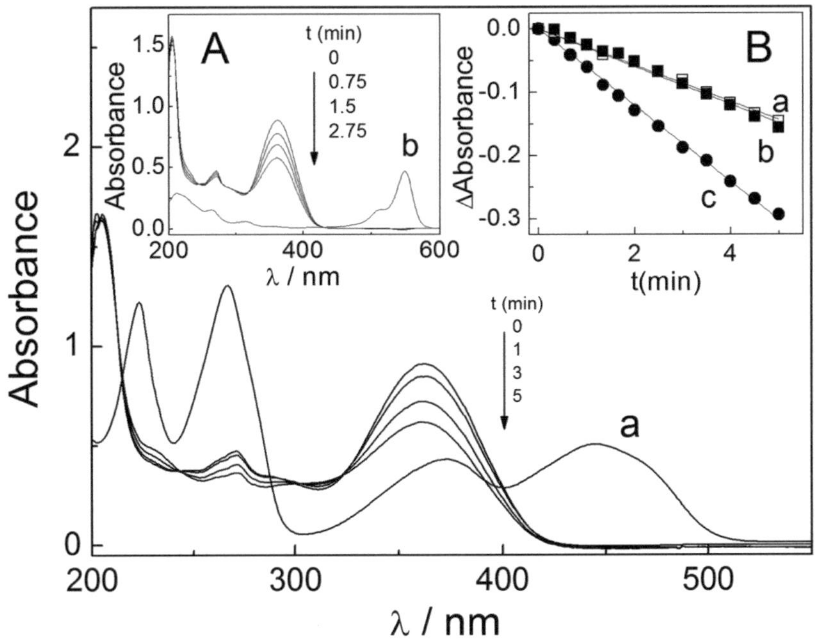

Figure 4. Changes in UV-vis absorption spectra of aqueous solution of 0.05 mM MEL plus 0.05 mM Rf upon photoirradiation taken vs. 0.05 mM Rf aqueous solution (spectrum **a**). Cut-off 450 nm interference filter, under air-saturated conditions. Numbers on the spectra represent photoirradiation time in minutes. (**Inset A)** Changes in UV-vis absorption spectra of aqueous solution of 0.05 mM MEL plus 0.05 mM RB upon photoirradiation taken vs. 0.05 mM RB aqueous solution (spectrum **b**). Cut-off 450 nm interference filter, under air-saturated conditions. Numbers on the spectra represent photoirradiation time in minutes. (**Inset B)** Oxygen consumption vs. photoirradiation time under air saturated conditions for the systems: a: Rf 0.05 mM plus TEN (0.5 mM) in MeOH-H_2O (buffer pH 7) 1:1 v/v; b: Rf 0.05 mM plus 0.5 mM *PIR* in MeOH-H_2O (buffer pH 7) 1:1 v/v; c: Rf 0.05 mM plus 0.5 mM MEL in aqueous buffer pH 7. $\lambda_{irr} > 480$ nm, cut-off filter. Reprinted from Ferrari et al. [11], © (2015), with permission from Elsevier B.V.

From all these preliminary findings, we assume that the transformations in NSAIDs can be attributed to interactions with electronically excited states of Rf with the possible participation of photogenerated ROS.

2.1.1. Kinetics and mechanism

The xantenic dye Rose Bengal (RB) is one of the most frequently employed photosensitizers that exclusively generate $O_2(^1\Delta_g)$, with a quantum yield of 0.7 in aqueous media [15, 16]. So, experiments performed in the presence of RB involved possible $O_2(^1\Delta_g)$-mediated oxidation of NSAIDs. In this case, eventual interferences of other ROS that could be generated by Rf were avoided. Comparing the rates of substrate consumption by Rf – photosensitization with those in the presence of RB it was possible to elucidate the relevance of $O_2(^1\Delta_g)$ in relation to other ROS also generated by Rf.

The combination of stationary and time-resolved experiments unambiguously demonstrates the participation of $O_2(^1\Delta_g)$ in NSAIDs' photooxidation processes. Using time-resolved phosphorescence detection (TRPD) [17], the overall quenching rate constant of $O_2(^1\Delta_g)$ by NSAIDs,

http://dx.doi.org/10.5772/66478

NSAID	$^1k_q \times 10^{10}(M^{-1}s^{-1})$	$^3k_q \times 10^9(M^{-1}s^{-1})$	$k_t \times 10^8(M^{-1}s^{-1})$	$k_r \times 10^8(M^{-1}s^{-1})$
IMT	0.89 ± 0.06 (a)	1.8 ± 0.3	2.6 ± 0.2	2.7 ± 0.2
DFN	0.90 ± 0.05 (a)	2.1 ± 0.5	1.7 ± 0.3	0.19 ± 0.1
MEL	2.84 ± 0.12	1.5 ± 0.3	1.15 ± 0.06 (b)	0.73 ± 0.04
TEN	0.88 ± 0.04	1.9 ± 0.4	1.00 ± 0.07 (c) (1.1) (d)	0.50 ± 0.03 (0.61) (d)
PIR	2.30 ± 0.06	1.7 ± 0.3	0.49 ± 0.05 (c)	0.48 ± 0.06 (1.6) (e)

(a) In MeOH; (b) in D_2O, pH 7; (c) in MeOH-D_2O (pD 7) 1:1 v/v; (d) in dioxane-water (molar fraction of water = 0.91) *Source*: [18]; (e) in MeCN *Source*: [19].

Table 1. Values for the rate constants for the interactions of each NSAID by quenching with electronically excited singlet (^1k_q), and triplet (^3k_q) of riboflavin; overall rate constants (k_t) **and reactive** (k_r) for the interaction of $O_2(^1\Delta_g)$ with each NSAID.

NSAID	k_r/k_t	RR_{Rf}	RR_{RB}
IMT	~1	1	1
DFN	0.11	0.26	0.07
MEL	0.63	1	1
TEN	0.52	0.48	0.68
PIR	~1.00	0.47	0.67

Source: [10, 11].

Table 2. Values for the ratio of the reactive and overall rates k_r/k_t, and relative rates of each NSAID consumption upon Rf (RR_{Rf}) and RB (RR_{RB}) photosensitization.

k_t (**Table 1**) was determined. Hence, k_t in the order of $10^7 M^{-1}s^{-1}$ allows the consideration of these substrates as good quenchers of $O_2(^1\Delta_g)$. The k_r/k_t ratio accounts for the fraction of the overall quenching of $O_2(^1\Delta_g)$ that produces chemical transformation in the substrate (**Table 2**). Low k_r/k_t values denote that $O_2(^1\Delta_g)$ removal will proceed without a significant loss of the present NSAIDs, which act as a scavenger [18, 19].

2.2. Interaction of NSAIDs with photogenerated ROS

Some compounds that are specific ROS quenchers have been used to elucidate which species are effectively involved in a given oxidative event [20, 21]. Catalase from bovine liver (CAT) reacts with H_2O_2, so the photodegradation via process in Eq. (11) is inhibited due to the process represented by Eq. (17).

$$2H_2O_2 + CAT \rightarrow 2H_2O + O_2(^3\Sigma_g^-) \quad (17)$$

The enzyme superoxide dismutase from bovine erythrocytes (SOD) dismutates the species $O_2^{\bullet-}$, as shown by Eq. (18).

$$2O_2^{\cdot -} + 2H^+ + SOD \rightarrow O_2(^3\Sigma_g^-) + H_2O_2 \tag{18}$$

Meanwhile, sodium azide (NaN_3) is a known physical quencher of $O_2(^1\Delta_g)$, with a reported rate constant k_q of 4.5 × 10^8 $M^{-1}s^{-1}$ in water at pH 7 (Eq. (14) with NaN_3 instead of NSAIDs) [22]. Several oxygen consumption experiments of NSAIDs upon Rf-photosensitization were performed adding each of these specific ROS interceptors. With DFN or IMT solutions different extent of decrease in the rates of oxygen consumption were observed upon using any of these three quenchers. This fact confirms a significant participation of $O_2(^1\Delta_g)$ in the degradation of

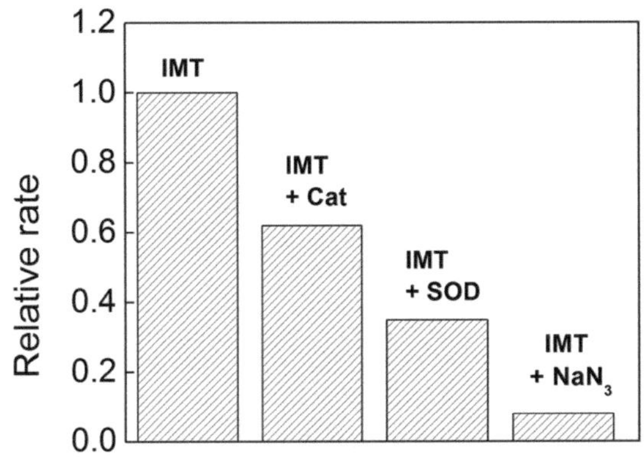

Figure 5. Bar diagrams for the relative rates of oxygen consumption with aqueous solutions pH 7, 0.5 mM IMT plus Rf (A_{445} = 0.5) as function of photoirradiation time (cut-off 400 nm): ITM: alone; IMT + CAT: in the presence of 1μg mL^{-1} CAT; IMT + SOD: in the presence of 1μg mL^{-1} SOD; IMT + NaN_3: in the presence of 1 mM NaN_3. Reprinted from Purpora et al. [10], © (2013), with permission from The American Society of Photobiology, a Wiley Company, John Wiley & Sons, Inc.

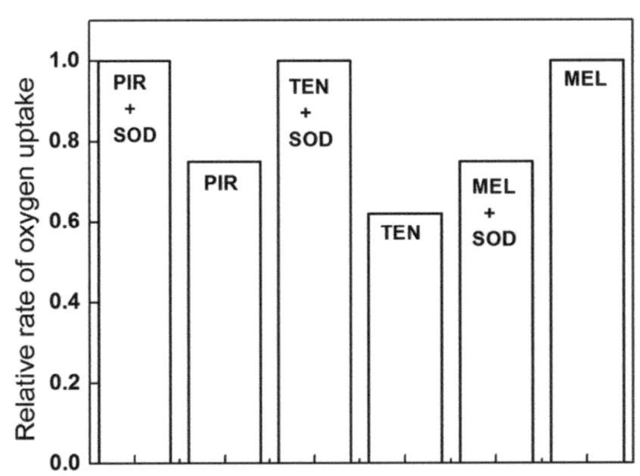

Figure 6. Bar diagrams for the relative rates of oxygen consumption upon photoirradiation as function of photoirration time (cut-off filter 400 nm) in the presence of Rf 0.05 mM with the following solutions: 0.5 mM PIR in MeOH-H_2O (buffer pH 7) 1:1 v/v plus 1 μg mL^{-1} SOD; 0.5 mM PIR in MeOH-H_2O (buffer pH 7) 1:1 v/v; 0.5 mM TEN in MeOH-H_2O (buffer pH 7) 1:1 v/v plus 1 μg mL^{-1} SOD; 0.5 mM TEN in MeOH-H_2O (buffer pH 7) 1:1 v/v; 0.5 mM MEL plus 1 μg mL^{-1} SOD in aqueous buffer pH 7; 0.5 mM MEL in aqueous buffer pH 7. Reprinted from Ferrari et al. [11], © (2015), with permission from Elsevier B.V.

http://dx.doi.org/10.5772/66478

the analgesics DFN and IMT, in which also $O_2^{\bullet-}$ and H_2O_2 take part. Bar diagram of the relative rates illustrates the results obtained with IMT solutions in the presence of each specific quencher (**Figure 5**); DFN solutions presented similar qualitative results.

Similar experiments were performed using solutions 0.5 mM of the three oxicams and *NaN*$_3$ NaN_3 or SOD. The participation of $O_2(^1\Delta_g)$ in the oxidation processes of these NSAIDs was revealed by the lower rates of oxygen uptake (**Figure 6**). As in the previous cases, for MEL the presence of SOD produced a decrease in the rates of oxygen consumption. Meanwhile for TEN and PIR it was the other way around. This fact can be due to the participation of $O_2^{\bullet-}$ with different mechanistic roles. The regeneration of $O_2(^3\Sigma_g^-)$ (Eq. (18)) at expenses of $O_2^{\bullet-}$ increases the $O_2(^1\Delta_g)$ leading to the detected rates increased.

3. Photoprotective effect of NSAIDs toward amino acids and peptides oxidation

In order to evaluate an eventual antioxidant/protective effect of NSAIDs towards biologically relevant substrates, amino acids (AA) and peptides may be employed as typical oxidizable targets in a proteinaceous medium.

Tryptophan (Trp) and tyrosine (Tyr) are AAs that can be affected by photo-damages through photodynamic activity [23, 24]. They are known quenchers of $^3Rf^*$ with ^3k_q of $2.5\times10^9 M^{-1}s^{-1}$ and $1.0\times10^9 M^{-1}s^{-1}$, respectively [13]. In order to evaluate the eventual protective effect of NSAIDs against photooxidation, Rf-photosensitized experiments were performed using each of these AA and the oxicam PIR. For comparative purposes, the trials were also performed replacing Rf by RB which ensures that the prevalent oxidation process is due to $O_2(^1\Delta_g)$. As a measure of the global photooxidative process, the rates of oxygen consumption were determined in each trial monitoring up to 10% conversion of the substrate under study.

PIR and Trp, as isolated substrates, are efficient $O_2(^1\Delta_g)$ chemical scavengers. Their k_r values are virtually identical, while the k_r/k_t relationship presents also very similar values. For the interaction Trp-$O_2(^1\Delta_g)$ it has been reported the rate constant values $k_t = 7.2\times10^7 M^{-1}s^{-1}$. and $k_t = 4.7\times10^7 M^{-1}s^{-1}$.[13, 25]. Using RB as the sensitizer, the rates of oxygen uptake for the mixture PIR + Trp were approximately equal to the rates of PIR and Trp individually considered, which may be due to the fact that they react through a pure $O_2(^1\Delta_g)$-mediated process (**Figure 7**). Employing Rf as the photosensitizer, the mixture PIR + Trp presented a rate of oxygen consumption significantly lower than the addition of the respective rates for each substrate. A possible explanation is that both compounds present a high ^3k_qvalue, so the simultaneous action of them may decrease the $O_2(^1\Delta_g)$ concentration leading to the lower rate observed with the presence of the mixture.

In neutral pH, Tyr is present in a very low reactive form. The interaction Tyr with $O_2(^1\Delta_g)$ mostly operates by physical deactivation of the ROS with a reported rate constant value

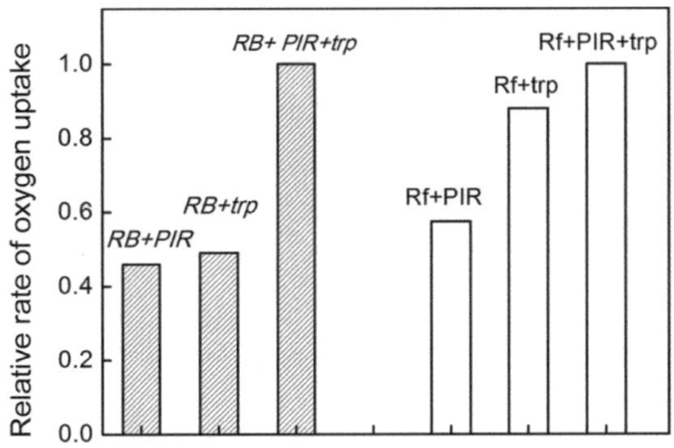

Figure 7. Bar diagrams for the relative rates of oxygen consumption upon RB (A_{560} = 0.4) photosensitization in pH 7 buffered aqueous solution by: 0.5 mM PIR; 0.5 mM Trp; 0.5 mM PIR plus 0.5 mM Trp. And upon Rf (A_{445} = 0.5) photosensitization in pH 7 buffered aqueous solution by: 0.5 mM PIR; 0.5 mM Trp; 0.5 mM PIR plus 0.5 mM Trp. Reprinted from Ferrari et al. [11], © (2015), with permission from Elsevier B.V.

$k_t = 1.5 \times 10^7 M^{-1}s^{-1}$ [22, 26]. The very low k_r/k_t may be due to the clear decrease in the rate of oxygen uptake by the mixture PIR + Tyr as compared to the one for the isolated PIR with RB as the photosensitizer. (**Figure 8**) With Rf as a sensitizer, the corresponding rates for PIR alone and the one for the mixture are practically equal.

A relevant result was that PIR in the presence of Rf showed an interesting degree of protection against Trp or Tyr oxidation by the *in situ*-photogenerated ROS. This fact has been revealed by

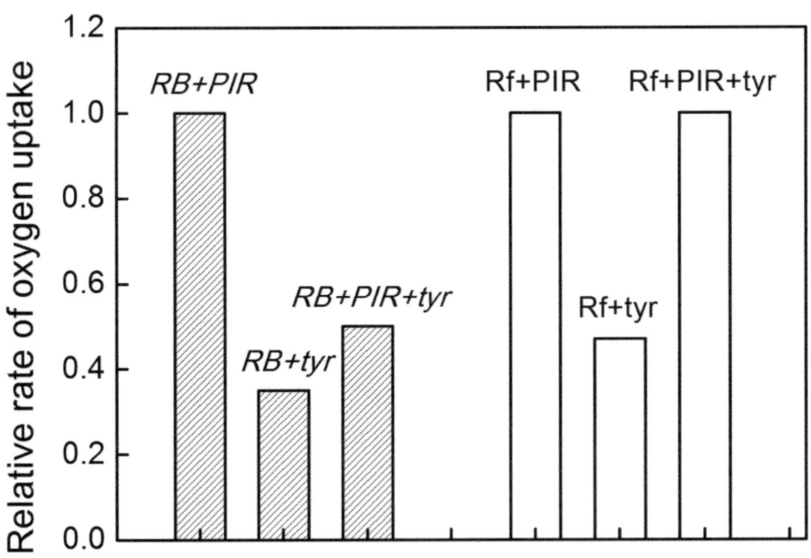

Figure 8. Bar diagrams for the relative rates of oxygen consumption upon RB (A_{560} = 0.4) photosensitization in pH 7 buffered aqueous solution by: 0.5 mM PIR; 0.5 mM Tyr; 0.5 mM PIR plus 0.5 mM Tyr. And upon Rf (A_{445} = 0.5) photosensitization in pH 7 buffered aqueous solution by: 0.5 mM PIR; 0.5 mM Tyr; 0.5 mM PIR plus 0.5 mM Tyr. Reprinted from Ferrari et al. [11], © (2015), with permission from Elsevier B.V.

the lower rates of oxygen consumption of the mixture oxicam-AA as compared to the ones for the individual substrates.

The dipeptide Trp-Tyr in a 0.5 mM aqueous solution was employed as a biologically relevant model compound, with RB or Rf as photosensitizers and IMT or DFN as potential photoprotective substrates. The $O_2(^1\Delta_g)$- mediated process of Trp-Tyr could be studied using RB alone. Its rate constant value $k_r = 5.9 \times 10^7 M^{-1} s^{-1}$ had already been reported [24]. The comparison of the relative rates of oxygen consumption in the presence and in the absence of 0.5 mM IMT showed that the value for the mixture Trp-Tyr + IMT was close to the simple addition of the respective individual rates (**Figure 9**).

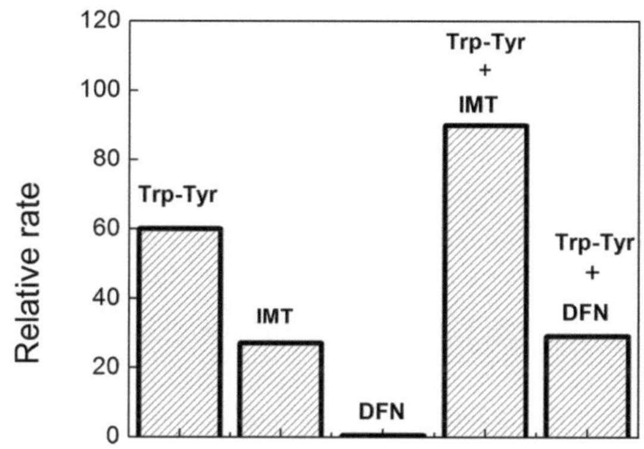

Figure 9. Bar diagram for the relative rates of oxygen consumption upon RB (A_{560} = 0.4) photosensitization in pH 7 buffered aqueous solution of: 0.5 mM Trp-Tyr; 0.5 mM IMT; 0.5 mM DFN; 0.5 mM Trp-Tyr plus 0.5 IMT; 0.5 mM Trp-Tyr plus 0.5 DFN. Reprinted from Purpora et al. [10], © (2013), with permission from The American Society of Photobiology, a Wiley Company, John Wiley & Sons, Inc.

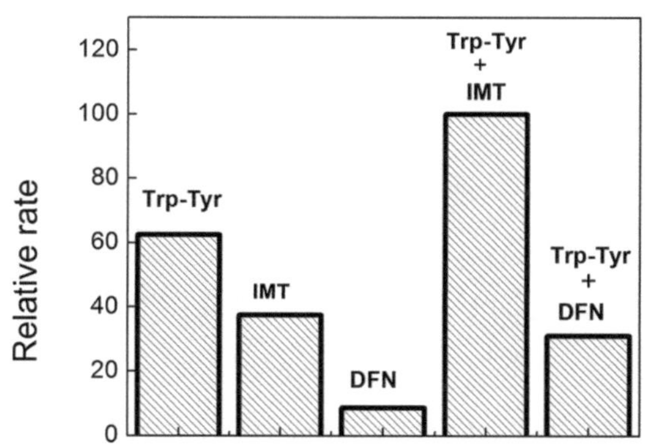

Figure 10. Bar diagram for the relative rates of oxygen consumption upon Rf (A_{445} = 0.5) photosensitization in pH 7 buffered aqueous solution of: 0.5 mM Trp-Tyr; 0.5 mM IMT; 0.5 mM DFN; 0.5 mM Trp-Tyr plus 0.5 IMT; 0.5 mM Trp-Tyr plus 0.5 DFN. Reprinted from Purpora et al. [10], © (2013), with permission from The American Society of Photobiology, a Wiley Company, John Wiley & Sons, Inc.

Meanwhile, the rate for the mixture Trp-Tyr + DFN decreased more than 50% of the one for the isolated dipeptide. Upon Rf-sensitization, similar results were obtained for DFN and IMT (**Figure 10**). This fact suggested that the photoxidation occurs mainly by reaction with the Rf-photogenerated $O_2(^1\Delta_g)$.

4. Conclusions

The results presented for the NSAIDs under study pointed out their efficiency as quenchers of photogenerated $O_2(^1\Delta_g)$. In Rf-photosensitized processes the dominant mechanism is the $O_2(^1\Delta_g)$-mediated, but also other ROS can be intercepted by most of them. The experiments here detailed showed that DFN and IMT can interact with H_2O_2 and $O_2^{\cdot-}$ whereas MEL is an effective quencher for the latter Rf-photogenerated species.

DNF could be considered as an ideal scavenger of $O_2(^1\Delta_g)$, as the oxidative process occurs by a physical mechanism without significant self-degradation of this NSAID. In the case of IMT or oxicams, their protective effect decline along the time. The reason is that these scavengers can also be targets of the oxidation ROS-mediated processes. Even though, the *in vivo* antioxidant effectiveness would be warranted by daily and prolonged intake. Generally, that is the form of administration in which these analgesics are employed in the treatment of serious detrimental inflammatory illness or chronic pains.

Based on the discussed results, the NSAIDs studied herein present, in principle, promising properties for medicinal use as bio-antioxidants against *in situ* generated ROS. Nevertheless, great care must be taken because at the same time different negative effects in the human body have been reported [27, 28]. The literature on this topic, in most cases, only mentions rare but possible gastrointestinal adverse effects [29]. In the case of DFN, the reported side effects are not so dramatic, but IMT and MEL have been connected to the pathogenesis of gastric and intestinal mucosal lesions with participation of ROS [30–32]. Those undesired effects must be thoroughly taken into account mainly because of the relative high doses necessary with some of them in order to guarantee the replenishment, ensuring the antioxidant effectiveness against ROS activity.

Author details

Norman A. García[1], Mabel Bregliani[2] and Adriana Pajares[2,3]*

*Address all correspondence to: apajares@live.com

1 Río Cuarto National University, Río Cuarto, Argentina

2 Austral Patagonia National University, Río Gallegos, Argentina

3 San Juan Bosco Patagonia National University, Comodoro Rivadavia, Argentina

References

[1] Page C., Curtis M., Sutter M., Walker M., Hoffman B.B. Integrated Pharmacology. 2nd ed. Maryland Heights, Missouri, USA: Mosby; 2002. 688 p.

[2] Dudley Hart F., Huskisson E.C. Non-steroidal anti-inflammatory drugs. Current status and rational therapeutic use. Drugs. 1984;**27**(3):232–255.

[3] Buer J.K. Origins and impact of the term "NSAID". Inflammopharmacol. 2014;**22**:263–267.

[4] McGeer E.G., McGeer P.L. Inflammatory processes in Alzheimer disease. Prog. Neuro-Psicoph. 2003;**27**:741–749.

[5] Dumont M., Flint Beal M. Neuroprotective strategies involving ROS in Alzheimer disease. Free Radic. Biol. Med. 2011;**51**:1014–1026.

[6] Lovell M.A., Markesbery W.R. Oxidative damage in mild cognitive impairment and early Alzheimer's disease. J. Neurosci. Res. 2007;**85**:3036–3040.

[7] Markesbery W.R., Lovell M.A. Damage to lipids, proteins, DNA, and RNA in mild cognitive impairment. Arch. Neurol. 2007;**64**:954–956.

[8] Choi W., Lee Y.J., Hong J.T., Lee H.J. Antioxidant properties of natural polyphenols and therapeutic to potentials for Alzheimer disease . Brain Res. Bull. 2012;**87**:2–3.

[9] Esposito E., Di Matteo V., Benigno A., Pierucci M., Crescimanno G., Di Giovanni G. Non-steroidal anti-inflammatory drugs in Parkinson's disease. Exp. Neurol. 2007;**205**:295–312.

[10] Purpora R., Massad W., Ferrari G., Reynoso E., Criado S., Miskoski S., Pajares A.M., García N.A. The NSAIDs indomethacin and diflunisal as scavengers of photogenerated reactive oxygen species. Photochem. Photobiol. 2013;**89**:1463–1470.

[11] Ferrari G., Natera J., Montaña M.P., Muñoz V., Gutierrez E., Massad W., Miskoski S., García N.A. Scavenging of photogenerated ROS by oxicams. Possible biological and environmental implications. J. Photochem. Photobiol. B: Biol. 2015;**153**:233–239.

[12] Heelis P.F. The photophysical and photochemical properties of flavins (isoalloxazines). Chem. Soc. Rev. 1982;**11**(1):15–39.

[13] Hellis P.F. Chemistry and Biochemistry of Flavoenzymes. Boca Ratón, FL: Muller F; 1991.

[14] Berlett B.S., Stadtman E.R. Protein oxidation in aging, disease, oxidative stress. J. Biol. Chem. 1997;**272**(33):20313–20316.

[15] Wilkinson F., Helman W.P., Ross A.B. Quantum yields for the photosensitized formation of the lowest electronically excited singlet state of molecular oxygen in solution. J. Phys. Chem. Ref. 1993;**22**:133–262. DOI: 10.1063/1.55593

[16] Lambert C.R., Kochevar I.E. Does rose bengal generate superoxide anion? J. Am. Chem. Soc. 1996;**118**:3297–3298.

[17] Neumann M., García N.A. . Kinetics and mechanism of the light-induced deterioration of lemon oil. J. Agric. Food Chem. 1992;**40**(6):957–960. DOI: 10.1021/jf00018a008

[18] Lemp E., Günther G., Zanocco S.A. Sensitized photooxigenation of piroxicam in neat solvents and solvent mixtures. J. Photochem. Photobiol. B: Biol. 2001;**65**:165–170. DOI: 10.1016/S1011-1344(01)00265-2

[19] Günther G., Lemp E., Zanocco S.A. Determination of chemical rate constants in singlet molecular oxygen reactions by using 1,4-dimethylnaphthalene endoperoxide. J. Photochem. Photobiol. A: Chem. 2002;**151**:1–5. DOI: 10.1016/S1010-6030(02)00175-2

[20] Silva E., Edwards D., Pacheco D. Visible light-induced photooxidation of glucose sensitized by riboflavin. J. Nutr. Biochem. 1999;**10**(3):181–185. DOI: 10.1016/S0955-2863(98) 00093-X

[21] Escalada J.P., Pajares A., Bregliani M., Biasutti A., Criado S., Molina P., et al. Kinetic aspects of the photodegradation of phenolic and lactonic biocides under natural and artificial conditions. In: Litter M.I., Candal R.J., Meitrich J.M., editors. Advanced Oxidation Technologies: Sustainable Solutions for Environmental Treatments. 2nd ed. The Netherlands: CRC Press; 2014. pp. 59–80.

[22] Wilkinson W.P., Helman W.P., Ross A.B. Rate constants for the decay and reactions of the lowest electronically excited state of molecular oxygen in solution. An extended and revised compilation. J. Phys. Chem. Ref. 1995;**24**(2):663–1021. DOI: 10.1063/1.555965

[23] Straight R.C., Spikes J.D. Photosensitized oxidation of biomolecules. In: Frimer A.A., editor. In Singlet O_2. Boca Ratón, FL, USA: CRC Press; 1985. pp. 91–143.

[24] Posadaz A., Biasutti A., Casale C., Sanz J., Amat-Guerri F., García N.A. Rose bengal-sensitized photooxidation of the dipeptides Trp-Phe, Trp-Tyr and Trp-Trp. Kinetics, mechanism and photoproducts. Photochem. Photobiol. 2004;**80**:132–138. DOI: 10.1562/2004-03-03-RA-097

[25] Görner H. Oxygen uptake after electron transfer from amines, amino acids and ascorbic acid to triplet flavins in air-saturated aqueous solution. J. Photochem. Photobiol. B: Biol. 2007;**87**(2):73–80. DOI: 10.1016/j.jphotobiol.2007.02.003

[26] García N. A. Singlet molecular oxygen mediated photodegradation of aquatic phenolic pollutants. A kinetic and mechanistic overview. J. Photochem. Photobiol. B: Biol. 1994;**22**(3):185–196. DOI: 10.1016/1011-1344(93)06932-S

[27] Takeiuchi K, Ueshima K., Hironaka Y., Fuyioka Y., Matsumoto J., Okabe S. Oxygen free radicals and lipid peroxidation in the pathogenesis of gastric mucosal lesions induced by indomethacin in rats. Digestion. 1991;**49**:175–184.

[28] Harirforoosh S., Asghar W., Jamali F. Adverse effects of nonsteroidal antiinflammatory drugs: An update of gastrointestinal, cardiovascular and renal complications. J. Pharm. Pharm. Sci. 2013;16(5):821–847.

[29] Evanson N. K. Diflunisal. xPharm: The Comprehensive Pharmacology Reference. 2007; pp. 1–5.

[30] Ganguly K., Kundu P., Banerjee A., Reiter R.J., Swarnakar S. Hydrogen peroxide-mediated down regulation of matrix metalloprotease-2 in indomethacin-induced acute gastric ulceration is blocked by melatonin and other antioxidants. Free Radic. Biol. Med. 2006;**41**:911–925.

[31] Yadav S. K., Adhikary B., Bandyopadhyay S.K., Chattopadhyay S. Inhibition of TNF-α, and NF-κB and JNK pathways accounts for the prophylactic action of the natural phenolic, allylpyrocatechol against indomethacin gastropathy. Biochim. Biophys. Acta. 2013;**1830**:3776–3786.

[32] Villegas I., Alarcón de la Lastra C., La Casa C., Motilva V., Martín M. J. Effects of food intake and oxidative stress on intestinal lesions caused by meloxicam and piroxicam in rats. Eur. J. Pharmacol. 2001;**414**:79–86.

Section 3

Alternative Therapies for Pain Relief

Chapter 13

Effect of Nonpharmacological Therapies on Pain and Health Perception in Patients with Knee Osteoarthritis

Paweł Lizis, Wojciech Kobza, Grzegorz Mańko,
Marcin Sitarz and Jarosław Pyka

Additional information is available at the end of the chapter

http://dx.doi.org/10.5772/66477

Abstract

Objective: Comparing the efficiency of ultrasound therapy (US) versus extracorporeal shock wave therapy (ESWT) on pain and perceived health in men with bilateral knee osteoarthritis (OA). **Design**: A pilot randomized trial with concealed allocation, assessor blinding and intention-to-treat analysis was conducted.

Participants: 60 men, 44–66 years old were randomized to an experimental (US) and a control (ESWT) group. **Intervention:** The participants in both groups attended 5-week treatments. The experimental group received continuous US and a series of 10 treatments two times per week. The control group received 5 ESWT treatments once per week. **Outcome measures:** The primary outcome was visual analogue scale (VAS) pain ratings. The secondary outcome measured perceived health using the Western Ontario and McMaster Universities Osteoarthritis Index (WOMAC). The examinations were taken before and after the treatment. **Results:** After 5-week treatment the experimental group had significantly worse scores than the control group on the VAS for pain, and on the WOMAC for perceived health. **Conclusion:** Patients with knee OA can achieve significant better health benefits caused by ESWT than by US.

Keywords: ultrasound, extracorporeal shock wave therapy, pain, perceived health, randomized trial

1. Introduction

Osteoarthritis (OA) is a chronic and degenerative disease and is considered to be one of the most common musculoskeletal disorders. Joints found in our body can be affected by OA. All the patients with OA have almost the same symptoms, including pain, stiffness, articular instability, limitation of motion and physical activity, and muscle weakness [1, 2]. Physiotherapy is one of the treatments that provides effective nonpharmacological interventions for people with knee OA, and procedures prescribed by physiotherapists are considered to be important and to play a fundamental role in patients' treatment. The most common types of electrotherapy are ultrasound (US), transcutaneous electrical nerve stimulation (TENS), and now more often appearing extracorporeal shock wave therapy (ESWT). US, as a noninvasive treatment is used to create a controlled, microtrauma to local affected tissue in order to stimulate a healing response and microvascularization [3, 4]. The first use of ESWT was not for musculoskeletal disorders but to break up kidney stones. It was a coincident that someone noticed an osteoblastic response pattern during studies at animals in the 1980s [5]. Recently, ESWT has been used for pain relief and musculoskeletal disorders' treatment. It turned out that ESWT is also a noninvasive treatment, and the effectiveness of this method is comparable to surgery. It has not yet been fully explained how it exactly works, but it probably involves microdestructions—the application of ESWT causes microbreaks in avascular or poorly vascularized tissue, thus stimulating appropriate revascularization and stem cell growth. It also induces the release of enzymes, which affect nociceptors, resulting in localized analgesia, giving the significant reduction of activity limitations and short duration of the treatment [6].

Despite the advances in the treatment, there is lack of comparative studies on the effects of US and ESWT in patients with knee OA. Therefore, the purpose of this study was to evaluate the effects of US versus ESWT protocol on pain measured by visual analogue scale (VAS), and on perceived health measured by WOMAC [7, 8] in men suffering from bilateral knee OA.

In our study we took hypothesis: there are differences between US and ESWT in reducing of pain, and improving perceived health in men suffering from bilateral knee OA.

Therefore the research question was

1. Is US more effective than ESWT on pain and perceived health in men with bilateral knee OA?

2. Method

2.1. Design

It was a randomized trial with concealed allocation, assessor blinding, and intention-to-treat analysis. The participants with knee OA were assessed for eligibility by an independent physician who was not involved into the study. The randomization into an experimental group (US) and a control group (ESWT) with a 1:1 ratio was generated by permuted block randomization using the website www.random.org. The randomization was achieved by having the participant selected one from 60 sealed opaque envelopes, each containing a group allocation, which had been prepared and shuffled by an independent investigator who was not involved into the recruitment or assessment of the participants. The researchers responsible for assessing the outcomes and analyzing the data were blinded to the type of the treatment procedure.

To keep the assessors blinded the participants were reminded before each measurement not to reveal the nature of their treatment. The participants were considered to be unaware of the group allocation because they were informed about the existence of two intervention groups but not about the study hypothesis. The data were obtained at baseline and 5 weeks later (immediately after the intervention period).

2.2. Participants and center

The inclusion criteria for participation in the study were: minimum age of 40, not currently receiving any physical therapy treatments for the knee OA condition, medication compliance (all patients were taking glucocorticoids at the time of the study), and the diagnosis of bilateral knee OA according to the American College of Rheumatology criteria [9].

The exclusion criteria were: any rheumatic disease (with the exception of bilateral knee OA), unilateral knee OA, skin changes, neurological disorders, mental illness, cancer, endocrinology disease, or previous knee surgery.

The evaluations of this study were conducted at the Physiotherapy Outpatient Department of the Regional Hospital in Zywiec, Poland. This study was designed with respect for the rules of conducting experimental studies with humans after the approval by the Bioethical Committee at the Holycross College in Kielce, and were consistent with the Helsinki Declaration of 1975 as revised in 2000. All participants signed consent forms knowingly participation in the study.

2.3. Intervention

The participants in both groups attended 5-week treatments. The experimental group received continuous US waves: intensity, 0.8 W/cm^2; 100% fill; carrier frequency, 1 MHz. The patients received a series of 10 treatments 2 times per week. The treatments were performed using a US 13 EVO Cosmogamma (Emildue, Italy). The patients lied in a supine position. The acoustic gel, that was applied, did not contain any pharmacologically active substance. The medial and lateral parts of the knee were treated with US applied in circular movements. To ensure the best absorption of the energy the probe was put at right angles. Each treatment session did not last longer than 10 minutes. During the treatment the patients received neither any anesthetic nor other physical actions. No adverse events were observed during the treatment. The same therapist made US to all the participants.

The control group received ESWT – 1000 pulses during the first treatment, 1500 during the second and the third treatments, and 2000 during the fourth and the fifth treatments, respectively (pressure, 2.5 bar; frequency, 8 Hz; energy density, 0.4 mJ/mm^2). The patients received 5 ESWT treatments once per week. The treatments were performed using a Rosetta ESWT (CR Technology, Korea). The patients were placed in a supine position with the affected knee unbent or flexed at 90°, and an acoustic gel that did not contain any pharmacologically active substance was applied. The shockwave probe was held stationary on a trigger point around the knee or at the patellofemoral and tibiofemoral borders of the target knee, avoiding direct placement on the peroneal nerve or vessel. Each treatment session did not exceed 10 minutes. During the treatments, the patients did not receive any other physical method.

No adverse events were observed during the treatment. The same therapist made ESWT to all the participants.

All of the treatments were performed at the Physiotherapy Outpatient Department of the Regional Hospital in Zywiec, Poland. Once a week for 5 weeks, the treatments were administered by an independent researcher who was not involved into this study. The same physiotherapist with a postgraduate degree in physiotherapy and 10 years' experience provided all the interventions to both (the experimental and the control) groups, and remained blind to primary and secondary outcome measures throughout the trial. The independent researcher analyzed the results/data also being blind to all of outcome measures throughout the trial.

2.4. Outcome measures

Primary outcome: The pain was assessed using a visual analogue scale (VAS), and a Laitinen scale. VAS is a line of 10 cm, the leftmost side is 0 = no pain and the far right is 10 = unbearable pain. The participants marked the scale of their current level of pain after their usual daily activities. The values in centimeters were recorded for statistical analysis. The same therapist administrated the measurements of all the participants and was blinded to the treatment.

Secondary outcome: In order to identify a specific index of disability there was used the WOMAC as a subjective measure of perceived health. It is a questionnaire that consists of three parts of questions and can be filled in a few minutes. There were 24 questions: about pain (5 questions), about stiffness (2 questions), and about physical function (17 questions) [10, 11]. In our study, we used a more detailed Likert scale version of the WOMAC, which includes a five-point scale for patients to mark (0 = none, 1 = mild, 2 = moderate, 3 = severe, and 4 = extreme). Achieving higher score means lower level of perceived health. All the scores were summed and coded. Answering the questions the patients described their stays during the past 3 days. The same therapist made the measurements to all the participants and was blinded to the treatment.

2.5. Data analysis

A priori sample size was determined in this study, giving the anticipated Cohen's d effect size of 0.8, the probability level of 5%, and the desired statistical test power level of 80%. We estimated that we needed minimum 26 participants in each group. The data were analyzed with descriptive as mean, standard deviation (SD) of two groups, mean (SD) within-group differences, 95% CI (95% confidence interval) of mean between-group differences, and inferential techniques. The mean within-group differences and the mean between-group differences (95% CI) were calculated for each of the outcomes based on the change scores (i.e., after minus before scores). The Shapiro-Wilk test identified the nonnormal distribution of the VAS and of the WOMAC data. The mean between-group differences for data was analyzed using the Mann-Whitney U test. To describe the differences in related treatments, the effect size between-group difference was calculated using Cohen's d, and classified as small (d = 0.2), moderate (d = 0.5), and large (d = 0.8) [12]. The level of statistical significance was set at a two-tailed p-value of 0.05. The analyses were performed by a blinded and independent statistician according to a prespecified statistical analysis plan on an intention-to-treat basis [13].

3. Results

3.1. Flow of participants through the study

A total of 75 participants that were admitted with bilateral knee OA between February and March 2016 were screened for inclusion. Fifteen patients were excluded based on the eligibility criteria. Therefore, the study reports the data of 60 participants. All of them agreed to participate and they were subsequently randomized: 30 in the experimental group (US) and 30 in the control group (ESWT), as presented in **Figure 1**. The baseline characteristics of participants are shown in **Table 1** and in the first two columns of data in **Table 2** and **Table 3**. No important differences in these characteristics were noted between the experimental and control groups.

3.2. Compliance with the study protocol

During the treatments the patients did not receive any anesthetic or any other physical actions. No participants received the wrong intervention. No adverse events were observed during the treatment. All the participants were analyzed in the group to which they had been randomly allocated.

3.3. Effect of intervention

Primary outcome: After the intervention in both, the experimental (US) and the control (ESWT), groups reduce of pain severity on VAS were identified. Pain severity decreased in the right knee, as well as in the left knee by the mean of 3 cm (±1) in the US group, whereas the ESWT group decreased in the right knee by the mean of 4 cm (±2), and in the left knee by the mean of 5 cm (±2). The significant between-group differences on the VAS score in the right knee and the left one were found. The ESWT group had lower score of pain severity on the VAS in the right and the left knees, by the mean of 2 cm (95% CI 1–3, $p < 0.001$, Cohen $d = 0.63$), and (95% CI 1–3, $p < 0.000$, Cohen $d = 1.26$), respectively. The effect size for pain on VAS was medium in the right knee and large in the left one, as presented in **Table 1**.

Secondary outcome: Regarding secondary outcomes, after the intervention in both, the experimental (US) and the control (ESWT), groups improvement of perceived health on WOMAC were identified. The domain "pain" (P) improved by the mean of 4 points (±2), the domain "stiffness" (ST) improved by the mean of 2 points (±2), the domain "physical function" (PF) improved by the mean of 17 points (±10), and the total score on WOMAC improved by the mean of 22 points (±11) in the US group. The ESWT group improved domain P by the mean of 10 points (±4), improved domain ST by the mean of 5 points (±1), improved domain PF by the mean of 29 points (±17), and improved the total score on WOMAC by the mean of 43 points (±20). The significant between-group differences were found. The ESWT group had better scores on the WOMAC for the domain P, by the mean of 6 points (95% CI 3–9, $p < 0.000$, Cohen $d = 1.90$), for domain ST, by the mean of 3 points (95% CI 2–5, $p = 0.002$, Cohen $d = 1.90$), for domain PF, by the mean of 12 points (95% CI 1–22, $p = 0.001$, Cohen $d = 0.86$). Consequently, a significant between-group difference on WOMAC was identified for total score of perceived health, with the mean of 20 points (95% CI 7 to 33, $p = 0.002$, Cohen $d = 1.30$) in favor for the

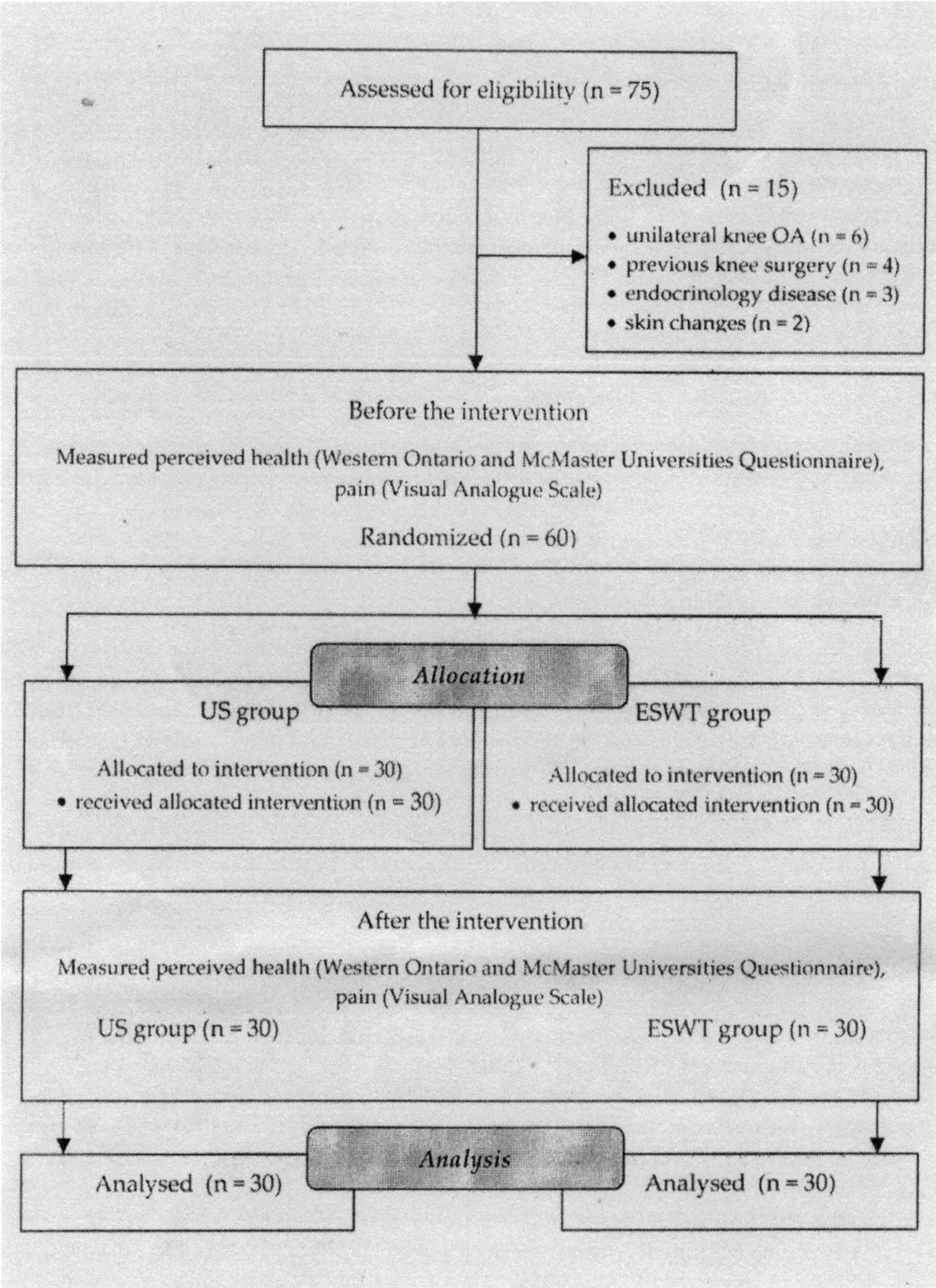

Figure 1. Recruitment and flow of participants through the trial.

Characteristic	Group Exp (n = 30)	Group Con (n = 30)
Age (yr) mean (SD)	55.2 (6.3)	55.8 (5.8)
Height (m) mean (SD)	1.75 (0.06)	1.77 (0.05)
Mass (kg) mean (SD)	74.5 (3.9)	75.8 (3.6)
BMI (kg/m^2) mean (SD)	24.15 (0.95)	24.35 (0.90)
Obese patients yes/no (n)	0/15	0/15
Level of education (n):		
Primary school graduates	3	5
Secondary school graduates	7	6
University graduates	5	4
Occupation:		
Physical worker/white-collar worker (n)	10/5	8/7
Duration of work (yr) mean (SD)	19.8 (6.1)	21.8 (5.6)
Duration of symptoms (yr) mean (SD)	8.9 (1.7)	8.3 (1.1)

Exp = ultrasound, US; Con = extracorporeal shock wave therapy (ESWT).

Table 1. Characteristics of the participants.

ESWT group. The effect size was large for perceived health on WOMAC, as presented in **Table 1**.

All of the outcomes show that greater reduce of pain severity leads to the better perceived health, which promotes generally better quality of life in the participants from the ESWT group than in the participants from the US group, as presented in **Tables 2** and **3**.

4. Discussion

A number of researches considered several aspects related to muscle function, such as strength and aerobic capacity as well as other clinical aspects, such as pain, stiffness, range of motion of the knee, and WOMAC in patients with OA [14–20].

Pain is one of the most common complaints and disability symptoms in patients with knee OA. The positive effects of nonpharmacologic management on knee pain and health status in OA patients were examined. Mascarin et al. [4] studied 40 patients and compared the TENS protocol with the US protocol. The TENS was applied using a frequency of 100 Hz, pulse width of 50 μs, intensity (mA) set at the individual subject's sensorial threshold, modulation up to 50% of variation frequency, quadratic biphasic symmetrical pulse and a length of application of 20 minutes. The US protocol consisted of continuous ultrasonic waves of 1

	Groups				Difference within groups		Difference between groups		
	Before		After		After–Before		After–Before		
	Exp (n = 30)	Con (n = 30)	Exp (n = 30)	Con (n = 30)	Exp (n = 30)	Con (n = 30)	Exp (n = 30)–Con (n = 30)	*p*	Effect size *(Cohen's d)*
VAS									
Right knee	6	6	3	2	–3	–4	2	0.001	0.63
	(1)	(2)	(1)	(2)	(1)	(2)	(1–3)		
Left knee	6	6	3	1	–3	–5	2	0.000	1.26
	(1)	(2)	(1)	(1)	(1)	(2)	(1–3)		

Exp = ultrasound, US; Con = extracorporeal shock wave therapy (ESWT); VAS = visual analogue scale.

Table 2. Mean (SD) of the groups, mean (SD) differences within the groups, and mean (95% CI) differences between the groups for VAS (in cm) outcomes.

http://dx.doi.org/10.5772/66477

	Groups				Difference within groups		Difference between groups		
	Before		After		After–Before		After–Before		
	Exp (n = 30)	Con (n = 30)	Exp (n = 30)	Con (n = 30)	Exp (n = 30)	Con (n = 30)	Exp (n = 30)–Con (n = 30)	*p*	Effect size *(Cohen's d)*
WOMAC									
P	14	14	10	4	–4	–10	6	0.000	1.90
	(4)	(5)	(5)	(2)	(2)	(4)	(3–9)		
ST	7	7	5	2	–2	–5	3	0.002	1.90
	(1)	(2)	(3)	(1)	(2)	(1)	(2–5)		
PF	52	52	34	23	–17	–29	12	0.001	0.86
	(14)	(18)	(15)	(13)	(10)	(17)	(1–22)		
Total	72	73	50	29	–22	–43	20	0.002	1.30
	(18)	(23)	(21)	(15)	(11)	(20)	(7–33)		

Exp = ultrasound, US; Con = extracorporeal shock wave therapy (ESWT); WOMAC = Western Ontario and McMaster Universities Osteoarthritis Index; *P* = pain; *ST* = stiffness; *PF* = physical function.

Table 3. Mean (SD) of the groups, mean (SD) differences within the groups, and mean (95% CI) differences between the groups for WOMAC (in points) outcomes.

wMHz frequency and 0.8 W/cm^2 power, applied with a 5-cm diameter applicator. The study results showed that TENS, as well as US, are effective for reducing pain and improving the WOMAC score. Ng et al. [21] studied 24 patients and compared electroacupuncture treatment and TENS, using the same parameters for both (low frequency = 2 Hz, continuous mode, pulsation of 200 μs for 20 minutes of application) and showed that either electroacupuncture treatment or TENS is effective in pain reduction because a prolonged analgesic effect maintained in the two groups.

Recently, ESWT has become one of the leading therapeutic alternatives. It can treat such diseases as chronic tendinopathies, nonunion of long bone fracture, and early stage of avascular necrosis of the formal head [22]. Moreover, ESWT diffused to the treatment of OA in animals [23, 24]. It improved the rats' walking ability [23]. It significantly improved the lameness degree in horses [24].

The results achieved in people only confirm these findings. Zhao et al. [25] used ESWT to treat knee OA over 12 weeks and compared it with placebo treatment. Seventy patients were randomized to receive either placebo (n = 36) or ESWT (n = 34). In the ESWT group, the patients received 4000 pulses of shockwave at 0.25 mJ/mm^2 a week during 4 weeks. In the placebo group, the patients got shockwave at 0 mJ/mm^2 in the same area for the same time. The authors found the effect on OA by pain on VAS and perceived of health on WOMAC. The evaluation was performed at baseline and after 1, 4, and 12 weeks. The authors found that ESWT was more effective than placebo in reducing pain and improving perceived of health at each time assessment of the research.

In our study following 5 weeks of the treatment the results were similar to the results of the other authors, although we applied another treatment protocol. We found that pain in knees decreased in both the experimental (US) and the control (ESWT) groups, but there were the significant between-group differences after the intervention in favor for ESWT, and also the effects sizes were always more far-reaching in the patients treated with ESWT, than those ones in the patients treated with US. In this study, we also found that both treatment methods improved the total score of WOMAC, but the health benefits in the patients treated with ESWT and their effect size were also more important than those ones in the patients from the US group.

Our study had as strengths as limitations. The strengths included the fact that the study was analyzed using the intention-to-treat principle, the patients were randomly assigned to the two groups—an experimental and a control one. The interventions were provided by the same blinded to outcome measures experienced physiotherapist. Also, they were administered by the same assistant, blind to the group allocation.

The major limitation was the short follow-up period. Therefore, the future study ought to be a minimal follow up of 1–2 years for all subjects, it would significantly increase the impact of this kind of the study, unfortunately we had no chances to prolong the study. The second limitation is the small sample size. Our findings are therefore to be read as preliminary ones in view of possible future long-term studies with a larger sample size to confirm these results and assess the impact of US and ESWT on pain and on perceived health in people suffering from knee OA.

5. Conclusion

Despite all the limitations of this study, the obtained results may be valuable for doctors, physiotherapists, and patients with knee OA in choosing the most appropriate types of treatment based on the patients' preference and convenience. Among the people, who were treated for knee OA, ESWT led to greater benefits in reduce pain and perception of health, than a protocol which included US.

Author details

Paweł Lizis[1*], Wojciech Kobza[2], Grzegorz Mańko[3], Marcin Sitarz[4], and Jarosław Pyka[5]

*Address all correspondence to: pawel_lizis@poczta.onet.pl

1 Education and Health Protection Department, Holy Cross College, Kielce, Poland

2 Physiotherapy Cabinet, Bielsko-Biała, Poland

3 Department of Ergonomics and Physiology of Physical Effort, Jagiellonian University, Cracow, Poland

4 NZOZ New Rehabilitation, Cracow, Poland

5 NZOZ Health Center Sanvita, Knurów, Poland

References

[1] Bennell KL, Hinman RS, Metcalf BR, Buchbinder R, McConnell J, McColl G, Green S, Crossley KM. Efficacy of physiotherapy management of knee joint osteoarthritis: a randomised, double blind, placebo controlled trial. Annals of the Rheumatic Diseases. 2005;6:906–912. DOI: 10.1136/ard.2004.026526

[2] Hunter DJ, Sharma L, Skaife T. Alignment and osteoarthritis of the knee. The Journal of Bone & Joint Surgery. 2009;1(Suppl 1):85–89. DOI: 10.2106/JBJS.H.01409

[3] Kozanoglu E, Basaran S, Guzel R, Guler-Uysal F. Short term efficacy of ibuprofen phonophoresis versus continuous ultrasound therapy in knee osteoarthritis. Swiss Medical Weekly. 2003;23–24:333–338. DOI: 2003/23/smw-10210

[4] Mascarin NC, Vancini RL, Andrade ML, Magalhães Ede P, de Lira CA, Coimbra IB. Effects of kinesiotherapy, ultrasound and electrotherapy in management of bilateral knee

osteoarthritis: prospective clinical trial. BMC Musculoskelet Disorders. 2012;13:182–189. DOI: 10.1186/1471-2474-13-182

[5] Vulpiani MC, Vetrano M, Trischitta D, Scarcello L, Chizzi F, Argento G, Saraceni VM, Maffulli N, Ferretti A. Extracorporeal shock wave therapy in early osteonecrosis of the femoral head: prospective clinical study with long-term follow-up. Archives of Orthopaedic and Trauma Surgery. 2012;132:499–508. DOI: 10.1007/s00402-011-1444-9.

[6] Wang CJ, Wang FS, Huang CC, Yang KD, Weng LH, Huang HY. Treatment for osteonecrosis of the femoral head: comparison of extracorporeal shock waves with core decompression and bone-grafting. The Journal of Bone & Joint Surgery. 2005;87: 2380–2387. DOI: 10.2106/JBJS.E00174

[7] Kutlay S, Küçükdeveci AA, Elhan AH, Oztuna D, Koç N, Tennant A. Validation of the World Health Organization disability assessment schedule II (WHODAS-II) in patients with osteoarthritis. Rheumatology International. 2011;3:339–346. DOI: 10.1007/s00296-009-1306-8

[8] Goggins J, Baker K, Felson D. What WOMAC pain score should make a patient eligible for a trial in knee osteoarthritis? The Journal of Rheumatology. 2005;3:540–542. PMID: 15742450

[9] Altman R, Asch E, Bloch D, Bole G, Borenstein D, Brandt K, Christy W, Cooke TD, Greenwald R, Hochberg M, Howell D, Kaplan D, Longley III S, Mankin H, McShane DJ, Medsger Jr. T, Meenan R, Mikkelsen W, Moskowitz R, Murphy W, Rothschild B, Segal M, Sokoloff L, Wolfe F. Development of criteria for the classification and reporting of osteoarthritis. Classification of osteoarthritis of the knee. Diagnostic and Therapeutic Criteria Committee of the American Rheumatism Association. Arthritis and Rheumatism. 1986;8:1039–1049. PMID: 3741515

[10] Bellamy N, Buchanan WW, Goldsmith CH, Campbell J, Stitt LW. Validation study of WOMAC: a health status instrument for measuring clinically important patient relevant outcomes to antirheumatic drug therapy in patients with osteoarthritis of the hip or knee. The Journal of Rheumatology. 1988;12:1833–1840. PMID: 3068365

[11] Soderman P, Malchau H. Validity and reliability of Swedish WOMAC osteoarthritis index: a self-administered disease-specific questionnaire (WOMAC) versus generic instruments (SF-36 and NHP). Acta Orthopaedica Scandinavica. 2000;1:39–46. PIMID: 10743991

[12] Cohen J. A power primer. Psychological Bulletin. 1992;112:155–159. PIMID: 19565683

[13] White IR, Horton NJ, Carpenter J, Pocock SJ. Strategy for intention to treat analysis in randomized trials missing outcome data. British Medical Journal. 2011;342:910–912. DOI: 10.1136/bmj.d40

[14] Tok F, Aydemir K, Peker F, Safaz I, Taşkaynatan MA, Ozgül A. The effects of electrical stimulation combined with continuous passive motion versus isometric exercise on symptoms, functional capacity, quality of life and balance in knee osteoarthritis: randomized clinical trial. Rheumatology International. 2011;2:177–781. DOI: 10.1007/s00296-009-1263-2

[15] Thorlund JB, Aagaard P, Roos EM. Muscle strength and functional performance in patients at high risk of knee osteoarthritis: a follow-up study. Knee Surgery, Sports Traumatology, Arthroscopy. 2011;6:1110–1117. DOI: 10.1007/s00167-011-1719-2

[16] Escalante Y, García-Hermoso A, Saavedra JM. Effects of exercise on functional aerobic capacity in lower limb osteoarthritis: a systematic review. Journal of Science and Medicine in Sport. 2011;3:190–198. DOI: 10.1016/j.jsams.2010.10.004

[17] Rosemffet MG, Schneeberger EE, Citera G, Sgobba ME, Laiz C, Schmulevich H, Artçanuturry P, Gagliardi S, Maldonado Cocco JA. Effects of functional electrostimulation on pain, muscular strength, and functional capacity in patients with osteoarthritis of the knee. Journal of Clinical Rheumatology. 2004;5:246–249. DOI: 10.1097/01.rhu.0000141831.40350.91

[18] Cammarata ML, Dhaher YY. Associations between frontal plane joint stiffness and proprioceptive acuity in knee osteoarthritis. Arthritis Care & Research. (Hoboken) 2012;5:735–743. DOI: 10.1002/acr.21589

[19] Holla JF, van der Leeden M, Roorda LD, Bierma-Zeinstra SM, Damen J, Dekker J, Steultjens MP. Diagnostic accuracy of range of motion measurements in early symptomatic hip and/or knee osteoarthritis. Arthritis Care & Research. (Hoboken) 2012;1:59–65. DOI: 10.1002/acr.20645

[20] Elbaz A, Debbi EM, Segal G, Haim A, Halperin N, Agar G, Mor A, Debi R. Sex and body mass index correlate with Western Ontario and McMaster Universities Osteoarthritis Index and quality of life scores in knee osteoarthritis. Archives of Physical Medicine and Rehabilitation. 2011;10:1618–1623. DOI: 10.1016/j.apmr.2011.05.009

[21] Ng MM, Leung MC, Poon DM. The effects of electro-acupuncture and transcutaneous electrical nerve stimulation on patients with painful osteoarthritic knees: a randomized controlled trial with follow-up evaluation. The Journal of Alternative and Complementary Medicine. 2003;5:641–649. DOI: 10.1089/107555303322524490

[22] Wang CJ. Extracorporeal shockwave therapy in musculoskeletal disorders. Journal of Orthopaedic Surgery and Research. 2012;7:11. DOI: 10.1186/1749-799X-7-11

[23] Ochiai N, Ohtori S, Sasho T, Nakagawa K, Takahashi K, Takahashi N, Murata R, Takahashi K, Moriya H, Wada Y, Saisu T. Extracorporeal shock wave therapy improves motor dysfunction and pain originating from knee osteoarthritis in rats. Osteoarthritis and Cartilage. 2007;15:1093–1096. DOI: 10.1016/j.joca.2007.03.011

[24] Frisbie DD, Kawcak CE, McIlwraith CW. Evaluation of the effect of extracorporeal shock wave treatment on experimentally induced osteoarthritis in middle carpal joints of horses. American Journal of Veterinary Research. 2009;70:449–454. DOI: 10.2460/ajvr.70.4.449

[25] Zhao Z, Jing R, Shi Z, Zhao B, Ai Q, Xing G. Efficacy of extracorporeal shockwave therapy for knee osteoarthritis: a randomized controlled trial. The Journal of Surgical Research. 2013;185(2):661–666. DOI: 10.1016/j.jss.2013.07.004

Chapter 14

Natural Products as a Source for Novel Analgesic Compounds

Rehab Fawzy Abdel-Rahman

Additional information is available at the end of the chapter

http://dx.doi.org/10.5772/66770

Abstract

Natural products have an important role in the discovery of analgesic drugs along with the determining of the complex mechanisms involved in pain transmission and pain relief. Lately, several substances with antinociceptive actions have been purified from natural sources and further identified, resulting in novel structural classes and more understanding of the underlying pharmacological mechanisms of actions. Yet, natural products still hold great potential for the discovery of novel agents for treatment of pain disorders and potentially drug addictions with exciting pharmacological profiles (i.e. no side effects, no addictive potential). The aim of this chapter is to highlight some active compounds derived from natural sources that possess analgesic properties. Additionally, the identification of new compounds derived from natural sources could lead to great understanding of the underlying pharmacological mechanisms of action, which will be addressed in this chapter as well.

Keywords: plant-derived compounds, analgesic properties, pharmacological mechanisms of action

1. Introduction

At the present time, many formulas for the relief of pain are present; among them, medicinal herbs are highlighted because of their wide popular use and availability. Many plant-derived compounds could offer valuable therapeutic effects for the treatment of chronic inflammatory conditions, which are likely associated with pain.

In the drug market today, about 40% of all medicines have been originated directly or indirectly from natural sources. It is estimated that about 25% being derived from plants, 13% from microorganisms and 3% from animals. For instance, morphine, salicin, artemisinin, capsaicin, atropine, pilocarpine, digitalis, quinine, scopolamine and captopril are examples of drugs derived from natural sources [1, 2].

2. Active compounds derived from natural sources possessing analgesic properties

Since ancient times, many active compounds originated from natural sources have been consumed for various medical purposes including the management of pain. Opium, for example, has been used since 7000 years ago. Up to the nineteenth century, other active components derived from different natural remedies were identified, purified and utilized. Since then, analogues have been made from natural sources, and completely synthetic compounds based on natural pharmacophores have been introduced into the market [3].

2.1. Aspirin

Aspirin or acetylsalicylic acid (**Figure 1**) is extracted from the bark of the Willow tree *Salix alba*, family *Salicaceae*. It is one of the most extensively used analgesic agents for the management of mild pain. Aspirin is considered the first nonsteroidal anti-inflammatory drug (NSAID) that inhibits the arachidonic acid pathway resulting in the synthesis of eicosanoids, which is a potent pain mediator [4]. Moreover, the inhibition of the cyclooxygenase (COX) enzymes by aspirin led to the discovery of other synthetic NSAIDs.

For instance, the study of the biochemical cascade of COX system led to the discovery of the COX-2 enzyme inhibitors. COX-2 inhibitors are believed to be safer than other NSAIDS that inhibit the COX-1 enzyme. Rofecoxib (Vioxx)® is an example of a compound that selectively targets the COX-2 enzyme, and it was voluntarily withdrawn by Merck and Co., Inc. on September 30, 2004, from the US drug market due to an increased risk of cardiovascular effects [5].

2.2. Opioids

Natural opiates and synthetic opioids are potent analgesics that bind to receptors for endogenous opiates in the central nervous system (CNS). Opioid is the common name for all com-

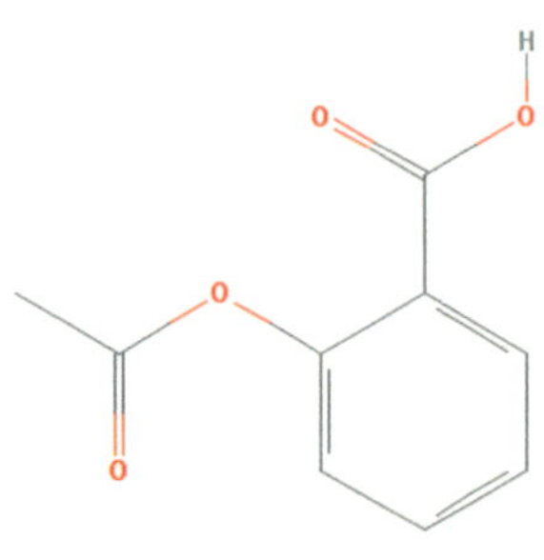

Figure 1. Aspirin.

http://dx.doi.org/10.5772/66770

pounds acting on opioid receptor as the constituents of opium, to produce morphine-like effects. *Papaver somniferum* (family: *Papaveraceae*) is one of the oldest medicinal plants known by mankind, and abuse of its opium juice has been known before history was recorded. Opium contains about 25 alkaloids, including morphine (**Figure 2**), codeine (**Figure 3**) and thebaine (**Figure 4**) [6]. Tramadol is a synthetic analogue of codeine that acts by binding to μ (mu) opiate receptors, added to that it inhibits norepinephrine and serotonin reuptake [7]. Whereas, by modifying the chemical structure of thebaine, a semisynthetic derivative is obtained, termed oxycodone [8]. The endogenous opioid receptor system includes four receptor subtypes designated as mu (μ), delta (δ), kappa (k) and opioid receptor like (ORL-1) receptors. These receptors are widely disseminated in the mammalian system and have been found in all vertebrates. Opioid receptors are highly distributed in the CNS, including the brain and spinal cord, but they are also found in the gastrointestinal system and in the cells of immune system [9].

Lately, newly discovered chemical structures have appeared in the literatures that interact either with opioid receptors directly or through some other mechanism of controlling opioid receptor signalling. These compounds are interesting from a drug design perspective as most of them do not contain nitrogen.

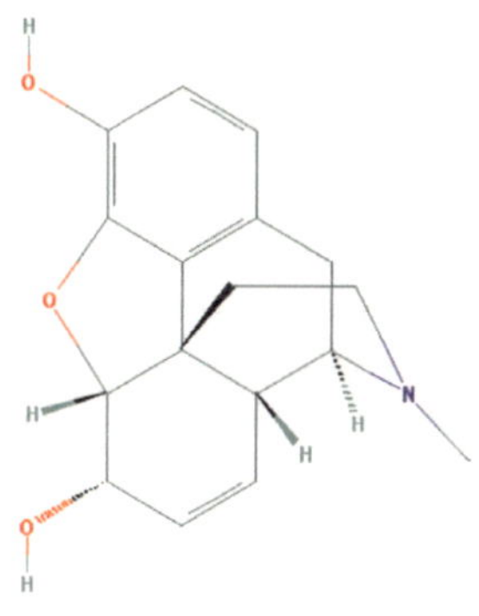

Figure 2. Morphine.

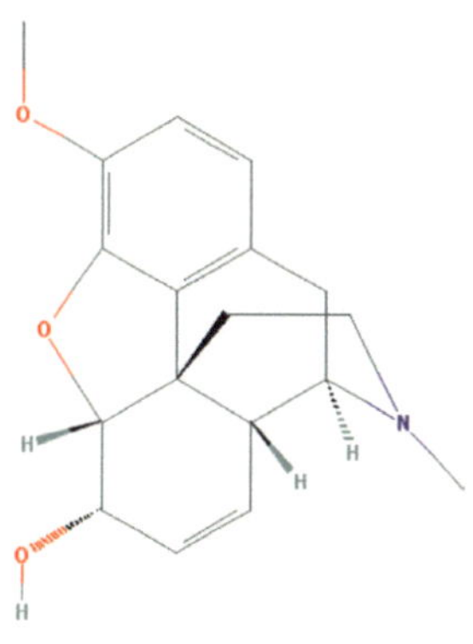

Figure 3. Codeine.

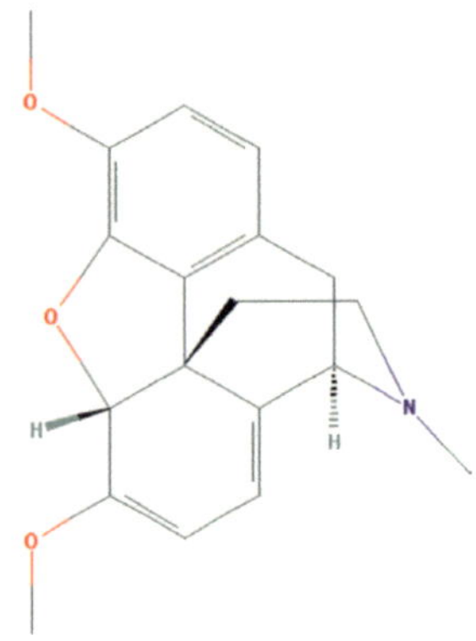

Figure 4. Thebaine.

2.2.1. Morphine

In the 1850s, morphine began to be used for chronic pain, in minor surgical operations and after surgery. Morphine is the most abundant opiate obtained from opium. It is the dried latex obtained by shallow slicing of the unripe seedpods of *Papaver somniferum*. Meperidine was the first synthetic opioid analgesic, with a completely different structure from that of morphine, and its analgesic properties were identified in 1939. Far ahead in 1942, nalorphine was obtained, as the first opioid receptor antagonist, by replacing the substituent group on the nitrogen atom. By replacing the allyl group with the methyl group, nalorphine (**Figure 5**) is obtained from morphine, and naloxone is obtained from oxymorphine (**Figure 6**) [10, 11].

Nalorphine acts as an antagonist at the μ and δ receptors, but it acts as a weak agonist at the k receptor, and thus gives slight analgesia. However, nalorphine has hallucinogenic side effects. Whereas, naloxone is an antagonist at the three opioid receptors (μ, δ and k receptors). This compound is used to elucidate the possible roles of opioids in response to stress [11, 12].

In spite of the remarkable efforts by researchers to discover safe, effective and nonaddictive opioids for pain treatment, morphine remains the most valuable painkiller in contemporary medicine [13].

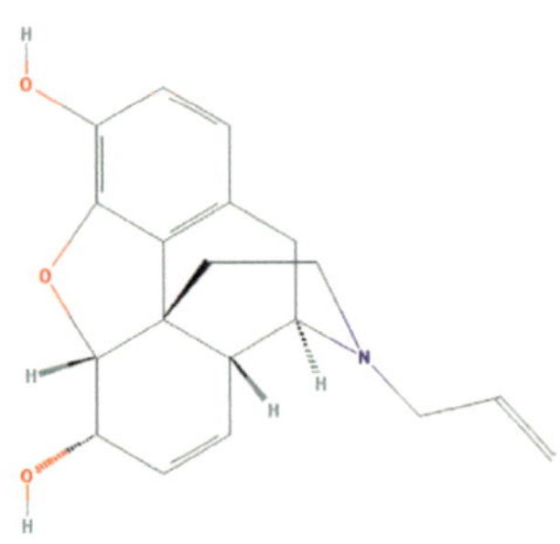

Figure 5. Nalorphine.

http://dx.doi.org/10.5772/66770

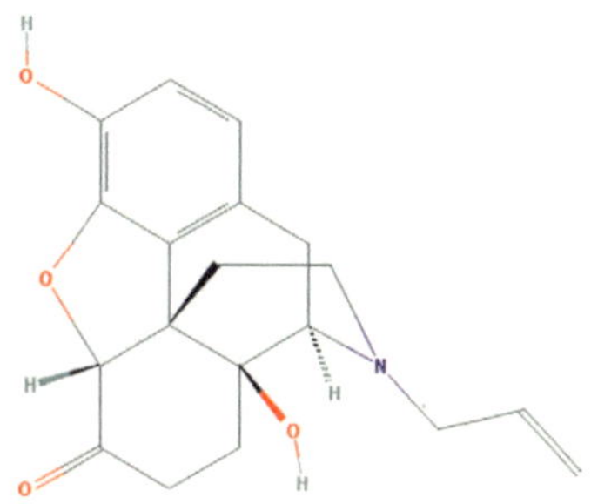

Figure 6. Naloxone.

The pharmacological properties of morphine are somewhat complex and varying according to the dose, site of action, route of administration and animal species. Morphine is mostly considered as pain perception modifier, resulting in an increase in the threshold of painful stimuli. Nowadays, analgesia induced by morphine is known to be mediated via activation of membrane opioid receptors, and consequently, it can be inhibited by opioid receptor antagonists, as naloxone. Furthermore, certain undesirable side effects of morphine as euphorogenic effect, inhibition of gastrointestinal transit time, constipation, loss of appetite, hypothermia, bradycardia and retention of urine seem to involve receptor-mediated actions [14].

As more chemical components of traditionally used plants for the treatment of pain are explicated, there is a great potential for the development of novel drug treatments acting through opioid receptors. Indeed, some newly discovered chemical structures have been published in the literatures that interact either directly with opioid receptors or through some other mechanisms of controlling opioid receptor signalling. In the next section, examples of some of those chemical structures will be reviewed.

2.2.2. Menthol

Menthol (**Figure 7**) is isolated from peppermint (*Menthapiperita,* family: *Lamiaceae*). For many centuries, menthol was utilized as an antipruritic, antiseptic and a coolant in topical preparations as it causes a feeling of coolness due to stimulation of 'cold' receptors by inhibiting Ca^{2+} currents of neuronal membranes. It has also been reported that modulation of Ca^{2+} currents is involved in the regulation of pain threshold. Indeed, the inhibition of Ca^{2+} currents by administration of voltage-sensitive Ca^{2+} channel blockers can produce antinociception in laboratory animals. Lately, it was evaluated in the hot plate and acetic acid writhing tests where it revealed potent activity through interaction with opioid receptors, and more selectively, kappa opioid receptors activation [15].

2.2.3. Salvinorin A

Salvinorin A (**Figure 8**), isolated from *Salvia divinorium* (*Lamiaceae,* formerly *Labiatae*), was first described in nonnitrogenous selective kappa opioid receptor ligand. Salvinorin A acts as k opioid receptors agonist in spinally mediated pain. There is a great attention for k opioid

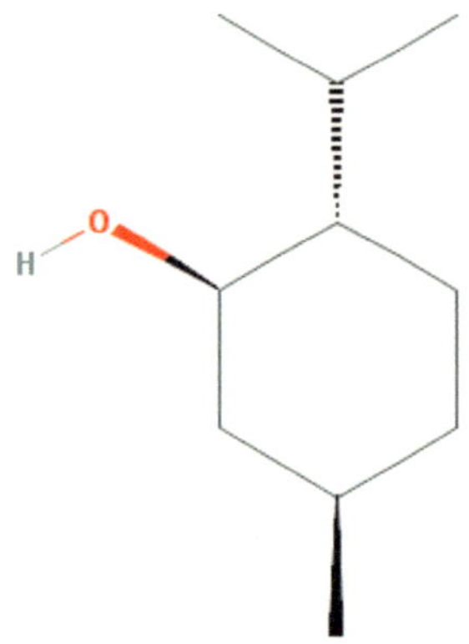

Figure 7. Menthol.

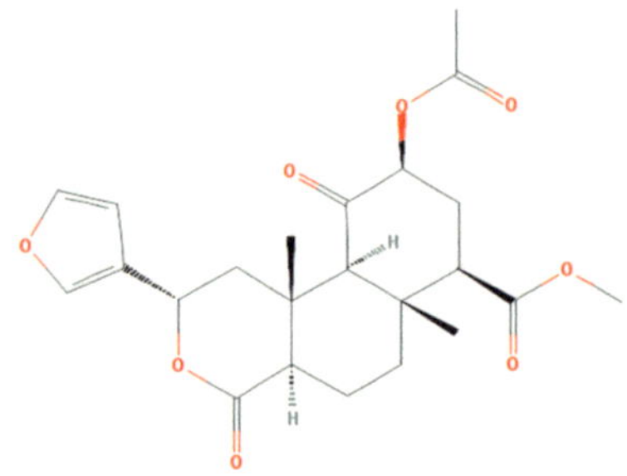

Figure 8. Salvinorin A.

receptor agonists among the pharmaceutical industry field [3, 16]. The ethnopharmacological uses of *Salvia divinorium* extract leaves being used to relief headaches, as a sedative, and for the treatment of some gastrointestinal disorders since the anatomical location of k opioid receptors in brain, spinal cord, GI tract, etc [17].

Unfortunately, k opioid receptor agonists produce unwanted side effects; thus, they are not commonly prescribed as analgesics. In this consent, salvinorin A has been reported to cause dysphoric hallucination when administered in human [18, 19]. Nonetheless, it is still listed as a chemical of concern by the United States Drug Enforcement Agency and is currently allowed to be marketed as alternative to other illegal hallucinogens.

2.2.4. *Mitragynine*

Mitragynine is a nitrogen-containing compound with a unique structure. It is derived from the traditional Thai herb *Mitragyna speciosa* (*Rubiaceae*). The herb has been used for many years in Thailand as a replacement for opium and used by drug addicts seeking for relief during opioid withdrawal stage. However, the use of *M. speciosa* is currently illegal in Thailand, Malaysia, South Korea and Australia, but widely available in the United States and UK [20–22].

At least two compounds have been identified in *M. speciosa* by Takayama "in Ref. [23]", both having opioid receptor activity. The first compound termed mitragynine (**Figure 9**) is one of the

http://dx.doi.org/10.5772/66770

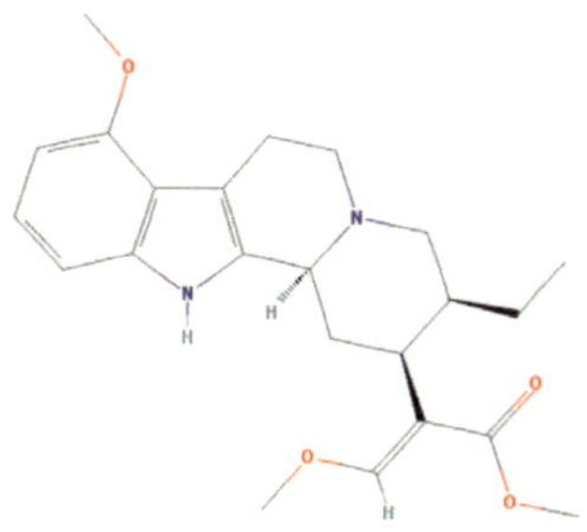

Figure 9. Mitragynine.

major alkaloidal components. It is a corynanthe based acting as a partial opioid receptor agonist, with about 26% the activity of morphine. The other and the more interesting compound is 7-hydroxymitragynine (mitragynine hydroxyindolenine) (**Figure 10**), with activity of 1000 times or more than that of morphine.

Mitragynine is ingested orally by chewing fresh leaves or by drinking a tea brewed with the substance. The medicinal properties of this plant had been previously described in combating fatigue and to tolerate hard work, due to its opium-like effect at high doses and cocain-like stimulant effect at low doses. However, death was reported as a result of mitragynine abuse [24, 25].

2.3. Capsaicin

Capsicum genus, which produces both chilli peppers and bell peppers, belong to the family of *Solanaceae*. Capsicum is originated in Central and South America and has more than 20 species that are widely spread around the world. Indeed, only five species are widely cultivated including: *C. annuum, C. chinense, C. frutescens, C. pendulum* and *C. pubescens* [26].

It seems that capsicum species are among the oldest cultivated plants in the world (5200–3400 BC). Scientists have found an evidence of people who consumed peppers in Mexico as early as 7000 BC; this was the oldest document of capsicum use [27]. Högyes (1878) was the first to make evident that the alcoholic extract of paprika (*Capsicum annuum*) resulted in hypothermia when administered systemically [28].

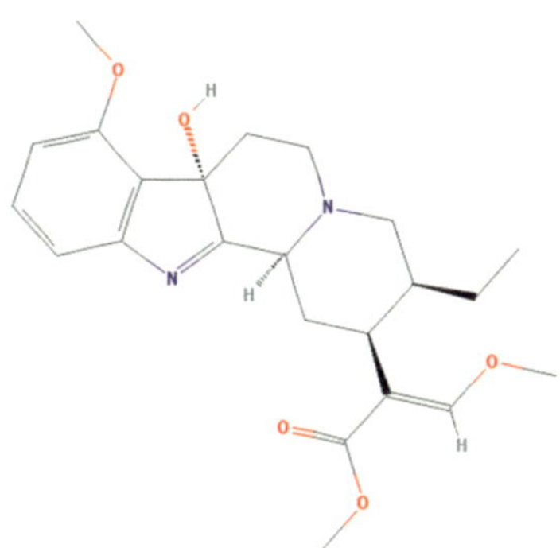

Figure 10. Mitragynine hydroxyindolenine.

Interestingly, the study of pungent principles began in the 1810s using the names "capsicol", "capsicin", "capsacutin", etc. Later, capsaicin is the active principle isolated from Capsicum species by Thresh in 1846 [29] (**Figure 11**). The exact chemical structure of capsaicin was identified after half a century by Nelson in 1919 [30]. Capsaicin is considered as the most prominent component in plants belonging to Capsicum species, with about 70% of the total pungent acid amides and 30% or less constituting dihydrocapsaicin, an analogue of capsaicin (capsaicinoid) [14, 31].

Despite the unwanted primary irritant effect of capsaicin to the mucous membranes and the eyes, it is used clinically for the management of neuropathic pain syndromes and arthritis [1, 3]. The Native Americans used Capsicum to treat cramps, diarrhoea and indigestion. Other folk medicinal uses of capsaicin include enhancement of appetite, treatment of gastric ulcers, rheumatism and restoration of hair growth [32].

The biological effects of capsaicin (8-methyl-*N*-vanillyl-6-nonenamide) are biphasic: first by the excitation of the primary afferents and the second phase involves desensitization or inactivation of neurons [33]. Capsaicin stimulates the afferent sensory neurons that conduct the nociceptive information to the central nervous system (CNS), precisely the C and Aδ fibres. The stimulatory effect is mainly through calcium influx, the release of several neuropeptides including tachykinins, calcitonin gene-related peptide (CGRP) and somatostatin. It also blocks the intra-axonal transport of macromolecules, such as the neural growth factor (NGF) [27]. Additionally, capsaicin is a vanilloid receptor -1 (VR1) agonist. It is known to have an inhibitory effect on nitric oxide (NOx) production in macrophages; this effect clarifies its implications in the pathogenesis of inflammatory diseases [3, 34].

2.4. Aconitum alkaloids

Aconitum species, family *Ranunculaceae*, known by different names such as aconite, monkshood, wolf's bane, women's bane, Devil's helmet or blue rocket. Aconitum plants (mainly *A. japonicum* Thunberg and *A. carmichaeli Debeaux*) have been used from the time of historic civilizations in Ayurvedic, Chinese, Tibetan and Greco-Roman medicines for their various

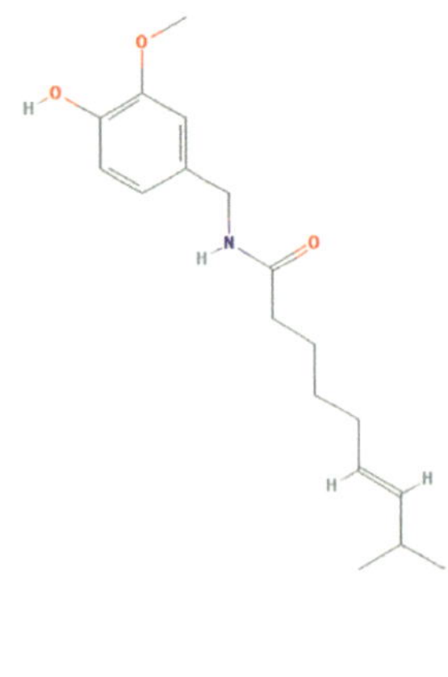

Figure 11. Capsaicin.

http://dx.doi.org/10.5772/66770

pharmacological effects. Plants of *Aconitum* genus were familiar in the European countries' medicine in the nineteenth century [35].

Leaves and roots of Aconitum plant were used to relieve neuralgic pain, particularly in the face to relieve the pain of sciatica. The root is extremely bitter; its paste is applied in acute rheumatism also on cuts and wounds as an anti-inflammatory and antiseptic agent [36].

There are two groups of Aconitum alkaloids revealing strong to moderate analgesic properties. The first group includes aconitine-like diester alkaloids with strong analgesic activity: aconitine (**Figure 12**), hypaconitine, mesaconitine, 3-acetylaconitine, bulleyaconitine, and yunaconitine. The second group involves less-toxic alkaloids having moderate analgesic effect. One of them, lappaconitine (**Figure 13**), it is believed that lappaconitine and its deacetylated analogue have lower toxicity than aconitine and, consequently, it is assumed to be safely used as analgesic or anaesthetic agents [35].

Aconitine, 3-acetylaconitine and hypaconitine revealed high affinity Na^+ channel ligands, thus having antinociceptive, strong arrhythmogenic effects and high acute toxicity, and induce a blockade of neuronal conduction by a permanent cell depolarization. In contrast, lappaconitine has lower affinity for Na^+ channel and thereafter has lesser antinociceptive and lesser cardiotoxic activity, acting as a local anaesthetic. Other alkaloids with lower Na^+ channel affinity such as lappaconidine and oxydelcorine have no antinociceptive effect

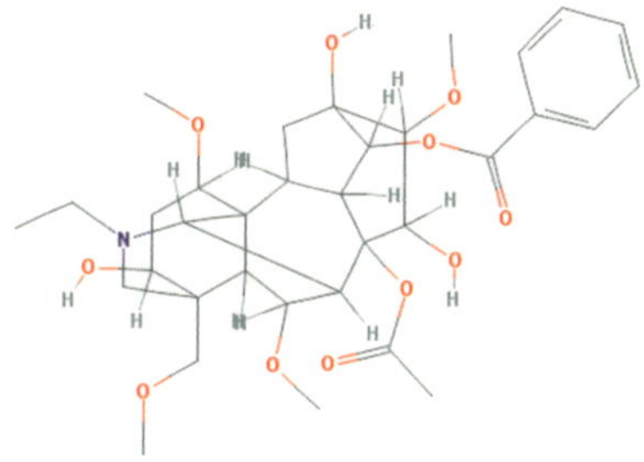

Figure 12. Aconitine.

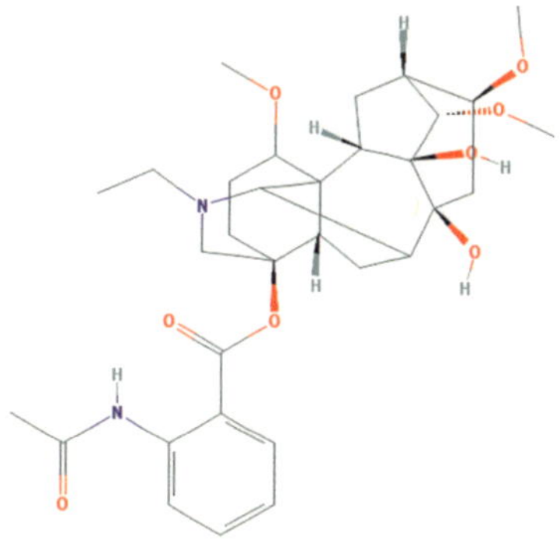

Figure 13. Lappaconitine.

[37]. Despite the large number of alkaloids isolated and identified from Aconitum sp. with antinociceptive effect, their cardiotoxic actions hindered their clinical use as analgesics [14].

2.5. Polygodial sesquiterpenes

Polygodial sesquiterpene is the major constituent present in the bark of *Drymis winteri* (*Winteraceae*) and related species, a well-known medicinal plant found in some South American countries such as Brazil. *Drymis winteri* is commonly used in folk medicine as an anti-inflammatory and for the treatment of asthma and allergy [38]. Phytochemical investigations of *D. winteri* demonstrated the occurrence of sesquiterpenes, lactones and flavonoids [39, 40].

As well, previous studies [40–42] indicated that a mixture of at least three sesquiterpenes, identified as being polygodial (**Figure 14**), 1-β-(ϱ-methoxycinnamoyl polygodial and drimanial (**Figure 15**), appear to be the main constituents present in the park of plant *D. winteri* that are accountable for the marked antinociceptive, anti-inflammatory and anti-allergic effects of the crude extract. With regard to the relatively high concentrations of polygodial and to a lesser extent, drimanial in the park of *D. winteri*, it can be proposed that the two sesquiterpenes are the most relevant active compounds and are responsible for the major pharmacological activities of the plant.

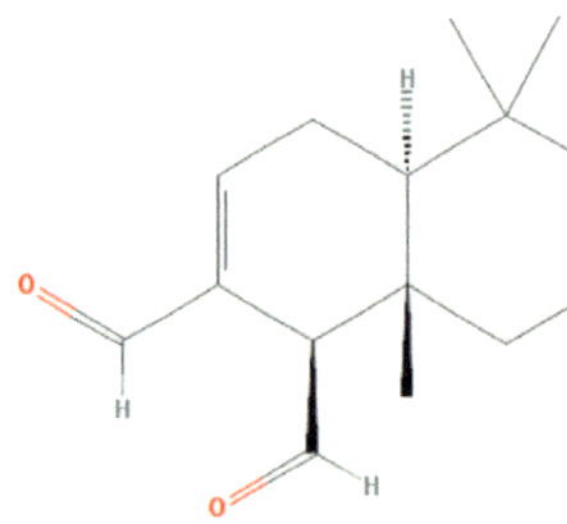

Figure 14. Polygodial.

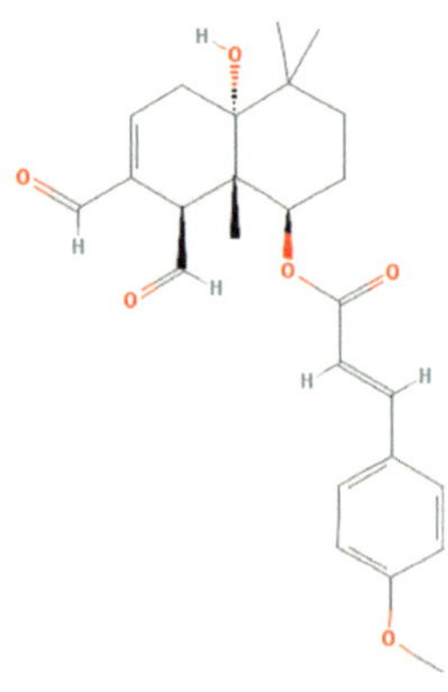

Figure 15. Drimanial.

The precise site of action by which polygodial induces antinociception is still under investigation. The modulatory role of polygodials as antinociceptives as proposed to be via the interaction with an opiate-like system through k and δ receptors, the α1-adrenergic receptor, the serotoninergic system, and an interaction with a Gi/o protein pertussis toxin-sensitive mechanism. Thus, polygodial or its derivatives might be concerned in the development of new analgesic drugs for controlling neurogenic pain [40, 43].

2.6. Caffeine

Caffeine is an alkaloid present in over 60 plant species. Caffeine (1,3,7-trimethylxanthine) is mainly in beverages derived from coffee beans, tea leaves and kola nuts (*Cola acuminate*, family: *Sterculiaceae*). Caffeine has been used medicinally together with ergotamine for migraine headaches and in combination with nonsteroidal anti-inflammatory drugs in analgesic preparations [44]. Moreover, caffeine is believed to be potentially effective cancer chemopreventive metabolite in terms of its antioxidant capacity [45].

Caffeine was isolated in 1820, but the precise structure of this methylxanthine was established in the last decade of the nineteenth century. Its properties were not fully recognized until 1981, when the stimulating properties of caffeine and its analogues by the blockade of adenosine receptors were allied [46].

Cola nut is native of West Africa, which has been introduced to the West Indies. It is used in large quantities in the soft drink industry. The active principles are caffeine (**Figure 16**) and theobromine (**Figure 17**), which are both stimulants [44].

Caffeine increases alertness, awareness and attention span, has stimulatory effects on mood and sense of wellbeing, and produces an increase in exercise tolerance. Other desirable physiologic effects involve protection of the cerebral vasculature by means of enhancing glucose metabolism. In this concern, it is believed that caffeine consumption has been associated with a reduced risk of Parkinson disease. It also constricts cerebral blood vessels, which is a highly desirable action in patients with migraine [47]. Caffeine is prescribed as a stimulant of the central nervous system and to treat postprandial hypotension and obesity, and also, it is indicated for treatment of apnoea in premature neonates [48].

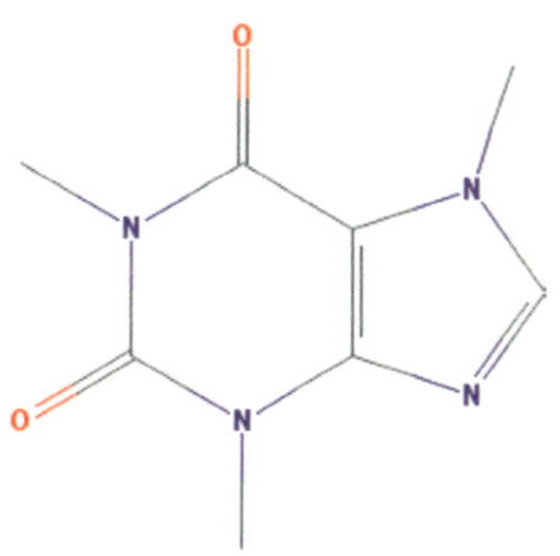

Figure 16. Caffeine.

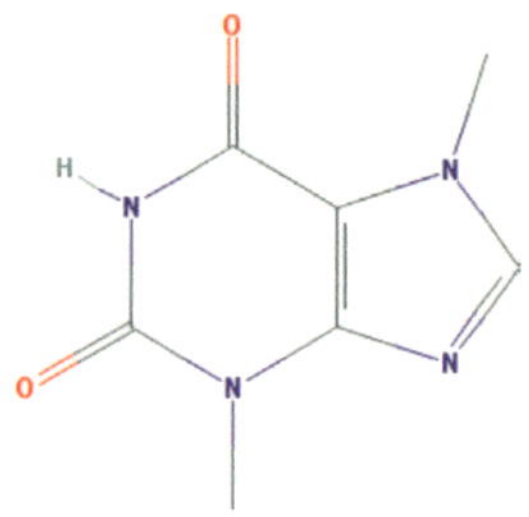

Figure 17. Theobromine.

Following oral intake, maximum plasma concentration arises between 30 min and 2 h, which may be prolonged with food ingestion. Caffeine is readily absorbed by the gastrointestinal tract, with 100% bioavailability and high solubility both in aqueous and nonpolar organic solvents. Caffeine is lipophilic with low protein binding. Its plasma protein binding—mainly albumin—is 10–35%. Caffeine rapidly crosses cell membranes, as well as the placental barrier, blood brain, producing drug levels in the brain and cerebrospinal fluid similar to those in plasma [46, 49].

In 1985, Burnstock and Kennedy cited that methylxanthines block purinergic receptors type 1 (P1) and have no effect on P2 receptors [50]. Added to that, the proposed mechanism of action of caffeine seems to be related to the blockade of peripheral and central adenosine receptors involved in the regulation of pain transmission, giving rise to its analgesic properties [14, 51].

2.7. Ginsenosides

Ginseng, the root of *Panax ginseng* (*Araliaceae*), has been reported to relieve a variety of ailments. Studies showed that ginseng saponins, which consist of various ginsenoids (**Figure 18**), are the most pharmacoactive constituent of ginseng root. Ginsenoids are believed to be involved in pain modulation as well as in opioid-induced antinociception and tolerance [52, 53].

In traditional folk medicine, ginseng has been used to relieve some types of pain such as toothache, abdominal pain, chest pain and neuralgia. A line of evidence also shows that ginseng

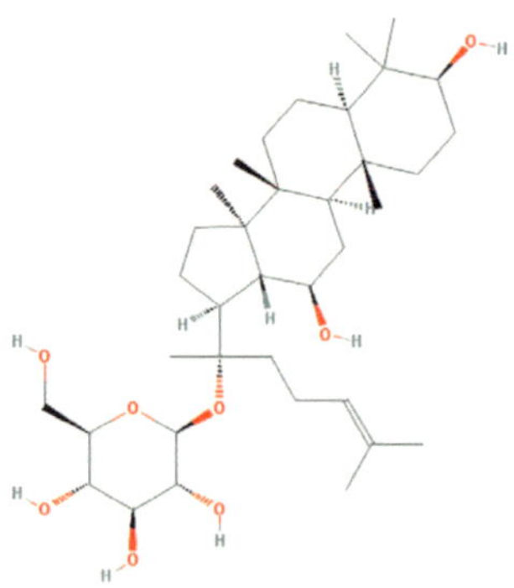

Figure 18. Ginsenosides.

http://dx.doi.org/10.5772/66770

saponins are responsible for relieving pain induced by chemicals or noxious heat in experimental animals [54].

Most ginseng species possess active naturally occurring constituents such as the ginsenosides, polysaccharides, peptides, polyacetylenic alcohols and fatty acids. From the ginseng saponin fraction, more than 30 triterpene ginsenoside derivatives containing sugars were isolated. Yet, there is a wide variation (2–20%) in the ginsenoside content among the different ginseng species [2].

Ginseng saponins inhibit voltage-dependent Ca^{2+} channels providing one possible explanation for its analgesic efficacy because sensory neurons transfer sensory information such as pain from the peripheral nervous system toward the central nervous system [55]. Furthermore, the regulation of voltage-dependent Ca^{2+} channels by ginseng saponins is not mediated through the inhibitory receptors such as opioids, α2-adrenergic, GABAergic, nor muscarinic receptors [53].

3. Pharmacological mechanisms of action for naturally derived analgesic drugs

Interestingly, the identification of new compounds derived from natural sources with potential antinociceptive effect could lead to great understanding of the underlying pharmacological mechanisms of action. Herein, the next section, we will review some targeted pharmacological mechanisms of action for naturally derived analgesic drugs.

3.1. Voltage-gated ion channels

Many natural products have been found to interact with voltage-gated ion channels. Some more recent natural products are to be studied at the Na^+, K^+ and Ca^{2+}channels. These compounds cause their effects through several mechanisms of action.

Voltage-gated Na^+ channels play a central role in the generation and dissemination of action potentials in neurons and other cells such as skeletal muscle and cardiac cells. Modulators of sodium channels are being used as local anaesthetics, antiarrhythmics, analgesics and antiepileptics, and for other disorders [56]. In this aspect, tetrodotoxin, isolated from the puffer fish, blocks sodium channels and causes great harm to those that ingest it leading to numbness in the lip and tongue within 20 min of ingestion followed by paralysis and may cause death. Consequently, the use of tetrodotoxin as a key compound for analgesic development has been limited by its toxic nature [3].

As well, voltage-gated K^+ channels have been shown to be involved in pain processes. Activation of potassium channels leads to membrane hyperpolarization then inhibition of cell excitability. Those pain signals may be transmitted either directly or indirectly depending on the location of these channels. Today, several anaesthetics are used clinically to work through interactions with potassium channels [57]. Certain peptides from natural sources have been identified to act through potassium channels. For instance, tertiapin, a peptide with 21 amino acids, isolated from the venom of the honey bee, has been shown to block inward rectifier potassium channels [58]. Moreover, administration of tertiapin in mice diminished the analgesic response evoked by spinal administration of high doses of morphine [59]. Further research in this area may result in better understanding of the pain modulation responses, managing drug addiction, and may lead to the discovery of new analgesic compounds.

Furthermore, voltage-gated Ca^{2+} channel activation directly affects membrane potential and contributes to the electrical excitability of neurons. Voltage-gated Ca^{2+} channels have an important role in the release of neurotransmitter from the presynaptic terminals in the dorsal horn in response to inward action potentials [60]. In this aspect, a peptide termed *N*-agatoxin isolated from the venom of the funnel web spider, and an American spider *Agelenopsis aperta* inhibits P/Q-type calcium channels that have been reported to play a role in migraine and headaches [61, 62]. Future research on the functional role of P/Q-type calcium channels may provide an additional target for the modulation of pain responses.

3.2. Acetylcholine receptors

Two classes of acetylcholine receptors are well-known, the muscarinic and the nicotinic acetylcholine receptors. Both classes were recognized through the utilization of the natural products, muscarine and nicotine, respectively. The role of these receptors in modulating the central nociception has been well-documented. The muscarinic acetylcholine receptors have several known natural product ligands including: hyoscyamine, atropine, scopolamine and Mamba snake toxins [3].

Epibatidin, an alkaloid isolated from the skin of the Ecuadorian dart-frog, *Epipedobates tricolor*, has been reported to be a potent nicotinic analgesic. It could be antagonized by mecamylamine, a nicotinic receptor antagonist [63]. Accordingly, it was established that epibatidine as a powerful tool for studying nicotinic pathways involved in pain perception. As well, its remarkable efficiency as an antinociceptive may be due to the selective effects on central antinociceptive pathways [64].

3.3. Cannabinoid receptors

Two cannabinoid receptors, CB1 and CB2, have been identified and subsequently cloned. They belong to G-protein coupled receptors family, sharing 44% amino acid sequence homology but vary in their anatomical distribution. Expression of CB1 receptor is mainly in the CNS and to a lesser extent in other tissues, while CB2 receptor is primarily expressed in peripheral tissues associated with immune functions, including macrophages, B and T cells, as well as in peripheral nerve terminals and on mast cells [65].

The endogenous family of ligands that interact with these receptors is known as the anandamides (*N*-arachidonoyl-ethanolamine). They are lipid in nature with antinociceptive activity but not as potent as tetrahydrocannabinol (THC) [66]. Interestingly, neurons in the brain produce, release and inactivate anandamide, confirming a role for this arachidonate derivative as an endogenous cannabinoid substance [67].

Remarkably, a nonnitrogenous lipophilic molecule, Δ^9-tetrahydrocannabinol (Δ^9-THC), isolated from *Cannabis sativa,* is the prototypical ligand, interacting with the cannabinoid G-protein coupled receptors [68]. It has also been reported that another constituent cannabidol isolated from *C. sativa* exerts important anti-inflammatory activity. Cannabinoid receptor agonists induce a number of unwanted CNS effects, which are supposed to be mediated mainly by the central distribution pattern of CB1 receptors [65].

3.4. Vanilloid receptors

Vanilloid receptors (VR), or vanilloid-gated ion channels, also known as capsaicin receptors, have been shown to be involved in nociception [69]. Nonetheless, their clinical potential remains to be proven. Vanilloid receptors are expressed almost exclusively by primary sensory neurons involved in nociception and neurogenic inflammation.

It is well established that the VR agonists give rise to excitatory effects characterized by nociception and neurogenic inflammation, followed by desensitization [14, 70]. Notably, many natural products are known as modulators of these receptors. Capsaicin, for example, is a VR1 receptor agonist and is marketed in the United States in topical preparations for the treatment of arthritis and inflammatory joint pain. At the present time, it is believed that VR1 receptor agonists can be good attractive therapeutic target. Interestingly, other "hot" spices, like piperine and zingerone, the active ingredients in black pepper and ginger, respectively, also appear to act through VR activation [71].

Peripheral fibres are the site of release of a variety of neuropeptides among which substance P (SP) and calcitonin gene-related peptide (CGRP) are defined. Depletion of SP and CGRP as well as of vanilloid receptors occurred following treatment with capsaicin, in the spinal and peripheral terminals of capsaicin sensitive neurons in almost 24 h [28].

Other naturally occurring compound acting at VR1 receptors is of fungal origin, a triprenyl phenol, termed scutigeral, a novel structural class of VR ligand. Scutigeral, isolated from the non-pungent edible mushroom *Albatrellus ovinus*, has been shown to stimulate rat dorsal root ganglion neurons by activation of vanilloid receptors [72].

3.5. Purinergic P2X receptors inhibitors

One pharmacological target in the area of analgesics and anti-inflammatory agents is purinergic P2X receptors (P2XR), which are important receptors in the modulation of inflammation and pain. In 1978, Burnstock [73] mentioned the existence of two classes of purinergic receptors, known as receptors P1 (adenosine) and P2 (adenosine 5′-triphosphate, ATP) [50]. Markedly, mammalian ATP-gated nonselective cation channels (P2XRs) consist of seven potential subunits; denoted P2X1 to P2X7 [74].

In 1995, a significant advance was made when the P2X3 ionotropic ion channel purinergic receptor was cloned and presented to be mainly localized on small nociceptive sensory neurons in dorsal root ganglia (DRG) [75]. Shortly, Burnstock [76] suggested a unifying purinergic hypothesis for the initiation of pain that ATP released as a co-transmitter with noradrenaline (NA) and neuropeptide Y from sympathetic nerve terminal varicosities probably that is involved in activating these receptors in three different pain conditions: as a co-transmitter from sympathetic nerves in sympathetic pain as causalgia and reflex sympathetic dystrophy; from endothelial cells in vascular pain, including migraine and angina; and from tumour cells in cancer.

Likewise, purinergic mechano-sensory transduction has been implicated for visceral pain. Meanwhile, ATP released from urothelial cells and epithelial cells lining intestine during the distension acts on P2X3 and P2X2/3, and perhaps P2Y, receptors on subepithelial sensory nerve fibres to initiate impulses in sensory pathways to the pain centres in the brain as well as triggering local reflexes. Besides, P1, P2X and P2Y receptors are possibly implicated in nociceptive neural pathways in the spinal cord, while P2X4 receptors on the spinal microglia are involved in allodynia [77].

Of the seven subtypes of P2XR, the types that are most related to the progression or control of pain status are the P2X3R, the heteromericeP2X2/3R, P2X4R, and the P2X7R [78].

An example of natural inhibitor of purinergic receptors is a product known as puerarin. Puerarin is an isoflavone isolated from a traditional Chinese herb (*Radix puerariae*). It was found to have an inhibitory effect on burn pain hyperalgesia through inhibiting the upregulation of the P2X3R protein expression in the dorsal root ganglion neurons [79].

Also, purotoxin, a peptide isolated from the venom of the Asian spider *Geolycosa*sp, also showed a potent and selective antagonist effect on P2X3R, inhibiting the ionic current in rat neurons and showing an analgesic effect on inflammatory pain [78].

4. Conclusion

Natural products are an extremely valuable source of novel compounds with potential analgesic properties. More research needs to be conducted on natural products to discover new compounds, and hereafter, new mechanisms of actions will be elucidated.

Lastly, the fields of pharmacognosy, medicinal chemistry and pharmacology are expected to work closely to ensure that novel naturally driven compounds are explored for their potential development as novel drugs as well as their pharmacological mechanisms of action.

Author details

Rehab Fawzy Abdel-Rahman

Address all correspondence to: rehabs2001@yahoo.com

Department of Pharmacology, National Research Centre, Giza, Egypt

References

[1] Yunes RA, Cechinel Filho V, Ferreira J, Calixto JB. The use of natural products as sources of new analgesic drugs. Studies in Natural Products Chemistry. 2005 Dec 31;30:191–212.

[2] Calixto JB, Scheidt C, Otuki M, Santos AR. Biological activity of plant extracts: novel analgesic drugs. Expert Opinion on Emerging Drugs. 2001 Oct 1;6(2):261–79.

[3] McCurdy CR, Scully SS. Analgesic substances derived from natural products (natureceuticals). Life Sciences. 2005 Dec 22;78(5):476–84.

[4] Vane JR. Inhibition of prostaglandin synthesis as a mechanism of action for aspirin-like drugs. Nature. 1971 Jun 23;231(25):232–5.

[5] Radwan MF, Dalby KN, Kaoud TS. Propyphenazone-based analogues as prodrugs and selective cyclooxygenase-2 inhibitors. ACS Medicinal Chemistry Letters. 2014 Jun 26;5(9):983–8.

[6] Trease GE, Evans WC. A textbook of pharmacognsy. Bailliere Tindall and Cox, London. 1978: p. 527–620.

[7] Lewis KS, Han NH. Tramadol: a new centrally acting analgesic. American Journal of Health-System Pharmacy. 1997 Mar 1;54(6):643–52.

[8] Pöyhiä R, Vainio A, Kalso E. A review of oxycodone's clinical pharmacokinetics and pharmacodynamics. Journal of Pain and Symptom Management. 1993 Feb 28;8(2):63–7.

[9] Dhawan BN, Cesselin F, Raghubir R, Reisine T, Bradley PB, Portoghese PS, Hamon M. International Union of Pharmacology. XII. Classification of opioid receptors. Pharmacological Reviews. 1996 Dec 1;48(4):567–92.

[10] Sabatowski R, Schafer D, Kasper SM, Brunsch H, Radbruch L. Pain treatment: a historical overview. Current Pharmaceutical Design. 2004 Mar 1;10(7):701–16.

[11] Zöllner and Stein. Opioids. In: Analgesia, Stein C, editor. Analgesia. Springer Science & Business Media; 2007 Jan 26.

[12] Ainsah O, Nabishah BM, Osman CB, Khalid BA. Effects of naloxone, glycyrrhizic acid, dexamethasone and deoxycorticosterone in repetitive stress. Clinical and Experimental Pharmacology and Physiology. 1999 May 1;26(5–6):433–7.

[13] Matthes HW, Maldonado R, Simonin F, Valverde O, Slowe S, Kitchen I, Befort K, Dierich A, Le Meur M, Dollé P, Tzavara E. Loss of morphine-induced analgesia, reward effect and withdrawal symptoms in mice lacking the μ-opioid-receptor gene. Nature. 1996; 383:819–23.

[14] Calixto JB, Beirith A, Ferreira J, Santos AR, Filho VC, Yunes RA. Naturally occurring antinociceptive substances from plants. Phytotherapy Research. 2000 Sep 1;14(6):401–18.

[15] Galeotti N, Mannelli LD, Mazzanti G, Bartolini A, Ghelardini C. Menthol: a natural analgesic compound. Neuroscience Letters. 2002 Apr 12;322(3):145–8.

[16] Roth BL, Baner K, Westkaemper R, Siebert D, Rice KC, Steinberg S, Ernsberger P, Rothman RB. Salvinorin A: a potent naturally occurring nonnitrogenous κ opioid selective agonist. Proceedings of the National Academy of Sciences. 2002 Sep 3;99(18):11934–9.

[17] Valdés LJ, Díaz J, Paul AG. Ethnopharmacology of skamariapastora (*Salvia divinorum,* Epling and Játiva-M.). Journal of Ethnopharmacology. 1983 May 1;7(3):287–312.

[18] Siebert DJ. *Salvia divinorum* and salvinorin A: new pharmacologic findings. Journal of Ethnopharmacology. 1994 Jun 30;43(1):53–6.

[19] Chavkin C. The therapeutic potential of κ-opioids for treatment of pain and addiction. Neuropsychopharmacology. 2011 Jan;36(1):369.

[20] Matsumoto K, Mizowaki M, Suchitra T, Takayama H, Sakai SI, Aimi N, Watanabe H. Antinociceptive action of mitragynine in mice: evidence for the involvement of supraspinal opioid receptors. Life Sciences. 1996 Aug 30;59(14):1149–55.

[21] Adkins JE, Boyer EW, McCurdy CR. *Mitragyna speciosa,* a psychoactive tree from Southeast Asia with opioid activity. Current Topics in Medicinal Chemistry. 2011 May 1;11(9):1165–75.

[22] Khor BS, Jamil MF, Adenan MI, Shu-Chien AC. Mitragynine attenuates withdrawal syndrome in morphine-withdrawn zebrafish. PLoS One. 2011 Dec 21;6(12):e28340.

[23] Takayama H. Chemistry and pharmacology of analgesic indole alkaloids from the rubiaceous plant, *Mitragyna speciosa*. Chemical and Pharmaceutical Bulletin. 2004;52(8):916–28.

[24] Moklas MA, Nurul Raudzah AR, Taufik Hidayat M, Sharida F, Farah Idayu N, Zulkhairi A, Shamima AR. A preliminary toxicity study of mitragynine, an alkaloid from *Mitragyna speciosa* Korth and its effects on locomotor activity in rats. Journal of Advanced Medical and Dental Sciences Research. 2008 Sep 1;2:56–60.

[25] Holler JM, Vorce SP, McDonough-Bender PC, Magluilo J, Solomon CJ, Levine B. A drug toxicity death involving propylhexedrine and mitragynine. Journal of Analytical Toxicology. 2011 Jan 1;35(1):54–9.

[26] Pickersgill B. Relationships between weedy and cultivated forms in some species of chili peppers (genus Capsicum). Evolution. 1971 Dec 1;25(4):683–91.

[27] Szallasi A, Blumberg PM. Vanilloid (capsaicin) receptors and mechanisms. Pharmacolog ical Reviews. 1999 Jun 1;51(2):159–212.

[28] Szallasi A. The vanilloid (capsaicin) receptor: receptor types and species differences. General Pharmacology: The Vascular System. 1994 Mar 1;25(2):223–43.

[29] Thresh LT. Isolation of capsaicin. Pharmaceutical Journal. 1846;6:941.

[30] Nelson EK. The constitution of capsaicin, the pungent principle of Capsicum. Journal of the American Chemical Society. 1919 Jul;41(7):1115–21.

[31] Suzuki T, Iwai K. Constituents of red pepper species: chemistry, biochemistry, pharmacology, and food science of the pungent principle of Capsicum species. The Alkaloids: Chemistry and Pharmacology. 1984 Dec 31;23:227–99.

[32] Szallasi A. Autoradiographic visualization and pharmacological characterization of vanilloid (capsaicin) receptors in several species, including man. Acta Physiologica Scandinavica. Supplementum. 1994 Dec;629:1–68.

[33] Dray A, Bettaney J, Forster P. Actions of capsaicin on peripheral nociceptors of the neonatal rat spinal cord-tail in vitro: dependence of extracellular ions and independence of second messengers. British Journal of Pharmacology. 1990 Nov 1;101(3):727–33.

[34] Oh GS, Pae HO, Seo WG, Kim NY, Pyun KH, Kim IK, Shin MK, Chung HT. Capsazepine, a vanilloid receptor antagonist, inhibits the expression of inducible nitric oxide synthase gene in lipopolysaccharide-stimulated RAW264. 7 macrophages through the inactivation of nuclear transcription factor-kappa B. International Immunopharmacology. 2001 Apr 30;1(4):777–84.

[35] Chodoeva A, Bosc JJ, Robert J. Aconitum alkaloids and biological activities. In Natural Products 2013 (pp. 1503–1523). Springer, Berlin Heidelberg.

[36] Khare CP. ed. Indian herbal remedies: rational Western therapy, ayurvedic, and other traditional usage, Botany. Springer Science & Business Media. 2004.

[37] Gutser UT, Friese J, Heubach JF, Matthiesen T, Selve N, Wilffert B, Gleitz J. Mode of antinociceptive and toxic action of alkaloids of Aconitum spec. Naunyn-Schmiedeberg's Archives of Pharmacology. 1997 Dec 1;357(1):39–48.

[38] Graves G. Medicinal plants: an illustrated guide to more than 180 herbal plants. Bracken Books, London; 1996: p. 116–118.

[39] Cechinel Filho V, Schlemper V, Santos AR, Pinheiro TR, Yunes RA, Mendes GL, Calixto JB, DelleMonache F. Isolation and identification of active compounds from *Drimys winteri* barks. Journal of Ethnopharmacology. 1998 Oct 31;62(3):223–7.

[40] Mendes GL, Santos AR, Malheiros A, CechinelFilho V, Yunes RA, Calixto JB. Assessment of mechanisms involved in antinociception caused by sesquiterpenes polygodial. Journal of Pharmacology and Experimental Therapeutics. 2000 Jan 1;292(1):164–72.

[41] Tratsk KS, Campos MM, Vaz ZR, Schlemper V, Yunes RA, Calixto JB. Anti-allergic effects and oedema inhibition caused by the extract of *Drymiswinteri*. Inflammation Research. 1997 Dec 1;46(12):509–14.

[42] Malheiros A, Cechinel Filho V, Schmitt CB, Santos AR, Scheidt C, Calixto JB, DelleMonache F, Yunes RA. A sesquiterpenedrimane with antinociceptive activity from *Drimys winteri* bark. Phytochemistry. 2001 May 31;57(1):103–7.

[43] Elisabetsky E and Etkin NL. Ethnopharmacology. Eolss Publishers Company Limited; 2009: Vol II, p. 47–48.

[44] Tan BK, Bay BH, Zhu YZ. Novel compounds from natural products in the new millennium: potential and challenges. World Scientific; 2004.

[45] Dubey NK. ed., Plants as a Source of Natural Antioxidants. CABI, Banaras Hindu University, India, 2014: p. 68.

[46] Tavares C and Sakata RK. Caffeine in the treatment of pain. Revista Brasileira de Anestesiologia. 2012;62(3):394–401.

[47] Goldstein J. Caffeine as an analgesic adjuvant. Inflammopharmacology. 2001;9(1):51–61.

[48] Sawynok J. Pharmacological rationale for the clinical use of caffeine. Drugs. 1995 Jan 1;49(1):37–50.

[49] Sawynok J, Yaksh TL. Caffeine as an analgesic adjuvant: a review of pharmacology and mechanisms of action. Pharmacological Reviews. 1993 Mar 1;45(1):43–85.

[50] Burnstock G, Kennedy C. Is there a basis for distinguishing two types of P 2-purinoceptor? General Pharmacology: The Vascular System. 1985 Dec 31;16(5):433–40.

[51] Sawynok, J. Adenosine receptor activation and nociception. European Journal of Pharmacology. 1998;347(1):1–11.

[52] Yoon SR, Nah JJ, Shin YH, Kim SK, Nam KY, Choi HS, Nah SY. Ginsenosides induce differential antinociception and inhibit substance P induced-nociceptive response in mice. Life Sciences. 1998 Apr 17;62(21):PL319–25.

[53] Shin YH, Jung OM, Nah JJ, Nam KY, Kim CY, Nah SY. Ginsenosides that produce differential antinociception in mice. General Pharmacology: The Vascular System. 1999 Jun 30;32(6):653–9.

[54] Nah JJ, Hahn JH, Chung S, Choi S, Kim YI, Nah SY. Effect of ginsenosides, active components of ginseng, on capsaicin-induced pain-related behavior. Neuropharmacology. 2000 Oct 31;39(11):2180–4.

[55] Nah SY, McCleskey EW. Ginseng root extract inhibits calcium channels in rat sensory neurons through a similar path, but different receptor, as μ-type opioids. Journal of Ethnopharmacology. 1994 Mar 31;42(1):45–51.

[56] Clare JJ, Tate SN, Nobbs M, Romanos MA. Voltage-gated sodium channels as therapeutic targets. Drug Discovery Today. 2000 Nov 1;5(11):506–20.

[57] Blednov YA, Stoffel M, Alva H, Harris RA. A pervasive mechanism for analgesia: activation of GIRK2 channels. Proceedings of the National Academy of Sciences. 2003 Jan 7;100(1):277–82.

[58] Jin W, Klem AM, Lewis JH, Lu Z. Mechanisms of inward-rectifier K^+ channel inhibition by tertiapin-Q. Biochemistry. 1999 Oct 26;38(43):14294–301.

[59] Marker CL, Stoffel M, Wickman K. Spinal G-protein-gated K^+ channels formed by GIRK1 and GIRK2 subunits modulate thermal nociception and contribute to morphine analgesia. The Journal of Neuroscience. 2004 Mar 17;24(11):2806–12.

[60] Okuse K. Pain signalling pathways: from cytokines to ion channels. The International Journal of Biochemistry & Cell Biology. 2007 Dec 31;39(3):490–6.

[61] Knight YE, Bartsch T, Kaube H, Goadsby PJ. P/Q-type calcium-channel blockade in the periaqueductal gray facilitates trigeminal nociception: a functional genetic link for migraine? The Journal of Neuroscience. 2002 Mar 1;22(5):RC213.

[62] Murakami M, Nakagawasai O, Suzuki T, Mobarakeh II, Sakurada Y, Murata A, Yamadera F, Miyoshi I, Yanai K, Tan-No K, Sasano H. Antinociceptive effect of different types of calcium channel inhibitors and the distribution of various calcium channel α 1 subunits in the dorsal horn of spinal cord in mice. Brain Research. 2004 Oct 22;1024(1):122–9.

[63] Spande TF, Garraffo HM, Edwards MW, Yeh HJ, Pannell L, Daly JW. Epibatidine: a novel (chloropyridyl) azabicycloheptane with potent analgesic activity from an Ecuadoran poison frog. Journal of the American Chemical Society. 1992 Apr;114(9):3475–8.

[64] Badio B, Shi D, Martin HM, Daly JW. Antinociceptive effects of the alkaloid epibatidine: Further studies on involvement of nicotinic receptors. Drug Development Research. 1995 Sep 1;36(1):46–59.

[65] Worm K, Zhou QJ, Saeui CT, Green RC, Cassel JA, Stabley GJ, DeHaven RN, Conway-James N, La Buda CJ, Koblish M, Little PJ. Sulfamoyl benzamides as novel CB 2 cannabinoid receptor ligands. Bioorganic& Medicinal Chemistry Letters. 2008 May 1;18(9):2830–5.

[66] Felder CC, Briley EM, Axelrod J, Simpson JT, Mackie K, Devane WA. Anandamide, an endogenous cannabimimetic eicosanoid, binds to the cloned human cannabinoid receptor and stimulates receptor-mediated signal transduction. Proceedings of the National Academy of Sciences. 1993 Aug 15;90(16):7656–60.

[67] Di Marzo V, De Petrocellis L, Fezza F, Ligresti A, Bisogno T. Anandamide receptors. Prostaglandins, Leukotrienes and Essential Fatty Acids (PLEFA). 2002 Feb 28;66(2):377–91.

[68] Gerard C, Mollereau C, Vassart G, Parmentier M. Nucleotide sequence of a human cannabinoid receptor cDNA. Nucleic Acids Research. 1990 Dec 11;18(23):7142.

[69] García-Martínez C, Humet M, Planells-Cases R, Gomis A, Caprini M, Viana F, De la Peña E, Sanchez-Baeza F, Carbonell T, De Felipe C, Pérez-Payá E. Attenuation of thermal nociception and hyperalgesia by VR1 blockers. Proceedings of the National Academy of Sciences. 2002 Feb 19;99(4):2374–9.

[70] Caterina MJ, Julius D. The vanilloid receptor: a molecular gateway to the pain pathway. Annual Review of Neuroscience. 2001 Mar;24(1):487–517.

[71] Szallasi A, Blumberg PM, Annicelli LL, Krause JE, Cortright DN. The cloned rat vanilloid receptor VR1 mediates both R-type binding and C-type calcium response in dorsal root ganglion neurons. Molecular Pharmacology. 1999 Sep 1;56(3):581–7.

[72] Szallasi A, Biro T, Szabo T, Modarres S, Petersen M, Klusch A, Blumberg PM, Krause JE, Sterner O. A non-pungent triprenyl phenol of fungal origin, scutigeral, stimulates

rat dorsal root ganglion neurons via interaction at vanilloid receptors. British Journal of Pharmacology. 1999 Mar 1;126(6):1351–8.

[73] Burnstock G. A basis for distinguishing two types of purinergic receptor. Cell membrane receptors for drugs and hormones: a multidisciplinary approach. 1978;107–18.

[74] Coddou C, Yan Z, Obsil T, Huidobro-Toro JP, Stojilkovic SS. Activation and regulation of purinergic P2X receptor channels. Pharmacological Reviews. 2011 Sep 1;63(3):641–83.

[75] Chen CC, Akopian AN, Sivilottit L, Colquhoun D, Burnstock G, Wood JN. A P2X purinoceptor expressed by a subset of sensory neurons. Nature. 1995 Oct 5;377(6548):428–31.

[76] Burnstock G. A unifying purinergic hypothesis for the initiation of pain. The Lancet. 1996 Jun 8;347(9015):1604–5.

[77] Burnstock G. Purinergic P2 receptors as targets for novel analgesics. Pharmacology & Therapeutics. 2006 Jun 30;110(3):433–54.

[78] Soares-Bezerra RJ, Calheiros AS, da Silva Ferreira NC, da Silva Frutuoso V, Alves LA. Natural products as a source for new anti-inflammatory and analgesic compounds through the inhibition of purinergic P2X receptors. Pharmaceuticals. 2013 Apr 29;6(5):650–8.

[79] Li X, Zhang J, Gao Y, Yang Y, Xu C, Li G, Guo G, Liu S, Xie J, Liang S. Puerarin alleviates burn-related procedural pain mediated by P2X3 receptors. Purinergic Signalling. 2011 Dec 1;7(4):489–97.

Footnotes

Chemical structures that cite in the current chapter are taken from those provided on submitted PubChem chemical compound records, as follows:

- **Aconitine**: National Center for Biotechnology Information. PubChem Compound Database; CID=2012, https://pubchem.ncbi.nlm.nih.gov/compound/2012.
- **Aspirin**: National Center for Biotechnology Information. PubChem Compound Database; CID=2244, https://pubchem.ncbi.nlm.nih.gov/compound/2244.
- **Caffeine**: National Center for Biotechnology Information. PubChem Compound Database; CID=2519, https://pubchem.ncbi.nlm.nih.gov/compound/2519.
- **Capsaicin:** National Center for Biotechnology Information. PubChem Compound Database; CID=1548943, https://pubchem.ncbi.nlm.nih.gov/compound/1548943.
- **Codeine**: National Center for Biotechnology Information. PubChem Compound Database; CID=5284371, https://pubchem.ncbi.nlm.nih.gov/compound/5284371.
- **Drimanial**: National Center for Biotechnology Information. PubChem Compound Database; CID=636975, https://pubchem.ncbi.nlm.nih.gov/compound/636975.

- **Ginsenosides**: National Center for Biotechnology Information. PubChem Compound Database; CID=9852086, https://pubchem.ncbi.nlm.nih.gov/compound/9852086.
- **Lappaconitine**: National Center for Biotechnology Information. PubChem Compound Database; CID=115161, https://pubchem.ncbi.nlm.nih.gov/compound/115161.
- **Menthol**: National Center for Biotechnology Information. PubChem Compound Database; CID=16666, https://pubchem.ncbi.nlm.nih.gov/compound/16666.
- **Mitragynine hydroxyindolenine**: National Center for Biotechnology Information. PubChem Compound Database; CID=44301524, https://pubchem.ncbi.nlm.nih.gov/compound/44301524.
- **Mitragynine**: National Center for Biotechnology Information. PubChem Compound Database; CID=3034396, https://pubchem.ncbi.nlm.nih.gov/compound/3034396.
- **Morphine**: National Center for Biotechnology Information. PubChem Compound Database; CID=5288826, https://pubchem.ncbi.nlm.nih.gov/compound/5288826.
- **Nalorphine**: National Center for Biotechnology Information. PubChem Compound Database; CID=5284595, https://pubchem.ncbi.nlm.nih.gov/compound/5284595.
- **Naloxone**: National Center for Biotechnology Information. PubChem Compound Database; CID=5284596, https://pubchem.ncbi.nlm.nih.gov/compound/5284596.
- **Polygodial**: National Center for Biotechnology Information. PubChem Compound Database; CID=72503, https://pubchem.ncbi.nlm.nih.gov/compound/72503.
- **Salvinorin A**: National Center for Biotechnology Information. PubChem Compound Database; CID=128563, https://pubchem.ncbi.nlm.nih.gov/compound/128563.
- **Thebaine**: National Center for Biotechnology Information. PubChem Compound Database; CID=5324289, https://pubchem.ncbi.nlm.nih.gov/compound/5324289.
- **Theobromine**: National Center for Biotechnology Information. PubChem Compound Database; CID=5429, https://pubchem.ncbi.nlm.nih.gov/compound/5429.

(All accessed Dec 4, 2016)

Chapter 15

Sweet Solution Analgesia

Khawla Nuseir, Manal Kassab and
Mohammed Al-Azzani

Additional information is available at the end of the chapter

http://dx.doi.org/10.5772/66596

Abstract

Mammals' first tasting experience is usually sweet solution. Whether it is milk (breast or formula), sugar water as in some cultures or even dates as advocated by Prophet Mohammed to his followers. Thus, it is no wonder the soothing, calming and even pain relieving effects of oral sweet solutions. Nevertheless, using sweet solution purposely for its pain-relieving effects for infants in the clinical setting is relatively recent; however, the discussion concerning sweet solution effectiveness, mechanism of actions and adverse long-term effects are still ongoing. In this chapter, we present an account of studies on both humans and animals that explored and examined the use of several sweet solutions for analgesia.

Keywords: premature, infants, pain, NICU, sucrose

1. Introduction

Young children are subjected to undergo many painful medical procedures early in their life. Althoughthese procedures are performed even in healthy children, they are more common in sick ones who need an admission to the hospital. Treating pain in the newborn is essential; firstly, for ethical reasons and, secondly, because pain can lead to several physiological and psychological effects. Not only such negative consequences are not related to repeated painful procedures but even short-term pain can have lasting negative effects [1]. Young children, including neonates, are more sensitive to nociceptive stimuli than adults [2]. Research findings emphasized that repeated exposure to painful stimuli during early stage of fundamental development of the nervous system leads to persistent behavioral and sensory changes [3]. Despite this fact, the use of appropriate pain relief interventions during potentially painful procedures is unusual in this population [4]. A paradox is still observed between the frequency of conditions that cause pain among young children and the use of appropriate pain relief intervention. The most often cited causes for this paradox are the several myths surrounding the painful experience in the neonatal population, particularly the perception that the newborn is too immature to feel pain [5]. It is known that the knowledge about the presence of pain in newborns has greatly increased among health providers who are responsible for neonatal care [6], but it is not known how each professional puts such knowledge into practice [7]. Young children including neonates do not have the ability to verbalize their pain thus health care providers must recognize their pain. Not only unmanaged pain causes distress and delayed recovery but pain in infancy also has short-term (physiological and behavioral) and long-term developmental consequences (increased or decreased behavioral responses to pain). Although infant's pain is not expressed as conscious memory, memories of pain may be recorded biologically and alter brain development and subsequent behavior. Some recent studies have reported that simple and benign interventions such as oral sweet solutions [5, 8, 9], milk [10] or sucking a pacifier [11] reduce pain in neonates during procedures. Pain relieving effects of sweet solutions such as sucrose have been examined in term and preterm neonates [12, 13]. Glucose and other sweet tasting solutions have also been found to have pain relieving effects [9]. The effect of sugar on calming a crying baby during painful procedure is not new but there are historical references pertaining to the analgesic and calming benefits of sweet substances dating back to AD 632, when Prophet Mohammed recommended giving infants a well-chewed date [14]. Also Thorek, in his textbook, *Modern Surgical Technique*, published in 1938, explained his ideas of acceptable pediatric anesthesia: "Often no anesthesia is required. A sucker consisting of a sponge dipped in some sugar water will often suffice to calm a baby" [15].

2. Sweet solutions in the clinical settings and guidelines

The implementation of sweet solution for minor painful and invasive procedures in the NICU has been documented in many studies and extensive review of studies showed that sweet solutions have analgesic effects in young children up to one-year-old [16].

Study findings show that giving sweet solutions to young infants during painful procedures reduces painful responses and crying time tends to be shorter [9]. Different concentrations and dose were examined and showed to have a pain relieving effect. The most widely used sweet solution is sucrose [17]. Glucose is the second most commonly used solution, as it is available as prepared solution at clinics and hospitals [9]. All sweet solutions are administered in the same way, on the infants' lateral side of the tongue prior to or 2 min before the procedure through a syringe slowly over 30 s [9, 18]. Another administration technique is through the use of non-nutritive sucking using pacifier to improve its effectiveness [11, 19].

Sweet solution is a fast acting pain-relief intervention (within 10 seconds) [20]. Although there is no evidence yet about the dose-response effects [21], dose ranging from 0.5 to 2 mL of 12–24% strength show pain-relief effect [11, 22]. For premature neonates, dose is calculated in accordance to their weight/volume ratio. **Table 1** displays the doses according to week's gestation and kilograms. In preterm neonates, it is recommended to use multiple dose regimens instead of given one dose to reduce any risk of adverse effects such as chocking. Several clini-

Age group	27–31 weeks	32 to terms	0–3 months
Suggested doses (single events)	0.2 mL	0.2–0.5 mL	0.2–2 mL
Suggested doses (24 hours)	1 mL	2.5 mL	5 mL
Suggested doses (in kg)	0.5 mL/kg/dose	0.5 mL/kg/dose	0.5 mL/kg/dose
Source: [23, 24].			

Table 1. Doses according to week's gestation and kilograms and the sweetener used.

cal guidelines included the use of sweet solution for analgesia particularly for minor painful procedures. Heel lance followed by venipuncture were the top benefiting procedures of this analgesic measure [25–27]. Sweet solution may be used in infants aged 27 or more-week gestation. The volume administered for each age group should be as follow: 27–31 weeks' gestation (0.1–0.5 mL); 32–36 weeks' gestation (0.5–1 mL) and greater than 37 weeks' gestation (1–2 mL)

• Infants with known sucrose or fructose intolerance
• Infants with sucrase-isomaltase deficiency (CSID)
• Infants with glucose-galactose malabsorption
• Infants who are less than 27 weeks' gestational age
• Infants who are critically ill
• Infants with confirmed or suspected GIT pathology, such as necrotizing enterocolitis
• Infants who are paralyzed or sedated
• Infants with altered gag or swallow reflex
Source: Refs. [28, 29].

Table 2. Contraindications for the use of sweet solution as analgesic.

[5, 8, 9]. Dosage is usually expressed in mg. It is recommended to record the given dose and time on the neonates' medication sheet. Sweet solution does not need a doctor's order but it could be given by a nurse as needed, which is prepared in the pharmacy if not readily available in sterile container at floors. Once the container is open, the solution may be kept at the bedside for 24 hours if not Contaminated. It is important to record the opening date and time on the container. Sweet solution should not be used on infants less than 27-week gestations, infants who have suspected or proven gastrointestinal dysfunction/abnormalities such as ileus, obstruction, necrotizing enterocolitis or who are postoperative. Sweet solution should not be used for unstable or compromised neonates. **Table 2** lists the contraindications for the use of sweet solutions for analgesia.

Around the world more and more hospitals and clinics are implementing the use of sweet substances to reduce pain and discomfort among premature and mature infants. Yet important knowledge and research gaps concerning long-term analgesic effects of repeated administration of sweet solutions still exist. One reason could be related to the fact that the mechanism of sweet-taste-induced analgesia is still not precisely understood, which prevented the uptake of such intervention using research evidence from being used in practice.

3. Sweet solution analgesia in human studies

Sweet solution as analgesic for painful events performed on premature and full term infants is a true revolutionary, novel and relatively current idea [30, 31]. It took long time for the clinical community to recognize and accept the fact that this special group of people does feel pain and this pain has short- and long-term negative consequences [32]. Moreover, available treatments such as opioids were considered unsafe and fear of their adverse effects lead to under treatment or even no treatment at all even for invasive practices [33]. Another obstacle was the lack of proper pain assessment measures for infants and nonverbal children [34]. Physiological and behavioral responses to pain were observed [34], and this lead to the development of pain assessment tools appropriate for measuring premature and infants pain, one of these tools is the premature infant pain profile (PIPP) that is utilized to assess pain and effectiveness of pain management among premature infants [35].

Sweet solution analgesia has been used for painful procedures performed in the NICU, for immunization, injections and circumcision. Heel lances performed quite often in the NICU provoked less physiological and behavioral responses of pain when proceeded with 2 mL of oral sucrose solution of 50% [36]. Same had been noticed for other routinely applied procedures such as intravenous or arterial line insertion, lumbar puncture, tape removal and venipuncture [37–39]. This analgesic effect also extends to even older infants; sucrose was also effective in lowering pain scores due to immunization for babies aged between 1 and 12 months [23, 40]. Sucrose was beneficial when paired with other analgesic for pain relief during circumcision, probably since circumcision is a more intensely painful procedure than other routine procedures undertaken at NICU, yet it gave a synergistic effect with other analgesic methods [41]. The concentration of the sweet agent also mattered; a more concentrated sugar solution was found to be a more effective analgesic than less concentrated ones [21].

Sucrose is the most widely used agent for sweet solution-induced analgesia, nevertheless, other sweeteners were also tried and found to be effective. Fructose, lactose, milk and non-caloric sweeteners had been used for analgesia, although less frequently [21]. Glucose 20–30% solution is effective for heel lance and venipuncture in preterm and term infants [42, 43]. Fructose was as effective as sucrose and both were more effective than glucose [31]. In humans, fructose is as sweet as sucrose and sweeter than glucose; this might explain why fructose and sucrose were more effective than glucose [44]. Non-caloric sweeteners were also as effective as sucrose in reducing pain due to procedures such as heel lance [45].

http://dx.doi.org/10.5772/66596

The effect of sweet solution in reducing pain and calming crying infants is restricted to oral administration [12], providing evidence that it is the taste of sweetness what causes analgesia and not the sugar itself. Further evidence comes from the observation that different sugars and even artificial sweeteners produce the same effect when given orally into the oral cavity. Activating sensory afferents in the oral cavity leads to pleasurable sensation or effect. This positive hedonic effect of sweet tasting substances induced analgesia further supports the theory that it is the taste of sweetness not the caloric value of the food [46].

The mechanism of this sweet-induced analgesia is not fully elucidated. While animal studies provided more convincing evidence for the involvement of the endogenous opioid system, human studies were equivocal [42, 47, 48]. Tolerance to repeated doses of glucose did not develop, and an opioid antagonist, naloxone, given before glucose did not diminish its analgesic effects. On the other hand, babies born to methadone-addict mothers did not respond to the calming effects of sucrose. Thus, so far the evidence support the idea that the mechanism of analgesia induction might be mediated via opioid and non-opioid pathways [8, 47].

This analgesic effect is short lived and repeat administration is needed for repeated procedures. Furthermore, this effect of sweet tasting solutions does not persist beyond infancy [21]. This sweet taste–induced analgesia does not extend to adults, and it seems to be related to the degree of sweetness; thus higher sucrose concentration were preferred by children compared to adults [49]. One explanation is that as we grow, the positive hedonic value of sweet tasting substances decreases thus evoking less pleasure and less analgesia.

Other non-pharmacological methods were also studied, kangaroo mother care KMC was found to be mildly effective at lowering pain responses to heel lance in full and preterm neonates [50]. Skin-to-skin contact between infant and mother alleviated pain occurrence during heel lance as well [51].

4. Sweet solution analgesia in animal studies

Animal studies have shown an analgesic effect of sweet solutions during infancy similar to that of humans [52]. Sweet components of milk including sucrose, glucose or fructose have shown to alleviate neonatal pain [53, 54]. The analgesic effect of sweet solutions is confined to the intraoral route as sucrose reduces pain sensation when administered orally not when applied via gastric gavage [12]. The antinociceptive actions of these solutions are not due to intraoral infusion alone because they are not produced by water or lactose [54, 55].

The most commonly studied is the natural sweetener sucrose. Sucrose has a long history of calming and analgesic effect especially for neonatal pain. The first observation of sucrose pain modulating effects was obtained by Blass et al. 1987 who reported that contact with a small amount of sucrose solution on the tongue of infant rats rapidly increased the paw withdrawal latency (a measure of pain threshold) in a hot-plate test [56]. Sucrose-induced analgesia during infancy develops rapidly and persists for several minutes [57]. In addition, sucrose ingestion for a relatively long period of time produces analgesia [58, 59]. Acute sucrose-induced analgesia is age-dependent that means it occurs mainly during the pre-weaning period in rats [57].

Artificial sweeteners have also shown analgesic actions when administered orally. Chronic saccharin intake decreases pain sensitivity and increases pain threshold as measured in hot-plate test [60]. Furthermore, acute saccharin administration for 5 hours resulted in analgesia that persists for 3 hours [61]. Aspartame, another sweetener, decreases pain sensitivity, and has shown to produce analgesic effects comparable with sucrose [62, 63].

Although the mechanisms behind sweet substances-induced analgesia are still not clearly defined; endogenous opioid system is implicated. Sweet palatable solutions augment morphine-induced analgesia [64–67], this has suggested that sweet solutions ingestion is associated with the release of endogenous opioids, a mechanism which involves stimulation of gustatory sweet receptors [68]. This mechanism was supported by the observation that sucrose reduces pain sensation when administered orally not when applied via gastric gavage [12, 69]. Furthermore, naltrexone and naloxone, opioid antagonists, were shown to abolish the analgesic effect of sweet-tasting solutions [56, 70–72] In addition, consuming palatable sweet substances increases endogenous β-endorphin activity in rat brain and in human plasma [69, 73–75]. Besides, endogenous opioid system, other neurotransmitters and receptors are probably involved. One study revealed a major involvement of nicotinic cholinergic receptors in the sweet substance-induced analgesia as atropine (cholinergic antagonist) diminished sucrose-induced analgesia [76]. Other studies have shown the involvement of noradrenaline, serotonin and their receptors in the central modulation sweet substance-induced analgesia [71, 77, 78].

Likewise, sweet solutions ability to prevent, decrease or reverse unfavorable long-term effects of neonatal pain had been explored. Unpublished data and a previous study from our lab indicate that early pain experience increases pain sensitivity and impairs spatial memory during adulthood in rats; the interventions using sucrose or saccharin solution prevented these long-term consequences of neonatal pain [75].

5. Short- and long-term effects of using sweet solutions during infancy

The fear of adverse effects following the use of nutritive sweet solutions for analgesia for premature and mature infants might be a hindrance to implementing this analgesic method. Among possible short-term effects are the fear of effect of sweet intake on milk feeding afterward. Also the effect on body weight, weather an increase due to development of sweet tooth or a decrease due to decrease in appetite for healthy food such as milk. Of the long-term effects are potential negative effects on growth and development. Of more concern would be the neurodevelopmental deficits, such as attention/orientation and motor tasks, that might result of higher intake of sugar during infancy, particularly infants who spend lengthier time at the NICU and are exposed to multiple painful procedures daily, thus requiring several doses of sweet solutions. It has been calculated that the amount of sugar a preterm infant will ingest over a period of a few weeks at the NICU will be equivalent to half a can of coke ingested by a 1-year-old [48]. Since few studies have examined the potential adverse effects of sweet solutions given at infancy, the word is still not out. Despite that, studies have shown no short-term adverse effects, however developmental effects were not examined thoroughly enough to arrive at a conclusive conclusion.

Studies have proclaimed sweet solutions as safe with no or minimum immediate or long-term negative effects [48]. A few on the other hand have challenged this notion and claimed that many long- and short-term adverse effects are associated with the use of sweet solutions for pain management during infancy [79].

In conclusion, oral sucrose (0.5 mL/kg of a 25% solution, 2 min prior to acute painful procedures) for pain relief in preterm neonates was effective and safe, exhibiting no short-term adverse effects in weight gain and feeding patterns, during hospitalization and post discharge [80].

6. Conclusion

Pain due to procedures applied to premature infants has shown to affect, in a negative way, brain development. Newborns, particularly premature infants have brains and nervous systems that are still under development and are very vulnerable to any insults. The plasticity of the brain at this early age makes it ideal for external stimuli to have long lasting effects [1]. Thus it is logical to put forward the hypothesis that managing this pain will in addition to its pain reducing effects be useful in inhibiting or at least reducing the long term unfavorable effects of untreated pain.

Despite availability of analgesia and knowledge about infants' pain, a gap still exists between theoretical knowledge and actual practice. Thus the availability of non-pharmacological analgesia is very important and might be the selling point for the use of analgesia for premature and mature infants [4].

In conclusion, using sweet solutions for pain management, particularly, for this special age group is probably effective and safe, and has the potential of reversing or decreasing long-term adverse effects of pain. More studies need to be done to further explore the safety and the dose of sweet solution for pain during infancy.

Author details

Khawla Nuseir[1]*, Manal Kassab[2] and Mohammed Al-Azzani[1]

*Address all correspondence to:kqnuseir@just.edu.jo

1 Clinical Pharmacy Department, Faculty of Pharmacy, Jordan University of Science and Technology, Irbid, Jordan

2 Maternal and Child Health Nursing, Faculty of Nursing, Jordan University of Science and Technology, Irbid, Jordan

References

[1] Brummelte S, Grunau RE, Chau V, Poskitt KJ, Brant R, Vinall J, et al. Procedural pain and brain development in premature newborns. Ann Neurol. 2012;71(3):385–96.

[2] Anand KJS, Scalzo FM. Can adverse neonatal experiences alter brain development and subsequent behavior? Biol Neonate. 2000;77(2):69–82.

[3] Grunau RE. Neonatal pain in very preterm infants: long-term effects on brain, neurodevelopment and pain reactivity. Rambam Maimonides Med J. 2013;4(4):e0025.

[4] Prestes ACY, Balda RDCX, Dos Santos GMS, Rugolo LMSDS, Bentlin MR, Magalhães M, et al. Painful procedures and analgesia in the NICU: what has changed in the medical perception and practice in a ten-year period? J Pediatr (Rio J). 2016;92(1):88–95.

[5] Stevens B, Yamada J, Lee GY, Ohlsson A. Sucrose for analgesia in newborn infants undergoing painful procedures. Cochrane Database of Systematic Reviews 2013, Issue 1. Art. No.: CD001069. DOI: 10.1002/14651858.CD001069.pub4.

[6] Akuma AO, Jordan S. Pain management in neonates: a survey of nurses and doctors. J Adv Nurs. 2012;68(6):1288–301.

[7] Lefrak L, Burch K, Caravantes R, Knoerlein K, DeNolf N, Duncan J, et al. Sucrose analgesia: identifying potentially better practices. Pediatrics. 2006;118(Supplement_2):S197–202.

[8] Harrison D, Beggs S, Stevens B. Sucrose for procedural pain management in infants. Pediatrics. 2012;130(5):918–25.

[9] Kassab M, Sheehy A, King M, Fowler C, Foureur M. A double-blind randomised controlled trial of 25% oral glucose for pain relief in 2-month old infants undergoing immunisation. Int J Nurs Stud. 2012;49(3):249–56.

[10] Blass EM, Watt LB. Suckling- and sucrose-induced analgesia in human newborns. Pain. 1999;83(3):611–23.

[11] Tsao JCI, Evans S, Meldrum M, Altman T, Zeltzer LK. A review of CAM for procedural pain in infancy: part I. Sucrose and non-nutritive sucking. Evidence-Based Complement Altern Med. 2008;5(4):371–81.

[12] Ramenghi L, Evans DJ, Levene MI. "Sucrose analgesia": absorptive mechanism or taste perception? Arch Dis Child Fetal Neonatal Ed. 1999;80:F146–7.

[13] Haouari N, Wood C, Griffiths G, Levene M. The analgesic effect of sucrose in full term infants: a randomised controlled trial. BMJ. 1995;310(6993):1498–500.

[14] Islamic Voice. Relief of pain: a medical discovery. [Internet]. 2002. Available from: http://www.islamicvoice.com/april.2001/quran.htm

[15] Thorek M. Modern surgical technique, Vol III. Monterial: Lippincott, 1938; 2021. As written by AM Unruh in her article, Voices from the past: ancient views of pain in childhood. Clin J Pain. 1992;8(249).

[16] Kassab M, Foster JP, Foureur M, Fowler C. Sweet-tasting solutions for needle-related procedural pain in infants one month to one year of age. Cochrane Database of Systematic Reviews 2010, Issue 3. Art.No.: CD008411. DOI: 10.1002/14651858.CD008411.

[17] Taddio A, Shah V, Hancock R, Basc RWS, Stephens D, Atenafu E, et al. Effectiveness of sucrose analgesia in newborns undergoing painful medical procedures. Can Med Assoc J. 2008;179(1):37–43.

[18] Taddio A, Appleton M, Bortolussi R, Chambers C, Dubey V, Halperin S, et al. Reducing the pain of childhood vaccination: an evidence-based clinical practice guideline (summary). CMAJ. 2010;182(18):1989–95.

[19] Pasek TA, Huber JM. Hospitalized infants who hurt: a sweet solution with oral sucrose. Crit Care Nurse. 2012;32(1):61–9.

[20] Buscemi N, Vandermeer B, Curtis S. The cochrane library and procedural pain in children: an overview of reviews. Evid Based Child Health. 2008;3:260–79.

[21] Harrison D, Bueno M, Yamada J, Adams-Webber T, Stevens B. Analgesic effects of sweet-tasting solutions for infants: current state of equipoise. Pediatrics. 2010;126(5):894–902.

[22] Stevens BJ, Abbott LK, Yamada J, Harrison D, Stinson J, Taddio A, et al. Epidemiology and management of painful procedures in children in Canadian hospitals. CMAJ. 2011; 183 (7): E403-E410.

[23] Harrison D, Stevens B, Bueno M, Yamada J, Adams-Webber T, Beyene J, et al. Efficacy of sweet solutions for analgesia in infants between 1 and 12 months of age: a systematic review. Arch Dis Child. 2010;95(6):406–13.

[24] Kassab, M, Foster, J, Foureur, M, Fowler, C. (2012). Sweet-tasting solutions for needle-related procedural pain in infants one month to one year of age. Cochrane Pain, Palliative Support Care Group. DOI:10.1002/14651858.CD008411

[25] Lago P, Garetti E, Merazzi D, Pieragostini L, Ancora G, Pirelli A, et al. Guidelines for procedural pain in the newborn. Acta Paediatr Int J Paediatr. 2009;98(6):932–9.

[26] Taddio A, McMurtry CM, Shah V, Riddell PR, Chambers CT, Noel M, et al. Reducing the pain of childhood vaccination: an evidence- based clinical practice guideline (summary). CMAJ. 2010; 182(18): 1989-95..

[27] Cincinnati Children's Hospital Medical Center. Reducing pain for children and adolescents receiving injections. 2013;1–9.

[28] Murki S and Subramanian S., "WHO | sucrose for analgesia in newborn infants undergoing painful procedures.RHL Commentary (Last Revised: 1 June 2011). The WHO Reproductive Health Library; Geneva: World Health Organization. World Health Organization, 2016.

[29] UW Health, Pain care fast facts: 5-mimute clinical inservice sucrose analgesia for infants. n.d., http://www.uwhealth.org/.

[30] Blass EM, Hoffmeyer LB. Sucrose as an analgesic for newborn infants. Pediatrics. 1991;87(2):215–8.

[31] Blass, EM, Smith BA Differential effects of sucrose, fructose, glucose, and lactose on crying in 1- to 3-day-old human infants: qualitative and quantitative considerations. Dev Psychol. 1992;28(5):804–10.

[32] Owens ME, Todt EH. Pain in infancy: neonatal reaction to a heel lance. Pain. 1984;20(1):77–86.

[33] Johnston CC, Collinge JM, Henderson SJ, Anand KJ. A cross-sectional survey of pain and pharmacological analgesia in Canadian neonatal intensive care units. Clin J Pain. 1997;13(4):308–12.

[34] Johnston CC, Strada ME. Acute pain response in infants: a multidimensional description. Pain. 1986;24(3):373–82.

[35] Stevens B, Johnston C, Petryshen P, Taddio A. Premature infant pain profile: development and initial validation. Clin J Pain. 1996;12(1):13–22.

[36] Bucher HU, Moser T, von Siebenthal K, Keel M, Wolf M, Duc G. Sucrose reduces pain reaction to heel lancing in preterm infants: a placebo-controlled, randomized and masked study. Pediatr Res. 1995;38(3):332–5.

[37] Elserafya FA, Alsaedi SA, Louwrensc J, Bin Sadiqd B, Mersal AY. Oral sucrose and a pacifier for pain relief during simple procedures in preterm infants: a randomized controlled trial. Ann Saudi Med. 2009;29(3):184–8.

[38] Stevens B, Yamada J, Beyene J, Gibbins S, Petryshen P, Stinson J, et al. Consistent management of repeated procedural pain with sucrose in preterm neonates: is it effective and safe for repeated use over time? Clin J Pain. 2005;21(6):543–8.

[39] Rouben N, Kaur R, Rao KLN. Effect of sucrose in pain during venipuncture in infants. Nurs Midwifery Res J. 2013;9(4):152–9.

[40] Barr RG, Young SN, Wright JH, Cassidy KL, Hendricks L, Bedard Y, et al. "Sucrose analgesia" and diphtheria-tetanus-pertussis immunizations at 2 and 4 months. Dev Behav Pediatr 1995;16(4):220–5.

[41] Bellieni CV, Alagna MG, Buonocore G. Analgesia for infants' circumcision. Ital J Pediatr. 2013;39(1):38.

[42] Eriksson M, Finnstro O. Can daily repeated doses of orally administered glucose induce tolerance when given for neonatal pain relief ? Acta Paediatr. 2004;93(18):246–9.

[43] Bueno M, Yamada J, Harrison D, Khan S, Ohlsson A, Adams-Webber T, et al. A systematic review and meta-analyses of nonsucrose sweet solutions for pain relief in neonates. Pain Res Manag. 2013;18(3):153–61.

[44] Fernstrom JD, Munger SD, Sclafani A, de Araujo IE, Roberts A, Molinary S. Mechanisms for sweetness. J Nutr. 2012;142(6):1134S–41.

[45] Ramenghi LA, Griffith GC, Wood CM, Levene MI. Effect of non-sucrose sweet tasting solution on neonatal heel prick responses. Arch Dis Child. 1996;4(74):129–32.

[46] Foo H, Mason P. Analgesia accompanying food consumption requires ingestion of hedonic foods. J Neurosci. 2009;29(41):13053–62.

[47] Gradin M, Schollin J. The role of endogenous opioids in mediating pain reduction by orally administered glucose among newborns. Pediatrics. 2005;115(4):1004–7.

[48] Holsti L, Grunau RE. Considerations for using sucrose to reduce procedural pain in preterm infants. Pediatrics. 2010;125(5):1042–7.

[49] Pepino MY, Mennella JA. Sucrose-induced analgesia is related to sweet preferences in children but not adults. Pain. 2005;119(1–3):210–8.

[50] Johnston CC, Filion F, Campbell-yeo M, Goulet C, Bell L, Mcnaughton K, et al. Kangaroo mother care diminishes pain from heel lance in very preterm neonates : a crossover trial. BMC Pediatr. 2008;9(13):1–9.

[51] Gray L, Watt L, Blass EM. Skin-to-skin contact is analgesic in healthy newborns. Pediatrics. 2000;105(1):e14.

[52] Fitzgerald M, Shaw A, MacIntosh N. Postnatal development of the cutaneous flexor reflex: comparative study of preterm infants and newborn rat pups. Dev Med Child Neurol. 1988;30(4):520–6.

[53] Blass EM, Fitzgerald E. Milk-induced analgesia and comforting in 10-day-old rats: opioid mediation. Pharmacol Biochem Behav. 1988;29(1):9–13.

[54] Blass EM, Shide DJ. Some comparisons among the calming and pain-relieving effects of sucrose, glucose, fructose and lactose in infant rats. Chem Senses. 1994;19(3):239–49.

[55] Ren K, Blass EM, Zhou Q, Dubner R. Suckling and sucrose ingestion suppress persistent hyperalgesia and spinal Fos expression after forepaw inflammation in infant rats. Proc Natl Acad Sci U S A 1997;94:1471–5.

[56] Blass E, Fitzgerald E, Kehoe P. Interactions between sucrose, pain and isolation distress. Pharmacol Biochem Behav. 1987;26(3):483–9.

[57] Anseloni VCZ, Weng HR, Terayama R, Letizia D, Davis BJ, Ren K, et al. Age-dependency of analgesia elicited by intraoral sucrose in acute and persistent pain models. Pain. 2002;97(1–2):93–103.

[58] Segato FN, Castro-Souza C, Segato EN, Morato S, Coimbra NC. Sucrose ingestion causes opioid analgesia. Braz J Med Biol Res 1997;30:981–4.

[59] Kanarek RB, Mandillo S, Wiatr C. Chronic sucrose intake augments antinociception induced by injections of mu but not kappa opioid receptor agonists into the periaqueductal gray matter in male and female rats. Brain Res. 2001;920(1–2):97–105.

[60] Bergmann F, Cohen E, Lieblich I. Biphasic effects of chronic saccharin intake on pain responses of healthy and diabetic rats of two genetically selected strains. Psychopharmacology (Berl). 1984;82(3):248–51.

[61] Suri M, Jain S, Mathur R. Pattern of biphasic response to various noxious stimuli in rats ingesting sucrose ad libitum. Physiol Behav. 2010;101(2):224–31.

[62] Rani S, Gupta MC. Evaluation and comparison of antinociceptive activity of aspartame with sucrose. Pharmacol Rep. 2012;64(2):293–8.

[63] Abdollahi M, Nikfar S, Abdoli N. Potentiation by nitric oxide synthase inhibitor and calcium channel blocker of aspartame-induced antinociception in the mouse formalin test. Fundam Clin Pharmacol. 2001;15(2):117–23.

[64] Kanarek RB, White ES, Biegen MT, Marks-Kaufman R. Dietary influences on morphine-induced analgesia in rats. Pharmacol Biochem Behav. 1991;38(3):681–4.

[65] D'Anci KE, Kanarek RB, Marks-Kaufman R. Beyond sweet taste: saccharin, sucrose, and polycose differ in their effects upon morphine-induced analgesia. Pharmacol Biochem Behav. 1997;56(3):341–5.

[66] Abdollahi M, Nikfar S, Habibi L. Saccharin effects on morphine-induced antinociception in the mouse formalin test. Pharmacol Res. 2000;42(3):255–9.

[67] Kanarek RB, Homoleski B. Modulation of morphine-induced antinociception by palatable solutions in male and female rats. Pharmacol Biochem Behav. 2000;66(3):653–9.

[68] Anseloni VCZ, Ren K, Dubner R, Ennis M. A brainstem substrate for analgesia elicited by intraoral sucrose. Neuroscience. 2005;133(1):231–43.

[69] Yamamoto T, Sako N, Maeda S. Effects of taste stimulation on beta-endorphin levels in rat cerebrospinal fluid and plasma. Physiol Behav. 2000;69(3):345–50.

[70] De Freitas RL, Kübler JML, Elias-Filho DH, Coimbra NC. Antinociception induced by acute oral administration of sweet substance in young and adult rodents: the role of endogenous opioid peptides chemical mediators and μ 1-opioid receptors. Pharmacol Biochem Behav 2012;101:265–70.

[71] Rebouças ECC, Segato EN, Kishi R, Freitas RL, Savoldi M, Morato S, et al. Effect of the blockade of mu1-opioid and 5HT2A-serotonergic/alpha1-noradrenergic receptors on sweet-substance-induced analgesia. Psychopharmacology (Berl). 2005;179:349–55.

[72] Shahlaee A, Farahanchi A, Javadi S, Delfan B, Dehpour AR. Sucrose-induced analgesia in mice: Role of nitric oxide and opioid receptor-mediated system. Indian J Pharmacol. 2013;45(6):593–6.

[73] Melchior JC, Rigaud D, Colas-Linhart N, Petiet A, Girard A, Apfelbaum M. Immunoreactive beta-endorphin increases after an aspartame chocolate drink in healthy human subjects. Physiol Behav. 1991;50(5):941–4.

[74] Dum J, Gramsch C, Herz A. Activation of hypothalamic β-endorphin pools by reward induced by highly palatable food. Pharmacol Biochem Behav. 1983;18(3):443–7.

[75] Nuseir KQ, Alzoubi KH, Alabwaini J, Khabour OF, Kassab MI. Sucrose-induced analgesia during early life modulates adulthood learning and memory formation. Physiol Behav 2015;145:84–90.

[76] Irusta AE, Savoldi M, Kishi R, Resende GC, Freitas RL, Carvalho AD, et al. Psychopharmacological evidences for the involvement of muscarinic and nicotinic cholinergic receptors on sweet substance-induced analgesia in *Rattus norvegicus*. Neurosci Lett. 2001;305(2):115–8.

[77] Miyase CI, Kishi R, De Freitas RL, Paz DA, Coimbra NC. Involvement of pre- and postsynaptic serotonergic receptors of dorsal raphe nucleus neural network in the control of the sweet-substance-induced analgesia in adult *Rattus norvegicus* (Rodentia, Muridae). Neurosci Lett. 2005;379(3):169–73.

[78] Kishi R, Bongiovanni R, De Nadai TR, Freitas RL, De Oliveira R, Ferreira CMDR, et al. Dorsal raphe nucleus and locus coeruleus neural networks and the elaboration of the sweet-substance-induced antinociception. Neurosci Lett 2006;395:12–7.

[79] Gaspardo CM, Miyase CI, Chimello JT, Martinez FE, Martins Linhares MB. Is pain relief equally efficacious and free of side effects with repeated doses of oral sucrose in preterm neonates? Pain. 2008;137(1):16–25.

[80] Harrison DM. Oral sucrose for pain management in infants: myths and misconceptions. J Neonatal Nurs. 2008;14(2):39–46.

[81] Linhares MBM, Gaspardo CM, Souza LO, Valeri BO, Martinez FE. Examining the side effects of sucrose for pain relief in preterm infants: a case-control study. Braz J Med Biol Res. 2014;47(6):527–32.

Chapter 16

Analgesics: New Target and Sources

Mohammad Saleem and Huma Naz

Additional information is available at the end of the chapter

http://dx.doi.org/10.5772/67853

Abstract

The aim of this chapter is to describe targets for analgesic drugs, including currently available target sites and possible future target sites for pain and information regarding analgesia for complete understanding of pain originating mechanism, pathways and related theories to recognize. This chapter fully describes methods for determination of analgesic effects of synthetic and natural substances by inducing pain in different models and methods of pain induction.

Keywords: pain, analgesics, targets, sources

1. Introduction

Pain is the measure of a cautious response against organ damage or unevenness in its capacities against conceivably unsafe stimulation. The rising pathway of pain incorporates the contralateral spinothalamic tract, lateral pons, mid brain to thalamus and at last, through the somatosensory cortex of the cerebrum that defines the zones, force and profundity of pain [1]. Pain is the most widely recognized experience reported by patients, and patient tension is a type of caution sign. It is an exotic and perceptual sensation, which causes enduring and enthusiastic condition of dangers associated with tension. Pain has numerous structures. It cautions against harm to the body, which is critical for maintaining a strategic distance from wounds and thus for survival. Pain not brought about by intense wounds can be insalubrious for the patient, or it can adjust a man's life, decrease the personal satisfaction and furthermore affect the patient's family. 'Pain' for the patient means malady and enduring, for the specialist, it is a side effect and for the physiologist, it is a sort of feeling that has its own particular anatomical and physiological framework which starts with the receptors and winds up in the cerebrum cortex. Feeling is a physical impression that can be affirmed by electrophysiological techniques, however, by and by, it is just a subjective sensation. Its force and quality go under different inside and outer elements; in this way, the same boost can be experienced distinctively in various circumstances and substantial and psychiatric conditions. The method for accepting pain is extremely individual and differs every once in a while in the same person. The force of pain is hard to quantify, and an individual's impression of nuisance relies upon the individual's enthusiastic state, circumstances under which the pain was obtained and whether it is seen as an undermining signal [2–4]. Before we understand that something harms, there are various physiological procedures in our body. Painful stimuli must be passed rapidly, in (milli) seconds. Intense pain cautions about looming or following risk while continual pain causes the burdened part of the body, for example, an immobilized and unused appendage, expanding the chance for healing. A solitary and sharp stimulus to pain can vanish and most likely not leave a track. Pain progression can be supported and inhibited by the adaptive changes in the central nervous system due to the repeated stimuli. Sense of pain is modified by the synthesis and activation of many receptor systems along with synthesis of numerous compounds in the brain and spinal cord. In this complicated process, glial cells perform a significant role in the preservation of the pain, even after the pain stimulus is disappeared [5].

In the peripheral and central nervous system, pain can also be generated without receptors. This sort of pain is always a pathological pain which ascends due to injury to the nervous system, and it has an altered nature from physiological pain and clinical presentation. Therefore, it is important to distinguish receptor pain—nociceptive, physiological pain from non-receptor pain—pathological, central and peripheral. In **Table 1**, different types of pain are defined.

Utilization of an intense harmful stimulus to ordinary tissue inspires intense physiological nociceptive pain. It shields tissue from being (further) harmed in light of the fact that withdrawal reflexes are typically inspired. Pathophysiological nociceptive pain happens when the tissue is excited or harmed. It might show up as unconstrained (pain without any deliberate incitement) or as hyperalgesia and/or allodynia. Hyperalgesia is a compelling pain force felt upon harmful incitement, and allodynia is the impression of discomfort inspired by stimuli that are ordinarily underneath pain edge. In non-neuropathic pain, a few creators incorporate the bringing down of the pain limit in the term hyperalgesia. While nociceptive pain is inspired by incitement of the tactile endings in the tissue, neuropathic pain results from harm or sickness of neurons in the peripheral or central nervous system. It does not essentially signal

Allodynia	Pain on account of a stimulation that does not customarily induce pain, e.g. pain brought on by a T-shirt patients with postherpetic neuralgia
Dysesthesia	An unpalatable anomalous sensation, whether unconstrained or evoked while paresthesia is not upsetting, e.g. in patients with diabetic polyneuropathy or lack of vitamin B1
Hyperalgesia	An expanded reaction to a jolt that is typically painful
Hyperesthesia	Expanded affectability to incitement, barring the exceptional senses, e.g. expanded cutaneous sensibility to warm sensation without agony/pain

Source: International Association for the Study of Pain.

Table 1. Types of pain.

noxious tissue stimulation and often feels abnormal. Its character is regularly smouldering or electrical, and it can be relentless or happen in short parts (e.g. trigeminal neuralgia), it might be consolidated with hyperalgesia and allodynia. Amid allodynia notwithstanding touching the skin can bring about serious pain. Reasons for neuropathic pain are various, including harm to central neurons (e.g. in the thalamus), axotomy, nerve or plexus harm, metabolic ailments such as diabetes mellitus or herpes zoster [6].

1.1. The nociceptive system

Nociception is the encoding and preparing of toxic boosts in the sensory system that can be measured with electrophysiological procedures. Neurons involved in nociception structure the nociceptive framework. Harmful boosts enact essential nociceptive neurons with 'free nerve endings' (Aδ and C strands, nociceptors) in the peripheral nerve. A large portion of the nociceptors reacts to toxic mechanical (e.g. crushing the tissue), warm (warmth or frosty) and substance jolts and in this manner is polymodal [7].

Nociceptors can likewise apply efferent capacities in the tissue by discharging neuropeptides (substance P (SP), calcitonin gene related peptide (CGRP)) from their tactile endings. Along these lines, they impel vasodilatation, plasma extravasation, attraction of macrophages or degranulation of mast cells and so on. This aggravation is called neurogenic inflammation [8].

Nociceptors and second-order neurons in the grey matter of the dorsal horn make synapses and nociceptors protrude towards spinal cord. A conscious pain response is produced due to the ascending axons of the second-order neurons and projection of brain stem or thalamocortical system upon noxious stimulation. Nociceptive motor reflexes include many spinal cord neurons that involve more unpredictable motor behaviour, such as hindrance in movements and generation of autonomic reflexes. The spinal nociceptive processing is reduced by descending tracts. These tracts are formed by pathways that originate from brain stem nuclei (in particular the periaqueductal grey, the rostral ventromedial medulla) and descend in the dorsolateral funiculus of the spinal cord. An intrinsic anti-nociceptive system involves this type of descending inhibition [9].

1.1.1. The peripheral pain pathway: primary afferent nociceptors

In skin, muscle and joint, numerous Aδ and C fibres thresholds have elevated for mechanical stimuli, along these lines going about as particular nociceptors that recognize possibly or really harming mechanical boosts. Mechano-receptors are fast-conducting Aβ afferents with corpuscular endings that react overwhelmingly to harmless mechanical boosts. An extent of Aδ and C strands results in warmth or frosty receptors encoding harmless warm and cold jolts yet not toxic warmth and cold. Notwithstanding polymodal nociceptors, joint, skin and instinctive nerves contain Aδ and C fibres that were named silent or initially mechano-insensitive nociceptors. These neurons are not enacted by harmful mechanical and warm boosts in typical tissue. Be that as it may, they are sharpened amid aggravation and after that begin to react to mechanical and warm jolts [10, 11]. This type of neurons produces enduring reaction to algogenic chemicals and also involved in intervening neurogenic inflammation in human beings [12]. They assume a noteworthy part in starting central sensitization [13]. These neurons have unmistakable axonal biophysical qualities isolating them from polymodal nociceptors [11].

1.1.1.1. Peripheral neuronal mechanisms of neuropathic pain

When nociceptive field is stimulated, action potentials are generated in the sensory endings of healthy sensory nerve fibres. Pathological ectopic discharges are expressed in damaged nerve fibres. At the site of nerve damage or in the cell body of DRG, action potentials are generated. The released designs shift from recurrent terminating to irregular blasts [14, 15].

Ectopic releases happen in Aδ and C fibres and in thick myelinated Aβ fibres. In this manner, after nerve damages both low-threshold Aβ and in addition high-threshold Aδ and C fibres might be included in the era of torment. The procedures of central sensitization have been experienced by Aβ fibres that may inspire misrepresented reactions in spinal cord neurons. It was recommended that pain is not created by the impaired nerve parts themselves but instead by nerve fibres in the region of harmed nerve elements. After an exploratory sore in the L5 dorsal root, unconstrained activity potential releases were seen in C fibres in the uninjured L4 dorsal root. These filaments might be influenced by the procedure of a Wallerian degeneration [16].

1.1.2. Central pain pathways

1.1.2.1. The spinothalamic pathway

Dorsal root ganglia are a door to spinal cord for the entrance of nerve fibres where these nerve fibres impregnate around the spinal cord (dorsolateral tract of Lissauer) as 1–2 sliced parts and interact with the nerve cells in Rexed lamina I (marginal zone) and lamina II (substantia gelatinosa) then arrive the spinal grey matter. Substantia gelatinosa layer of the spinal cord is for the innervation of C fibres and marginal zone is for the innervation of Aδ fibres. These innervation of nerve cells is proceeded in the nucleus proprius (an area of spinal cord grey matter involving Rexed layers IV, V and VI), which remains continue to spinal midline then come up (in the anterolateral or ventrolateral part of the spinal white matter) through the medulla and pons and finally reaches the thalamus particular zone.

In this way, pain information and normal thermal stimuli ($<45°C$) are transmitted through spinothalamic pathway. The thalamic pathway encountering anomaly represents as a cradle of pain; this can be seen in patients with central pain or thalamic pain after stroke in the region of paralysis. In **Figure 1**, bradykinins, K^+ and prostaglandins are released by tissue injury thus stimulates nociceptors and subsequent release of substance P and histamine produce vasodilation and swelling.

1.1.2.2. The trigeminal pathway

Trigeminal ganglion and cranial nuclei VII, IX and X are the sites for the nerve cells to recognize the harmful stimuli through the nerve fibres where nerve fibres cross the threshold to the brainstem as well as medulla. Across the neural midline, these nerve fibres ascend to the contralateral side of the thalamic nerve cell. Trigeminal neuralgia is defined as the spontaneous firing of trigeminal nerve ganglion (In the positive results of Janetta's trigeminal decompression

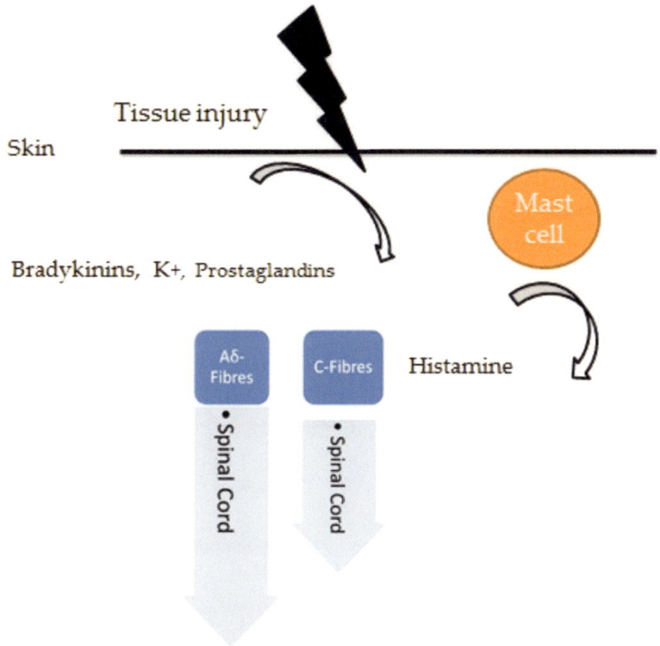

Figure 1. Nociceptor stimulation by tissue damage and vasodilation and swelling by the release of histamine (modified from Patel [17]).

surgery, cerebellar artery and local trigeminal nerve damage by mechanical lesion is thought to be cause).

The range of the thalamus that gets the pain data from the spinal cord and trigeminal nuclei is additionally the territory that gets data about normal sensory stimuli, for example, touch and pressure. From this territory, nerve fibres are sent to the surface layer of the cerebrum (cortical regions that arrangement with sensory data).

In this way, evidence on the area and the intensity of the pain can be handled to wind up a 'confined painful feeling' by having both the nociceptive and the normal somatic sensory information focalize on the same cortical territory.

In certain situations, e.g., after limb amputations, cortical representation may change into two types of painful ('phantom pain') and non-painful sensations ('telescoping phenomena') [18]. In **Figure 2**, the raphe nucleus provides serotoninergic (5-HT), and locus ceruleus provides adrenergic modulation. Therefore, selective serotonin reuptake inhibitors (SSRIs) and tricyclic antidepressants (e.g., amitriptyline) may exhibit analgesic properties.

1.1.3. Pain theories

1.1.3.1. Specificty theory

In this theory, Descartes suggested that harmful and non-harmful perceptions can be distinguished by the decoding of specific pain fibres [19].

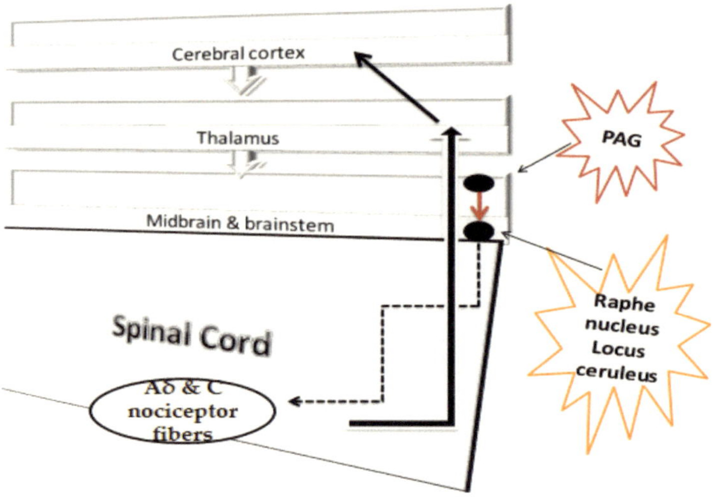

Figure 2. Serotoninergic (5-HT) and adernergic modulation by the raphe nucleus and locus ceruleus. PAG—periaqueductal grey matter, part of endogenous opioid system (modified from Patel [17]).

1.1.3.2. Intensity theory

Sydenham proposed that the peripheral stimulus acts as a signal whose intensity determines which type of sensation should be percieved [20].

1.1.3.3. Gate control theory

Melzack and Wall recommended that second-order spinal neurons (Dorsal horn transmission cell or wide dynamic range (WDR) neuron are stimulated by sensory fibers of divergent specificity that, unpredictably fire, subject to their degree of facilitation or inhibition. Inhibitory substantia gelatinosa (SG) cells are stimulated by large sensory fibres because in dorsal horn transmission cells are triggered by both large and small diameter afferents [21]. In the substantia gelatinosa, neuron and integrated circuits regulate the opening and closing of 'gate' [22].

Direct suppression of transmission cells by SG cells close the gate. On the other hand, the SG cells suppressive effect declines due to the amplified activity in small diameter fibres which can also be increased by the peripheral nerve damage and cause the opening of gate and also face decrease in inhibition of large fibres [23].

2. Target of pain: central and peripheral

2.1. Peripheral targets

At the peripheral terminal, pro-inflammatory mediators are released from the mast and schwann cells, macrophages and neutrophils which are resident and migrating cells, respectively, due to the injury to cells and blood vessels in return of stimuli, for example, a tissue damage or infection. Dorsal root ganglion (DRG) cells hold receptors for these mediators, which upon activation initiates a cascade of event from the intracellular kinases. In turn, receptor phosphorylation causes the terminal sensitization, amplified afferent movement and stimulation at lower threshold.

2.2. Central targets

The spinal primary afferents due to cell insult, such as tissue injury, inflammation or nerve injury activate the primary afferents and induce voltage gated calcium cannels (CaV) and soluble N-ethylmaleimide-sensitive factor activating protein receptor (SNARE) Protein-dependent release of neurotransmitters, growth factors and neuropeptides. The resident glial and migrating cells (T cells, macrophages and neutrophils) in the spinal cord along with the second-order neurons are activated by the release of these substances, which in turn release a collection of pro-inflammatory and anti-inflammatory molecules to further act on the second-order neurons activating several protein kinases responsible for the phosphorylation of several membrane bound receptors, thus initiating and maintaining the hyperexcitable state of these neurons, and further sending the nociceptive signals to higher brain centres. The second-order neurons facilitate the excitability of dorsal horn projection neurons and scheme onto raphe-spinal serotonergic neurons through the bulbospinal pathway which dismiss in dorsal horn neurons [24]. In **Table 2**, central and peripheral pain targets are shown along with their source of cell insult/stimuli and inflammatory mediators and receptors which are and may be the future targets for pain alleviation.

2.3. Pain targets with molecular mechanisms of activation and sensitization of nociceptors

In **Figure 3**, Nociceptors direct ion channels for generation of transduction and action potential, and a large number of receptors for inflammatory and other mediators are either coupled to ion channels or, more often, activate second messenger systems that influence ion channels.

2.3.1. Transient receptor protein (TRP) channels

The transient receptor protein subfamily V member 1 is an individual receptor from the TRP (transient receptor protein) family. Other TRP individuals might be transducers of temperature boosts in different extents [26]. Capsaicin, the compound in hot pepper, opened the ion channel that grounds burning pain. Specifically, Ca^{2+} moves through this channel and depolarizes the cell. The TRPV1 receptor is opened by heat (>43°C) thus measured one of the transducers of noxious heat. In TRPV1 knock-out mice, the heat response is not eradicated but the mice do not display thermal hyperalgesia throughout inflammation, presenting the significance of TRPV1 for inflammatory hyperalgesia [27, 28]. Up-regulation of TRPV1 transcription during inflammation explains longer lasting heat hypersensitivity. The TRPV2 receptor in nociceptors is assumed to be a transducer for exciting heat (threshold >50°C). TRPA1 could be the transducer molecule in nociceptors reacting to frosty. It is actuated by impactful mixes, e.g. those present in cinnamon oil, mustard oil and ginger. By differentiation, TRPV3 and/or TRPV4 might be transduction molecules for harmless warmth in warm receptors and TRPM8 may transduce chilly jolts in harmless cold receptors. Despite the fact that the putative warmth transducer TRPV4 demonstrates some mechano-sensitivity, it is still in vague whether TRPV4 is included in the transduction of mechanical stimuli [29–31].

Type of targets	Peripheral targets		Central targets		
Stimulus	Tissue injury, inflammation or infection		Tissue injury, inflammation or nerve damage		
Source	**Local/resident cells**	**Migrating cells (Local/ DRG)**	**Resident cells**	**Spinal neurons**	**Migrating cells**
	Endothelial cells	Macrophages	Astrocytes		T cells
	Keratinocytes	Neutrophils	Microglia		Macrophages
	Mast cells	Bacteria			Neutrophils
	Schwann cells				
Inflammatory mediators and receptors	DNA, RNA, HMGB1 →	TLRs	**Pro-analgesics**	**Anti-analgesics**	
			Chemokines	**Cytokines**	
			CCL21	IFNy, IL-4, IL-10, IL-14	
			CCL2	**Lipid mediators**	
			Cytokines	Resolvins	
			TNF, IL-1β, IL-6	Protectins	
			Growth factors	Lipoxins	
			ATP	**Epoxy fatty acids**	
				Epoxyeicosatrienoic acids	
			↘	↙	
	FPS	FPR1	**Second-order neurons**		
	Bradykinins, 5-HT, CGRP, Prostaglandins, Lipoxygenases, proteinases	GPCRs	↓	↓	
			Protein kinases	Receptors	
	ATP	Purinergic Receptors	CaMK	NK-1	
	NGF, BDNF	TRK	PKA	NMDA	
	Chemokines (e.g. CCL2, CXCL1)	Chemokines Receptors	PKC	AMPA-CP	
	Cytokines (e.g TNF, IL-1β)	Cytokines Receptors	MAPK	mGluR1	
	sP	NK1		mGluR5	

Type of targets	Peripheral targets		Central targets	
	H+	ASIC		P2X
	Lipids	TRPV1		GABA-A
		TRPA1		Glycine
			5HT3R	

Source: Yaksh et al. [24].

Table 2. Schematic representation of peripheral as well as central targets from the point of insult to cells, sources of cell insult and inflammatory mediators and receptors for the current and future analgesics.

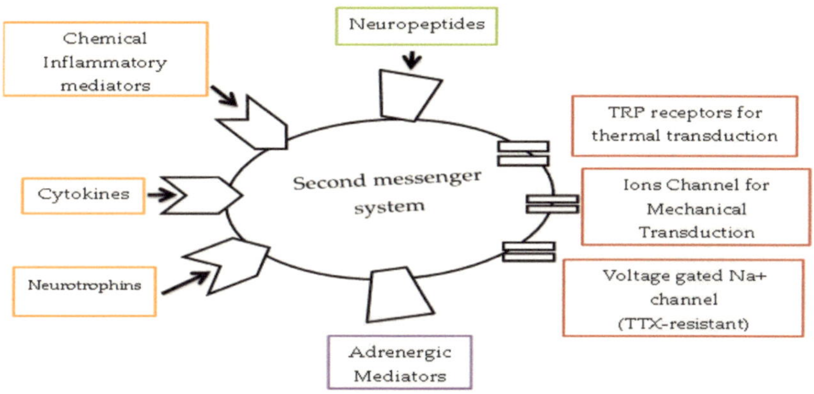

Figure 3. Ion channels for transduction of thermal and mechanical stimuli and action potential generation and metabotropic receptors subserving chemosensitivity involving sensory ending of nociceptor (modified from Schaible [25]).

2.3.2. *Voltage-gated sodium channels and acid sensing ion channels*

Tetrodotoxin (TTX) hindered many voltage-gated Na+ channels and numerous small dorsal root ganglion (DRG) cells direct TTX-resistant (R) Na+ channels, notwithstanding TTX-sensitive (S) Na+ channels. Both TTX-S and TTX-R Na+ channels pay to the Na+ influx during the action potential. Excitingly, inflammatory mediators pre-disposed TTX-R Na+ currents. Nociceptors are sensitized by boosted prostaglandin E2 (PGE2). This raises the likelihood that TTX-R Na+ channels likewise assume a part in the transduction procedure of poisonous boosts. SNS−/− knock-out mice (SNS is a TTX-R Na+ channel) show declared mechanical hypoalgesia, however just little shortages in the reaction to thermal incitements [32, 33]. Low pH values cause opening of acid sensing ion channels (ASICs) and are Na+ channels. In general, ASIC family comprises of six subunits (1a, 1b, 2a, 2b, 3, and 4). This is of interest because many inflammatory exudates exhibit a low pH. Protons straightforwardly initiate ASICs with ensuing generation of action potentials. The ASIC family expressed in peripheral neurons is ASIC 1b and ASIC 3 subunits which possess a high degree of selectivity in sensory neurons [34, 35].

2.3.3. Receptors of inflammatory mediators (chemosensitivity of nociceptors)

The chemosensitivity of nociceptors permits inflammatory and trophic intermediaries to follow up on these neurons. Inflammatory cells and non-neuronal tissue cells are their cradles. In the activation and sensitization of neurons, two types of receptors either ionotropic (the mediator opens an ion channel) or metabotropic (the mediator activates a second messenger cascade that influences ion channels and other cell functions) are encompassed. Numerous receptors are coupled to G proteins, which signal by means of the generation of the second messenger cyclic adenosine monophosphate (cAMP), cyclic guanosine monophosphate (cGMP), diacylglycerol and phospholipase C. The receptors are having intrinsic protein tyrosine kinase domains that associate with cytosolic tyrosine kinases and protein serine/threonine kinases [31, 36]. There are several functions of mediators, which may involve the direct activation of neurons (e.g. the bradykinin induces action potentials by itself) and/or sensitization of neurons for mechanical, thermal and chemical stimuli (e.g. bradykinin and prostaglandins increase the excitability of neurons so that mechanical stimuli arouse action potentials at a lower threshold than under switch circumstances occur). PGE2, for example, activates G protein-coupled EP receptors that cause an increase of cellular cAMP. This second ambassador actuates protein kinase A, and this pathway impacts ion channels in the membrane, prompting an improved edginess of the neuron with brought down limit and expanded action potential recurrence inspired amid suprathreshold incitement. Bradykinin receptors are of awesome interest on the grounds where bradykinin enacts various Aδ and C fibres and sharpens them for mechanical and warm boosts [37]. Freund's complete adjuvant induced mechanical hyperalgesia of the rat knee joints and thermal hyperalgesia can be reversed by the bradykinin receptor antagonists. A few reports recommend that specifically bradykinin B1 receptors are up-controlled in sensory neurons taking after tissue or nerve damage, and that B1 antagonist diminishes hyperalgesia. Up-regulation of B2 receptors during inflammation also found by some authors [38, 39].

2.3.4. Neuropeptide receptors and adrenergic receptors

Receptors for a few neuropeptides have been recognized in primary afferent neurons, including receptors for the excitatory neuropeptides SP (neurokinin 1 receptors) and CGRP, and receptors for inhibitory peptides, in particular for opioids, somatostatin and neuropeptide Y (NPY) [40, 41].

3. Current strategies for pain control

The treatment of constant pain ought to be multi-directional. There are pharmacological strategies for treatment, physical, rehabilitation, neuromodulation, psychological techniques and now and again, surgical methods. It is critical to guarantee careful and exhaustive nurture of the patient, and to elucidate and acquire acknowledgment of the picked strategy for treatment from the patient.

3.1. Pharmacotherapy

Pharmacotherapy should always be chosen independently be chosen exclusively, in light of the fact that what helps one individual does not as a matter of course help another, and may even be unsafe. The decision of medication ought to be founded on fitting finding and presently utilized pain relieving treatment. It is critical to consider conceivable symptoms which happened amid the past utilization of the medications. It is additionally critical to consider conceivable association of the proposed drug with different pharmaceuticals utilized by patient for different illnesses. To get a viable pain control, a blend of medications with various components of activity is utilized. They are additionally accessible as prepared details containing a mix of two or more active ingredients. In **Table 3**, some nociceptive conditions are described which can be managed by the drugs interfering neurotransmission.

3.1.1. Classification of Non-steroidal anti-inflammatory drugs

Currently used non-steroidal anti-inflammatory drugs with their mechanism of actions, indications, therapeutic advantages and disadvantages are listed in the **Table 4**.

3.2. Physical therapy and rehabilitation

A supporting technique is utilized as a part of the treatment of pain. The most well-known strategies for physical treatment are thermotherapy (heat), cryotherapy (cool), laser treatment, electrotherapy, manual methods, restorative concentrates and kinesiotherapy. These techniques, utilized as a part of a fitting way, may enhance life and portability of a few patients.

3.3. Neuromodulation

Neuromodulating treatments are aimed at stimulating the pain systems. Currently, several neuromodulation methods are used: percutaneous nerve electrostimulation (TENS), peripheral nerve stimulation, acupuncture and vibration. Neuromodulation supports pain treatment

Conditions	Pain management
Inflammatory states	NSAIDs, act on COX-1, COX-2 and opiate receptors
Nerve injury	Antidepressants, MAO Inhibitors, e.g. Amitriptyline, Duloxetine, Venlafaxine
Neuropathic pain	Sodium channel blockers (Lidocaine, Carbamazepine)
	Calcium channel blockers (Ziconotide, Gabapentin)
	Increasing extracellular level of inhibitory transmitter (GABA), e.g. Tigabin
	Opioids (lesser extent)
Topical medication for cutaneous allodynia and hyperalgesia	Lidocaine, Capsaicin

Source: Sinatra [42].

Table 3. Pain conditions and Current analgesics for pain management.

NSAID	Mechanism of action	Therapeutic advantages	Therapeutic disadvantages	Indications
Salicylates				
Aspirin	Irreversibly inhibit COX-1 and COX-2	Low cost; long history of safety	Upper GI disturbances are common	Fever, pain, anti-inflammatory and anti-platelet
Diflunisal			No anti-pyretic effect	
Acetic acids				
Indomethacin	Reversible inhibitors of COX-1 and COX-2		Upper GI disturbances are common Very potent should be used only after less toxic agents have proven ineffective	Anti-pyretic, analgesic, anti-inflammatory
Sulindac		Long half-life permit once or twice daily dosing	Same as indomethacin but less sever	Fever, pain inflammation, RA, ankylosing spondylitis, osteoarthritis of hip
Propionic acids				
Ibuprofen	Reversible inhibitors of COX-1 and COX-2	Lower toxicity and better acceptance in some patients	Headache, patent ductus arteriosis, tinnitus, dizziness, prolong bleeding time	Fever, pain, anti-inflammatory, anti-platelet, osteoarthritis, rheumatoid arthritis
Fenoprofen				
Flurbiprofen				
Ketoprofen				
Naproxen		Naproxen is considered by some experts as one of the safest NSAID		
Oxaprozin		Long half-life permit once daily dosing		
Oxicams				
Piroxicam	Inhibits both COX-1 and COX-2, with preferential binding for COX-2	Long half-life permit once or twice daily dosing	GI disturbance in 20% patients	osteoarthritis, rheumatoid arthritis, ankylosing spondylitis
Meloxicam		Long half-life permit once or twice daily dosing	Less GI irritation than Piroxicam	
Fenamates				
Mefenamic acid			Diarrhoea, inflammation of bowel, haemolytic anaemia	
Meclofenamic acid				
COX-2 inhibitors				
Celecoxib	More selectively inhibit COX-2	Less GI irritation than aspirin	Potential for increasing myocardial infarctions	RA, rheumatoid arthritis, acute to moderate pain

http://dx.doi.org/10.5772/67853

NSAID	Mechanism of action	Therapeutic advantages	Therapeutic disadvantages	Indications
			and strokes, headache, diarrhoea	
Heteroaryl acetic acids				
Diclofenac	Selective COX-2 inhibitor	Employed in long-term therapy		osteoarthritis, rheumatoid arthritis, ankylosing spondylitis
Tolmetin				Anti-inflammatory, anti-pyretic, analgesic
Ketorolac			Fatal peptic ulcer, GI Bleeding, Perforation of the stomach or intestine	Moderate to Severe pain, moderate inflammation, allergic conjunctivitis

Source: Clark et al. [43].

Table 4. Classification of currently used Non-steroidal anti-inflammatory drugs along with mechanism and indications.

methods, and by activating the pain inhibitory mechanisms, one can reduce pain and improve the quality of life of patient with chronic pain.

3.4. Psychological therapies

Psychological factors have a big influence on the perception of pain, as well as the effectiveness of the treatment. Therefore, all patients with chronic pain should be able to take advantage of professional psychological help, which can affect the emotional aspect of pain. Among the psychological methods that can be effective as a technique supporting the treatment of chronic pain, the most commonly used are cognitive therapy, behavioural therapy, relaxation techniques and hypnotherapy.

3.5. Invasive methods

These procedures of pain management should be executed and administered by experienced specialists in specific cases. Numbers of methods are available, i.e. individual nerves block, intrathecal administration of drugs (e.g. epidural anaesthesia during childbirth) to neurodestructive

Scientific name/common name	Family	Parts used	Medicinal used	References
Berberis calliobotrys	Berberidaceae	Stem	Analgesic for Rheumatoid arthritis	[44, 45]
Manilkara zapota	Sapotaceae	Leaves	Analgesic	[46]
Clerodendrum phlomidis	Verbenaceae	Stem bark	Analgesic	[47]
Bach	Araceae	Rhizome	Analgesic	[48]
Ocimum suave	Lamiaceae		Analgesic	[48]
Lippia adoensis	Verbenaceae	flower	Analgesic	[48]
Ajuga remota /bugle	Lamiaceae		Analgesic	[48]
Pimpinella anisum	Umbellifera	Seeds	Narcotic analgesic	[49]

Scientific name/common name	Family	Parts used	Medicinal used	References
Myrtus communis	Myrtaceae	Leaves	Narcotic analgesic	[50]
Tribulus terrestris	Zygophyllaceae	Aerial	Narcotic analgesic	[51]
Sinapis arvensis	Solanaceae	Aerial	Narcotic analgesic	[51]
Withania somnifera	Solanaceae	Leaves and fruit	Narcotic analgesic	[51]
Peganum harmala	Zygophyllaceae	Whole plant	Narcotic analgesic	[51]
Hibiscus rosa sinensis	Malvaceae	leaves	Analgesic	[52]
Stylosanthes fruticosa	Papilionaceae	Whole plant	Analgesic	[53]
Polyalthia longifolia	Annonaceae	Leaves	Analgesic	[53]
Ficus glomerata	Moraceae	Bark and leaves	Toothache, analgesic	[53]
Baugainvillea spectabilis	Nyctaginaceae	Leaves	Analgesic	[53]
Toona ciliata	Meliaceae	heart wood	Analgesic	[53]
Sida acuta	Malvaceae	whole plant	Analgesic	[53]
Chococca brachiata	Rubiaceae	Root	Anti-inflammatory, analgesics	[54]
Bauhinia racemosa	Caesalpiniaceae	Stem bark	Analgesic	[54]
Casearia sylvestris Swartz. (wild coffee)	Flacurtiaceae	Leaves and bark	Anti-inflammatory, analgesics	[54]
Elephantopus scaber	*Elephantopus scaber*	Leaves	Anti-inflammatory, analgesics	[54]

Table 5. Some plant sources under study to develop new analgesics.

procedures (neurolysis, thermo lesion,) and neurosurgery. Advance medicine provides many different methods for the management of pain.

4. Plant sources of analgesics

Due to obvious adverse effect of synthetic drugs, herbal medicinal plants are focusing to develop newer analgesic agents with fewer side effects. Some plants having analgesic activity are given in **Table 5**.

5. Experimental models for screening of analgesic substances

The animal models employed for screening of analgesic agents include

5.1. Pain-state models using thermal stimuli

For the activation of cutaneous receptors, heat is a suitable stimulus. Nociceptive stimulation origin can be far apart from its target, for example radiant heat from a lamp in a direct touch

http://dx.doi.org/10.5772/67853

with the skin. Comparatively, radiant heat comprises a selective stimulus for nociceptors; moreover, it has an advantage of producing no tactile stimulus over the other ways of thermal stimulation.

5.1.1. The tail-flick model using radiant heat/immersion of the tail in hot water

It is one of the most simplified procedures used in human subjects with radiant heat [55]. In fact, Hardy et al. finally used this method in rats [56]. After the exposure to thermal radiation of the tail of an animal it takes out the tail by a brief dynamic movement [57]. This separation of the tail from the heat source is termed as 'tail-flick latency'. In this method, a timer is started at the time of application of heat and the time taken for the rat to withdraw its tail from heat source is recorded. Withdrawal time is usually within 2–10 s. It is advisable to not to lengthen the exposure to radiant heat more than 20 s as the skin of the tail may be burnt. In order to control the intensity of the current passing through the filament, a rheostat is inserted in the apparatus which further controls the intensity of radiant heat. Some investigators have used cold as a substitute of hot stimuli; this test can be used on monkeys as well. The use of immersion of the tail is apparently a variant of the test described above [58].

5.1.2. Paw-withdrawal test

This test is completely comparable to the test of D'Amour and Smith [59] but have the benefit that it does not involve the pre-eminent organ of thermoregulation in rats and mice, i.e. the tail [60]. In this test, a paw is exposed to radiant heat that had previously been swollen by a subcutaneous injection of carrageenan. By exposure to ultraviolet rays, inflammation can also be produced. Heat applied to a freely moving animal is an advantage of these types of tests [61].

5.1.3. Hot-plate model

In this test, a mouse or rat is presented into an open-ended cylindrical space with a floor composed of metallic plate that is heated by boiling liquid or a thermoderm [62]. Two behavioural components are produced by heating the plate at constant temperature that is calculated in terms of their reaction times, namely jumping and paw licking. In terms of analgesic chemicals, the paw licking behaviour is influenced only by opioids. On the contrary, by using less powerful analgesics, for example, paracetamol or acetylsalicylic acid, the jumping reaction time can be increased, especially when the temperature of the plate is 50°C or less or if the temperature is changing incrementally and in linear fashion, e.g. from 43 to 52°C at 2.5°C/min [63]. The behaviour is more complex in the rat and relatively stereotyped in the mouse like it sniffs, licks its forepaws, licks its hind paws, straightens up, and stamps its feet, starts and stops washing itself, among other things. These behaviours have been labelled 'chaotic defensive movements' [64].

5.1.4. Pain-state models using cold stimuli

For stimulation and measurement of pain in mice, a new animal model has been developed and designed. This laboratory model (M-model) basically consists of four parts (i) perspex-box,

(ii) M-Zone, (iii) ice-tray and (iv) ice floor. At the start, the mouse is exposed to different parts of the M-model mainly M-Zone for about 60 s, so that the mouse is sensitive of the existence of M-Zone prior to the initiation of the experiment. From the top/ceiling of the perspex box, the animal is inserted. The ice tray containing of ice block is slide onto the floor of the perspex box. When the animal is not able to bear the cold surface of ice floor, it escapes to M-Zone. The time taken by the animal to run away into the M-Zone (Flight-Zone) when placed on the ice-floor is called endurance time. This time is recorded with the help of a stopwatch. In general, mice take about 4–6 s to escape into the M-Zone to evade ice floor. Separate groups of animals are pre-treated with narcotics such as butorphanol (partial opioid agonist, 2 mg/kg, s. c), tramadol (opioid agonist, 5 mg/kg, s. c), pentazocine (10 mg/kg, s. c) and non-narcotic analgesics such as ketoprofen (non-selective COX inhibitor, 5 mg/kg, p. o), diclofenac (non-selective COX inhibitor, 15 mg/kg, i. p) and meloxicam (preferential COX-2 inhibitor, 5 mg/kg, s. c) to determine their effect on endurance time. This time is recorded at 0, 15, 30, 45, 60, 120 and 180 min after administration of the standard drugs [65].

5.2. Pain-state models using mechanical stimuli

5.2.1. Strain gauges

In this test, an increasing amount of pressure is applied to a punctiform area on the hind paw or, far less frequently, on the tail. The tail or paw is wedged between a plane surface and a blunt point mounted on top of a system of cog wheels with a cursor that can be moved in the direction of length of a graduated beam [66]. When the pressure increases, following step wise reactions occurs, i.e. the reflex removal of the paw or a complex movement of the animal to free its captured limb and at last a vocal response is noticed. Randall and Selitto with the aim of enhancing the sensitivity of the test offer comparison of thresholds seen with an inflamed paw and with a healthy paw [67].

5.2.2. von-Frey filaments

The key method for the study of pain in animal models is the assessment of mechanosensitivity. This is frequently executed with the use of von-Frey filaments in an up-down testing model. This is the most commonly used method for measuring pain in animals described by Vivancos [68] for mechanosensitivity testing in rodents. Though, in this method, animals are getting a changeable amount of stimuli which may direct the animals in distinctive groups getting diverse testing experiences that affect their subsequent responses. In order to standardize the measurement of mechano-sensitivity, a simplified up-down method (SUDO) for reckoning paw withdrawal threshold (PWT) with von-Frey filaments has been developed that uses a constant number of five stimuli per test [69].

5.3. Pain-state models using electrical stimuli

5.3.1. Electrical stimulation of the tail

Progressively escalating strength of electrical stimuli can be applied in range (lasting for some milliseconds) through subcutaneous electrodes positioned in the tail of the mouse or the rat. One can see the following: when such slowly increasing intensities of electrical stimuli are applied from invariable voltages 40–50 V, i.e., the impulse movement of the tail, vocalization occurs at the time of stimulation, and then, utterance continuing ahead for the period of stimulation. Due to the electrical current, the animal may be died. Morphine or morphine-like drugs are useful in this model [70].

5.3.2. *Grid-shock test*

Approximately weighing of 18–20 g of male mice is put into the clear plastic chambers. The floor of box spaced about 1 mm apart is wired firmly with stainless steel wire. In the form of square wave pulses, the stimulus is given 30 cycles/s with a period of 2 ms/pulse. By escalating shock intensities, the mice gasp, show a frightening reaction, increase movement or effort to jump. Pain threshold response is defined as the behaviour correctly reflected on the oscilloscope by marked vacillation of the displayed pulse. Prior to administration of the test drug the pain thresholds are find out in each individual mouse twice at 15, 30, 60, 90 and 120 min subsequent dosing [71].

5.3.3. *Stimulation of the tooth pulp*

In this method, electric current is applied to stimulate the tooth-pulp of the animal. Pain symbol is exhibited as biting, chewing, licking and head flicking.

Rabbits of either sex are used as animal model. Thiopental 15 mg/kg or fentanyl-citrate 0.2 mg/kg i.v. produces anaesthesia. A high-speed dental drill is used to create pulp chambers in the lateral margins of the two front upper incisors.

Rectangular current with a frequency of 50 Hz for 1 s is applied. The 0.2-mA electrical current produces the phenomenon of licking [72].

5.3.4. *Monkey-shock titration test*

This model carries monkeys as animal model and kept them in restraining chairs. The monkey shock titration is a final evaluation of a new compound before administration to man. Electrical current is conveyed by a Coulbourn Instrument programmable stunner through cathodes coupled to two test tube clasps, which are connected to a shaved bit of the tail. The current ranges from 0 to 4 mA through 29 progressive steps. This current is suppressed by a bar pressed by monkey. On the day before the drug administration, a stable baseline shock level is recognized for each monkey. Drugs in different doses like 3.0 mg/kg i.m. morphine, 1.7 mg/kg i.m. methadone, and 10 mg/kg i.m. pentazocine were used. However, this test is time consuming [73].

5.3.5. *Stimulation of the limbs*

For pharmacological studies of analgesia, electromyographic recordings of nociceptive limb reflexes have been used for, but they are far less common than behavioural tests. These electromyographic studies have permitted the measurement of reactions paying little heed to whether there is any development.

5.4. Pain-state models using chemical stimuli

The experimental models in which chemical stimulation is done with the administration of algogenic agents represent an irreversible, slow, and progressive form of stimulation, which are nearby in nature to clinical pain.

5.4.1. Formalin test

The formalin test in rats, a chronic pain model is used to assess the centrally active analgesic agents. In this test, excessive licking and biting of the paw is recorded as response after the administration of formalin (37% solution of formaldehyde) into the front paw. Both paws resting on the floor indicated the analgesic response or protection of the test drug. The response as painful behaviour can be evaluated on a four-level scale related to posture: 0 represents normal texture; 1 represents the injected paw not supporting the animal but leftovers on the ground; 2 represents animal raised up the injected paw visibly; and 3 represents animal shows responses like licking, nibbling or shaking of injured paw [74].

5.4.2. Acetic acid induced writhing test

In this method, pain is indicated as a characteristic behaviour of contraction of abdominal muscles and stretching of hind paws along with twisting of dorso-abdominal muscles, and motor in co-ordination in rats or mice (called writhing) after the administration of allogenic agents like phenyl quinone or acetic acid into the peritoneal cavity which irritate the serous membrane; therefore, this test is called 'writhing test'. These writhings are counted as per unit of time [74].

5.4.3. Stimulation of hollow organs

In hollow organs such as rat colon, formalin is injected, and a complex biphasic type of 'true visceral pain' is exhibited in two phases. In first phase, contraction and stretching of body and in second phase, abdominal licking and nibbling behaviour is shown by the animal. Intravesical administration of capsaicin or turpentine produce bladder pain, glycerol produces abdominal constrictions and intrauterine injections of mustard oil show complex behaviour patterns in a number of models including rats. Another mean of stimulus for colorectal distension in rat is an inflatable balloon [75, 76].

6. Conclusion

The ASIC family is a potential target for new analgesics. In rheumatoid arthritis and vascular ischemia, as well as in the routine perioperative settings, inflammation and ischemic pain conditions are a sign mark of acidic nociception which can be reduce by the NSAIDs and by direct inhibition of sensory neuron ASIC current [77].

Work is currently in progress on a more selective and potent ASIC blocker and could potentially be an effective agent in the treatment of inflammatory and ischemic acute or chronic pain in the future [78]. Key regulators of membrane excitability are inflammatory mediators and key receptors (kinins, mPGEs), ion channels (TRPV1, NaV 1.7), and neurotrophins (NGF).

http://dx.doi.org/10.5772/67853

Similarly, α(2A)-adrenoceptor agonists also proven to be effective in various pain conditions, in the spinal dorsal horn, by inhibitory action on α(2A)-adrenoceptors on central terminals of primary afferent nociceptors (presynaptic inhibition), by direct α2-adrenergic action on spinal pain-relay neurons (post-synaptic inhibition) noradrenaline released from descending pathways originating in the pontine A5–A7 cell groups decreases pain and by α1-adrenergic activation of inhibitory interneurons. Furthermore, α(2C)-adrenoceptors on axon terminals of excitatory interneurons might subsidize to spinal control of pain [79]. These targets are currently under work to establish new analgesics with minimum side effects as exhibited by the currently used COX inhibitors.

Author details

Mohammad Saleem* and Huma Naz

*Address all correspondence to: saleem2978@hotmail.com

Faculty of Pharmaceutical Science, Government College University, Faisalabad, Pakistan

References

[1] Brune K. New Pharmacological and Epidemiological Data in Analgesics Research. Basel, Switzerland: Birkhauser Verlag; 1990

[2] Domżał T. Kliniczne podstawy badania i oceny bólu wprowadzenie do tematu. Polski Przegląd Neurologiczny. 2007;**3**(4):211-215

[3] Thor P. Podstawy patofizjologii człowieka. In: Nowak Ł, Wordliczek J, Dobrogowski J, editors. Mechanizmy bólu. 2nd ed. Kraków; Publisher Medical PZWL, 2007. pp. 63-97 (in Polish)

[4] Neural Plasticity and Disorders of the Nervous System. Cambridge University Press. 2006. pp. 149-240

[5] Świeboda P, Filip R, Prystupa A, Drozd M. Assessment of pain: types, mechanism and treatment. Annals of Agricultural and Environmental Medicine. 2013;(Special Issue 1):2-7

[6] Cervero F, Laird JMA. One pain or many pains? A new look at pain mechanisms. News Physiological Sciences. 1991;**6**:268-273

[7] Belmonte C, Cervero E. Neurobiology of Nociceptors. Oxford: Oxford University Press; 1996

[8] Schaible HG, Del Rosso A, Matucci-Cerinic M. Neurogenic aspects of inflammation. Rheumatic Disease Clinics of North America. 2005;**31**:77-101

[9] Fields HL, Basbaum AI. Central nervous system mechanisms of pain modulation. In: Wall PD, Melzack R, editors. Textbook of Pain. London: Churchill Livingstone; 1999. pp. 309-329

[10] Schaible HG, Schmidt RF. Time course of mechanosensitivity changes in articular afferents during a developing experimental arthritis. Journal of Neurophysiology. 1988;**60**:2180-2219

[11] Weidner C, Schmelz M, Schmidt R, Hansson B, Handwerker HO, Torebjork HE. Functional attributes discriminating mechano-insensitive and mechano-responsive C nociceptors in human skin. Journal of Neuroscience. 1999;**19**:10184-10190

[12] Ringkamp M, Peng B, Wu G, Hartke TV, Campbell JN, Meyer RA. Capsaicin responses in heat-sensitive and heat-insensitive A-fiber nociceptors. Journal of Neuroscience. 2001;**21**:4460-4468

[13] Klede M, Handwerker HO, Schmelz M. Central origin of secondary mechanical hyperalgesia. Journal of Neurophysiology. 2003;**90**:353-359

[14] Han HC, Lee DH, Chung JM. Characteristics of ectopic discharges in a rat neuropathic pain model. Pain. 2000;**84**:253-261

[15] Liu CN, Michaelis M, Amir R, Devor M. Spinal nerve injury enhances subthreshold membrane potential oscillations in DRG neurons: relation to neuropathic pain. Journal of Neurophysiology. 2000;**84**:205-215

[16] Wu G, Ringkamp M, Hartke TV, Murinson BB, Campbell JN, Griffin JW, Meyer RA. Early onset of spontaneous activity in uninjured C-fiber nociceptors after injury to neighbouring nerve fibers. Journal of Neuroscience. 2001;**21 RC**(140):1-5

[17] Patel NB. Physiology of pain. Guide to Pain Management in Low-Resource Settings. 2010.

[18] Westmoreland BE, Benarroch EE, Daude JR, Reagan TJ, Sandok BA. Medical Neuroscience: An Approach to Anatomy, Pathology, and Physiology by Systems and Levels. 3rd ed. Boston: Little, Brown and Co.; 1994. pp. 146-154

[19] Sabatowski R, Schafer D, Kasper SM, Brunsch H, Radbruch L. Pain treatment: a historical overview. Current Pharmaceutical Design. 2004;**10**(7):701-716

[20] Melzack R, Wall PD. Pain mechanisms: A new theory. Science (New York, NY). 1965;**150** (699):971-979

[21] Ataka T, Kumamoto E, Shimoji K, Yoshimura M. Baclofeninhibits more effectively C-afferent than Adelta-afferent glutamatergic transmission in substantia gelatinosa neurons of adult rat spinal cord slices. Pain. 2000;**86**(3):273-282

[22] Basbaum AI. A new way to lose your nerve. TheScience of Aging Knowledge Environment. 2004;**2004**(15):15

[23] Mendell LM, Wall PD. Responses of single dorsal cord cells to peripheral cutaneous unmyelinated fibres. Nature. 1965;**206**:97-99

[24] Yaksh TL, Woller SA, Ramachandran R, and Sorkin LS. The search for novel analgesics: Targets and mechanisms. F1000 Prime Reports. 2015;**7**:56

[25] Schaible HG. Peripheral and central mechanisms of pain generation. Analgesia, 2006;**177**: 3-28.

[26] Papapoutian A, Peier AM, Story GM, Viswanath V. ThermoTRPchannels and beyond: Mechanisms of temperature sensation. Nature Review Neuroscience. 2003;**4**:529-539

[27] Davis JB, Gray J, Gunthorpe MJ, Hatcher JP, Davey PT, Overend P, Harries MH, Latcham J, ClaphamC, Atkinson K, Hughes SA, Rance K, Grau E, Harper AJ, Pugh PL, Rogers DC, Bingham S, Randall A, Sheardown SA. Vanilloid receptor-1 is essential for inflammatory thermal hyperalgesia. Nature. 2000;**405**:183-187

[28] Caterina MJ, Leffler A, Malmberg AB, Martin WJ, Trafton J, Petersen-Zeitz KR, Koltzenburg M, Basbaum AI, Julius D. Impaired nociception and pain sensation in mice lacking the capsaicin receptor. Science. 2000;**288**:306-313

[29] Peier AM, Moqrich A, Hergarden AC, Reeve AJ, Andersson DA, Story GM, Earley TJ, Dragoni I, McIntyre P, Bevan S, Patapoutian A. A TRP channel that senses cold stimuli and menthol. Cell. 2002;**108**:705-715

[30] Bandell M, Story GM, Hwang SW, Viswanath V, Eid SR, Petrus MJ, Earley TJ, Patapoutian A. Noxious cold ion channel TRPA1 is activated by pungent compounds and bradykinin. Neuron. 2004;**41**:849-857

[31] Marchand F, Perretti M, McMahon SB. Role of the immune system in chronic pain. Nature Review Neuroscience. 2005;**6**:521-532

[32] Akopian AN, Souslova V, England S, Okuse K, Ogata N, Ure J, Smith A, Kerr BJ, McMahon SB, Boyce S, Hill R, Stanfa LC, Dickenson AH, Wood JN. The tetrodotoxin-resistant sodium channel SNS has a specialized function in pain pathways. Nature Neuroscience. 1999;**2**:541-548

[33] McCleskey EW, Gold MS. Ion channels of nociception. Annual Review of Physiology. 1999;**61**:835-856

[34] Voilley N, et al. Nonsteroid anti-inflammatory drugs inhibit both the activity and the inflammation-induced expression of acidsensing ion channels in nociceptors. Journal of Neuroscience**.** 2001;**21**(20):8026-8033

[35] Sutherland SP, Benson CJ, Adelman JP, McCleskey EW. Acid-sensing ion channel 3 matches the acid-gated current in cardiac ischemia-sensing neurons. Proceedings of the National Academy of Sciences of the United States. 2001;**98**:711-716

[36] Gold MS. Molecular basis of receptors. In: Merskey H, Loeser JD, Dubner R, editors. The paths of pain 1975-2005. Seattle: IASP Press; 2005. pp. 49-67

[37] Liang YF, Haake B, Reeh PW. Sustained sensitization and recruitment of cutaneous nociceptors by bradykinin and a novel theory of its excitatory action. Journal of Physiology. 2001;**532**:229-239

[38] Banik RK, Kozaki Y, Sato J, Gera L, Mizumura K. B2 receptor-mediated enhanced bradykinin sensitivity of rat cutaneous C-fiber nociceptors during persistent inflammation. Journal of Neurophysiology. 2001;**86**:2727-2735

[39] Segond von Banchet G, Petrow PK, Brauer R, Schaible HG. Monoarticular antigeninduced arthritis leads to pronounced bilateral upregulation of the expression of neurokinin and bradykinin 2 receptors in dorsal root ganglion neurons of rats. Arthritis Research. 2000;**2**:424-427

[40] Bar KJ, Schurigt U, Scholze A, Segond von Banchet G, Stopfel N, Brauer R, Halbhuber KJ, Schaible HG. The expression and localisation of somatostatin receptors in dorsal root ganglion neurons of normal and monoarthritic rats. Neuroscience. 2004;**127**:197-206

[41] Brack A, Stein C. Potential links between leukocytes and antinociception. Pain. 2004;**111**:1-2

[42] Sinatra RS. Acute Pain Management. Cambridge: Cambridge University Press. 2011.

[43] Clark MA, Finkel R, Rey JA, Whalen K. (2012). Lippincott's Illustrated Reviews. Pharmacology, 5th ed., Baltimore, MD: Wolters Kluwer Health/Lippincott Williams and Wilkins, 2012.

[44] Alamgeer, Umme HH, Ambreen MU and Shahid R. Evaluation of in vitro and in vivo anti-arthritic potential of Berberis calliobotrys. Bangladesh Journal of Pharmacology. 2015;**10**:807-819

[45] Alamgeer, Huma N, Shahid R, Sayed AR, Taseer A, Haseeb A, Muhammad NM, Hira A, Zahid K, Nabeela N, Ambreen MU, Umme H-H. Anti-inflammatory, analgesic and anti-pyretic activities of the aqueous methanolic extract of *Berberis Calliobotrys* in albino mice. Acta Poloniae Pharmaceutica ñ Drug Research. 2016;**73**(3):717-723

[46] Jain PK, Soni P, Upmanyu N, Shivhare Y. Evaluation of Analgesic Activity of *Manilkara Zapota* (Leaves). European Journal of Experimental Biology. 2011;**1**(1):14-17.

[47] Srinivasa U, Neelakanta, Shabaraya AR, Rao VJ. Analgesic activity of Clerodendrum phlomidis stem bark. Indain Drugs. 2010;**47**(2):57-59

[48] Makonnen E, Debella A, Abebe D, Teka F. Analgesic properties of some ethiopian medicinal plants in different models of nociception in mice. Phytotherapy Research. 2003;**17** (9):1108-1112

[49] Sathisha A, Udupa L, Raathanakar UP, Pai PG, Acharya SD, Shastry R. Anti-inflammatory and Analgesic activity of *Phyllanthus niruri* in Rodent models. Indian Drugs. 2009;**46** (12):50-53

[50] Silva J, Abebe W, Sousa SM, Duarte VG, Machadoand MIL, Matos MJA. Analgesic and anti-inflammatory effects of essential oils of Eucalyptus. Journal of Ethnopharmacology. 2003;**89**(2-3):277-283

[51] Podder MK, Das BN, Saha A, Ahmed M. Analgesic activity of bark of *Murraya paniculata.* International Journal of Medicine and Medical Sciences. 2011;**3**(4):105-108

[52] Nikajoo Lt. Analgesic activity of aqueous and alcohol root extracts of pergularia Daemia (Forsk.) Chiov. International Journal of Pharmacy and Pharmaceutical Sciences. 2009;**1**(1):33-37

[53] Twaij H, El-Jalil HA. Evaluation of narcotic (Opioid Like) analgesic activities of medicinal plants. European Journal of Scientific Research. 2009;**33**(1):179-182

[54] Ruppett BM, Peveria EFR, Gonccalves LC, Pereira NA. Pharmacological screening of plants recommended by Folk medicine as anti-snake venom-1, analgesic and Anti-inflammtory activities. Mem.Inst. Oswaldo Cruz, Rio de Janeiro. 1991;**86**(II):203-205

[55] Hardy JD, Wolff HG, Goodell H. Studies on pain. A new method for measuring pain threshold: Observation on spatial summation of pain. Journal of Clinical Investigation. 1940;**19**:649-657

[56] Hardy JD, Stoll AM, Cunningham D, Benson WM, Greene L. Responses of the rat to thermal radiation. American Journal of Physiology. 1957;**189**:1-5

[57] Smith DL, D'Amour MC, D'Amour FE. The analgesic properties of certain drugs and drug combinations. Journal of Pharmacology and Experimental Therapeutics. 1943;**77**:184-193.

[58] Parle M, Yadav M. Laboratory models for screening analgesics international research. Journal of Pharmacy. 2013;**4**(1)

[59] D'Amour FE, Smith DL. A method for determining loss of pain sensation. Journal of Pharmacology and Experimental Therapeutics. 1941;**72**:74-79

[60] Hargreaves K, Dubner R, Brown F, Flores C, Joris J. A new and sensitive method for measuring thermal nociception in cutaneous hyperalgesia. Pain. 1988;**32**:77-88

[61] Perkins MN, Campbell E, and Dray A. Antinociceptive activity of the bradykinin B1 and B2 receptor antagonists, des-Arg9,(Leu8)-BK and HOE 140, in two models of persistent hyperalgesia in the rat. Pain. 1993;**53**:191-197

[62] Eddy NB, Leimbach D. Synthetic analgesics: II. Dithenylbutenyl and dithienyl- butylamines. Journal of Pharmacology and Experimental Therapeutics. 1953;**107**:385-393

[63] Hunskaar S, Hole K. The formalin test in mice: dissociation between inflammatory and non-inflammatory pain. Pain. 1987;**30**:103-114

[64] Knoll J, Kelemen K, Knoll B. Experimental studies on the higher nervous activity of animals. I. A method for the elaboration of a nonextinguishable conditioned reflex in the rat. Acta Physiologica Academiae Scientiarum Hungaricae. 1955;**8**:327-344

[65] Yadav M, Parle M. A simple laboratory model for inducing and measuring pain in small experimental animals. International Journal of Pharmacy and Pharmaceutical Sciences. **8** (7):156-162

[66] Green AF, Young PA, Godfrey EI. A comparison of heat and pressure analgesimetric methods in rats. British Journal of Pharmacology. 1951;**6**:572-585

[67] Randall LO, Selitto JJ. A method for measurement of analgesic activity on inflamed tissue. Arch Int Pharmacodyn Ther. 1957;**111**:409-419

[68] Vivancos GG, Verri Jr WA, Cunha TM, Schivo IRS, Parada CA, Cunha FQ, Ferreira SH. An electronic pressure-meter nociception paw test for rats. Brazilian Journal of Medical and Biological Research. 2004;**37**(3):391-399

[69] Wang Y, Zhang R, Xie J, Lu J, Yue Z. Analgesic activity of catalpol in rodent models of neuropathic pain, and its spinal mechanism. Cell Biochemistry and Biophysics. 2014;**70** (3):1565-1571

[70] Laster MJ, Liu J, Eger E, Taheri S. Electrical stimulation as a substitute for the tail clamp in the determination of minimum alveolar concentration. Anesthesia and Analgesia. 1993;**76** (6):1310-1312

[71] Blake L, Graeme ML, Sigg EB. Grid shock test for analgesics in mice. Journal of Experimental Medicine. 1996;**9**:146-150

[72] Steinfels GF, Cook L. Antinociceptive profiles of mu and kappa opioid agonists in a rat tooth pulp stimulation procedure. Journal of Pharmacology and Experimental Therapeutics. 1986;**236**(1):111-117

[73] Bloss JL, Hammond DL. Shock titration in the rhesus monkey: effects of opiate and nonopiate analgesics. Journal of Pharmacology and Experimental Therapeutics. 1985;**235**:423-430

[74] Joshi P, Priya B, Gahlot M. Anti-inflammatory and analgesic activities of methanol extract of vallaris solanacea leaves. International Journal of Pharmacy and Pharmaceutical Sciences. **6**(Suppl 2):622-624

[75] Craft RM, Carlisi VJ, Mattia A, Herman RM, Porreca F. Behavioral characterization of the excitatory and desensitizing effects of intravesical capsaicin and resiniferatoxin in the rat. Pain. 1993;**55**:205-215

[76] Wesselmann U, Czakanski PP, Affaitati G, Giamberardino MA. Uterine inflammation as a noxious visceral stimulus: behavioral/ characterization in the rat. Neuroscience Letters. 1998;**246**:73-76

[77] Voilley N, et al. Nonsteroid anti-inflammatory drugs inhibit both the activity and the inflammation-induced expression of acidsensing ion channels in nociceptors. Journal of Neuroscience. 2001;**21**(20):8026-8033

[78] Jones NG, et al. Acid-induced pain and its modulation in humans. Journal of Neuroscience. 2004;**24**(48):10974-10979

[79] Pertovaara A. The noradrenergic pain regulation system: a potential target for pain therapy. European Journal of Pharmacology. 2013;**716**(1-3):2-7

Chapter 17

Analgesic Potential of Extracts and Derived Natural Products from Medicinal Plants

Abdur Rauf, Noor Jehan, Zarka Ahmad and
Mohammad S. Mubarak

Additional information is available at the end of the chapter

http://dx.doi.org/10.5772/intechopen.68631

Abstract

Since ancient times, plants have always been a reliable and important source of bioactive compounds used to treat several diseases, and thus play a central role in human health. In addition, medicinal plants are a rich source of bioactive secondary metabolites that have a wide range of medicinal uses. This is the reason why, currently, 90% of drugs come from natural or semisynthetic origins. Chemical diversity of plants made them one of the main sources for the extraction and purification of secondary metabolites. On the other hand, pain has always been a cause of concern to humans who searched for a remedy from natural sources, mostly from plants. In this respect, substances that relieve pain (algesia) can be described as analgesics (painkillers). Chemically diverse structures have been identified as pain relievers; they relieve pain through various mechanisms and act either centrally (opioids receptor agonism) or peripherally. Therefore, this chapter is intended to summarize the literature pertaining to plants and their constituents discovered with analgesic potential in the last four decades.

Keywords: medicinal plants, analgesics, extract, derived natural products

1. Introduction

Medicinal plants are a rich source for making phytochemicals with great efficiency and selectivity. Since the middle of the nineteenth century, many natural products were obtained in a pure form from plants; most of these products are available to be used as active agents in modern medication. Despite the significant advances in synthetic drugs, side effects remain that necessitate the search for effective, inexpensive, and more accessible drugs. Medicinal plants may provide such valuable therapeutic alternatives. Use of traditional medicinal plants with analgesic effects has recently gained popularity worldwide because of their natural origin and fewer side effects [1]. Moreover, medicinal plant extracts and their fractions are used by 80% of the world population for their simple health care necessities. They are the significant source of natural drug molecules and secondary metabolites which can be used in modern medicine for the cure of various diseases. Throughout history, people relied on an old-style traditional system of medicine to cure diseases and disorders, which with time has gained popularity and global significance. Present approximations suggest that in numerous developing countries, a large proportion of the population seriously trusts traditional specialists and local healers in addition to trusting medicinal plants and medicinal plants-derived drugs to cure diseases, though modern drugs may be accessible in these countries. However, herbal medicines must be approved by local authorities before being prescribed.

Native people and early civilizations tested different plants and animal parts to determine what effect they have. Using trial and error methods, local healers and shamans found that particular plants or parts had therapeutic activity. These indicated the first crude drugs and this knowledge was passed down through the generations and arranged similar to the old-style Chinese medicine as well as Ayurveda [2, 3]. Many traditional medicines have actual and useful effects, and extracts of these medicines have led to the discovery of bioactive molecules and to the growth of current chemically active pure drug discovery [3].

Recently, several people in developed countries have turned to complementary treatments including the use of therapeutic herbs [2]. In this context, the term Ayurvedic medicine has been introduced which is mainly in the form of a crude extract that consists of a mixture of several compounds; however, when the active agents are isolated and purified, they individually fail to give the desired activity. Therefore, pharmacological data on several medicinal plants and isolated compounds are required to regulate active compounds with the desired biological potency. Furthermore, modern methods of production, purification, and standardization should be followed to obtain plant-derived materials of high quality [3]. In ancient times, humans extracted chemicals from plants for treatment of various diseases, and kept records of useful properties and uses of medical plants, such as willow bark and *Papaver somniferum*, used as a pain killers. It is now documented that willow bark contains acetylsalicylic acid, the active ingredient in aspirin [3].

Due to its frequent occurrence, pain is a public health problem with considerable socioeconomic effects. It is an indication of several illnesses and it is predicted that about 80–100% of the population will experience, for example, back pain once in life [4]. Pain treatment requires analgesics including, anti-inflammatory medicines, which at maximum doses have analgesic properties. In this respect, inhibition of nitric oxide (NO) and prostaglandin E2 production has been reported as a potential therapy for different inflammatory disorders [5]. Though several anti-inflammatory and analgesics drugs exist on the shelves, current drug therapy is related to certain adverse effects such as gastrointestinal irritation [6], bronchospasm, fluid retention, and extension of bleeding time. Consequently, it is necessary to discover new drugs with fewer adverse effects. Accordingly, people resort to medicinal plants for discovery and development of new drugs [7]. In addition, scientists discovered that extracts from medicinal plants can be a significant source of natural and safer new drugs for the treatment of inflammation and pain [8, 9].

http://dx.doi.org/10.5772/intechopen.68631

2. Analgesic (painkiller)

Analgesics drugs include paracetamol (acetaminophenol), in addition to the nonsteroidal anti-inflammatory drugs (NSAIDs) such as salicylates, and morphine and oxycodone isolated from opium. There are many classes of drugs available for treatment of pain. Each class has a dissimilar history of uses for treatment of different types of pain and in different types of people.

Analgesic selection is governed by the type of pain. For example, for neuropathic pain, traditional analgesics are less effective, whereas drugs that are not normally mentioned as analgesics, such as tricyclic antidepressants and anticonvulsants medicine, are more effective as pain killers [10]. In general, pain killers are not used if there have other serious side effects. For pain relief, drugs are classified based on either their chemical structures or on their uses for different classes of medical illnesses. Moreover, some drugs are arranged according to the requirements of people who use them. In other cases, these drugs are listed based on accessibility in a geographical zone, possibly to stop obtaining drugs which are prohibited there.

2.1. Acetaminophen

Acetaminophen (paracetamol) is a common medication to treat fever and pain [11]; this medicine is mostly used for slight and moderate body pain. On the other hand, paracetamol in combination with opioid are used for severe pain, such as pain after surgery [12]. Acetaminophen is used orally or taken intravenously [12] and its effect lasts between 2 and 4 hours. Acetaminophen is classified as slight analgesic [13] and is harmless at the recommended doses [13, 14].

2.2. NSAIDs as analgesics drug

Nonsteroidal anti-inflammatory drugs (NSAIDs) are a class of medications that provide anti-pyretic and analgesic effects, and in higher doses have anti-inflammatory potential. They are among the most commonly used analgesics for arthritic pain worldwide. The prominent members of this group of drugs are ibuprofen, aspirin, and naproxen, which are available and used in most countries [15]. Analgesic NSAIDs are nonnarcotic and are used as a nonaddictive alternate to narcotics.

2.3. Archetypal opioids

The archetypal opioids (morphine) and all similar extracts, as well as other opioids, affect the cerebral opioid receptor coordination [16, 17]. Tramadol is a serotonin-norepinephrine reuptake inhibitor (SNRI) through feeble μ-opioid receptor agonist actions, whereas buprenorphine is a partial agonist of the μ-opioid receptor [18]. Tramadol and venlafaxine are structurally very close to codeine that exerts analgesia not by individual opioid-like properties but through less agonism of the μ-opioid receptor and by acting as a serotonin-releasing agent and a norepinephrine reuptake inhibitor [19–22]. Opioids, though very active analgesics, might have certain unfriendly side effects. Those patients starting morphine might experience vomiting and nausea [23].

2.4. Alcohol compounds as analgesics

Alcohol compounds are also documented to treat pain [24]; however, alcohols have biological, mental, and social properties that affect the significance of their use for treatment of pain [25]. Although reasonable usage of alcohol can reduce certain kinds of pain under certain conditions [26], the use of alcohol to cure pain, however, is encountered by the negative effects of extreme drinking [27].

2.5. Cannabis and cannabinoids as analgesic

Cannabis or medical marijuana is related to the use of cannabis and isolated cannabinoids to cure diseases and relieve pain [28]. In addition, cannabis and its compounds are used to treat chronic pain. The best-known analgesic of these cannabinoids for treatment of pain is tetrahydrocannabinol, or the best known as THC [29–31].

In comparison, numerous mixtures of analgesic drugs have been determined to have insufficient effectiveness compared to similar doses of their separate mechanisms. Furthermore, these analgesic mixtures frequently result in consequences such as unintentional overdoses, often owing to misperceptions that arise from the many mentioned compounds and combinations [32]. Countless people use alternative medicine for pain relief. There are indications that some medications relieve some kind of pain more efficiently than others [33]; however, additional research would be essential to improve comprehension of the uses of many alternative medicine [34].

2.6. Plants as new sources of pain killers

Numerous medicinal plants and their derived phytochemicals were evaluated for their analgesic and anti-inflammatory effects. For example, extracts of bark as well as terpenoids obtained from *Combretum molle* (Combretaceae), β-glucopyranosyl, and other isolated compounds have been documented to have an excellent potential against carrageenan-induced paw edema in rats [7]. Similarly, *Millettia versicolor* crude extract and its isolated phytochemicals were found to inhibit 12-*O*-tetradecanoylphorbol-13-acetate (TPA)-induced acute ear edema and phospholipase A_2 acute mouse paw edema [8]. Furthermore, chemical constituents isolated from various parts of *Millettia griffoniana, Erythrina addisoniae,* and *Erythrina mildbraedii* have been reported to exhibit significant anti-inflammatory activity on induced-paw edema and induced-ear edema in mice [8], whereas compounds isolated from *Erythrina sigmoidea* have been shown to possess anti-inflammatory activity against 12-*O*-tetradecanoylphorbol-13-acetate (TPA)-induced ear edema [8]. Based on the above facts, the present chapter will focus on documenting the recent literature pertaining to medicinal plants and their phytochemicals and extracts as analgesics and in the treatment of inflammation.

2.7. Other natural products with analgesic properties

Natural products play a key role for living organisms. Primary metabolites are defined by Kossel as the main components of metabolic paths that are compulsory for life. Primary metabolites are related to important cellular roles, such as energy production, assimilation of nutrients, and development/growth. Secondary metabolites, in contrast to primary, are not essential and not required for the survival of living organisms [35–38].

Interestingly, secondary metabolites possess a broad range of functions. They comprise pheromones, which can act as community gesturing molecules with additional individuals of the same species [39–41]. Communication molecules entice and stimulate a symbiotic organism and agents to solubilize and transport various nutrients, including siderophores, as well as good arms such as venoms, repellants, and toxins, which are used as a prey and predators competitors [42]. It has been documented in the literature that nearly 10 million organic compounds have been discovered and many new and novel compounds are still being isolated and characterized in various parts of the world.

Regarding these compounds, one hypothesis is that they present a good benefit to the living organism which makes them. Another view says that these compounds have similarity to the immune system of living organisms, and although they have no function, yet they can afford assorted bioactive compounds which have important biological activity [42].

Naturally obtained agents such as aspirin, morphine, codeine, thebaine, and others have been reported to have analgesic activity. Aspirin derived from salicylic acid extracted from barks of the willow tree (*Salix alba*) is one of the most extensively used compounds for the managements of mild pain. On the other hand, morphine codeine and thebaine isolated from plants are used as analgesics (**Figure 1**) [43, 44].

Different types of active phytochemicals, such as steroids, alkaloids, tannins, phenol, and polyphenols are produced by medicinal plants [45–49]. In addition, a large number of plants that have been investigated are reported to have less pharmacologically active secondary metabolites identified. Plant-derived molecules are mainly reported for their medical importance; this includes morphine, nicotine, quinine, steroidal, and many others [50]. A large number of presently recommended drugs have been derived from natural medicinal plants; some characteristic examples are given in next sections.

2.7.1. *Salicin*

It has been reported in the literature that extracted natural products possess analgesic activity. The bark of willow trees has been recognized for pain-relieving properties. It has been further reported that willow bark contains a bioactive compound, salicin, which hydrolyses into salicylic acid. As we know that derivative acetylsalicylic acid is known as aspirin and is used as a pain killer, the main mechanism of its action is inhibition of the cyclooxygenase enzyme (COX). There are two types of cyclooxygenase-2 enzyme isozymes; COX-1 (PTGS1) and COX-2 (PTGS2). It is nonselective and permanently inhibits both form, but it is weakly more selective for COX-1. COX produces prostaglandins most of them are pro-inflammatory and thromboxanes, which promote clotting [51].

Nonsteroidal anti-inflammatory drugs (NSAIDs) act via inhibition of cyclooxygenase enzyme (COX). Research findings suggest the opposing effects of nonsteroidal anti-inflammatory

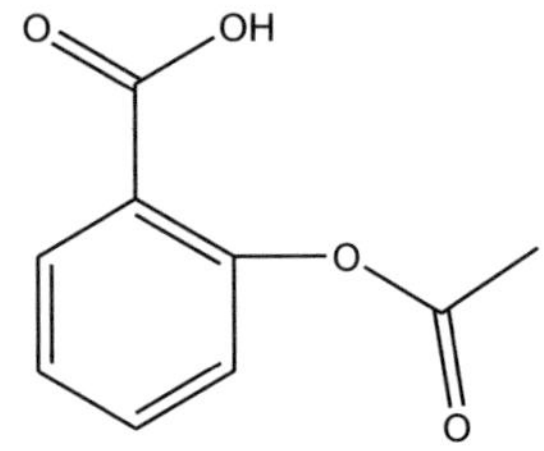

Aspirin (1)

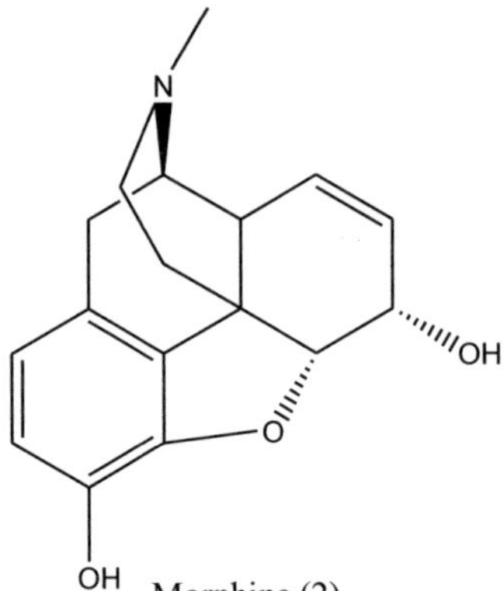

Morphine (2)

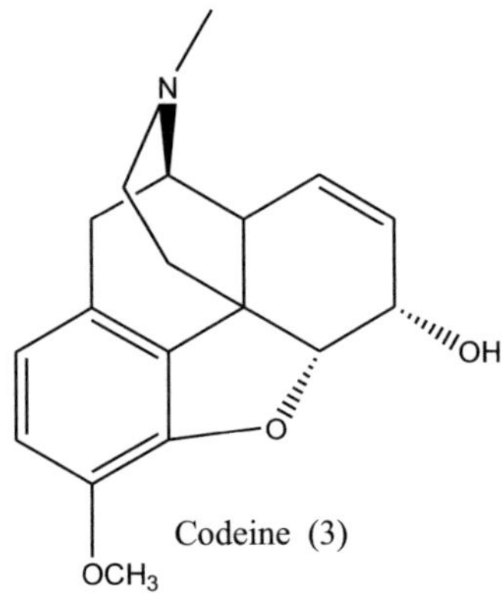

Codeine (3)

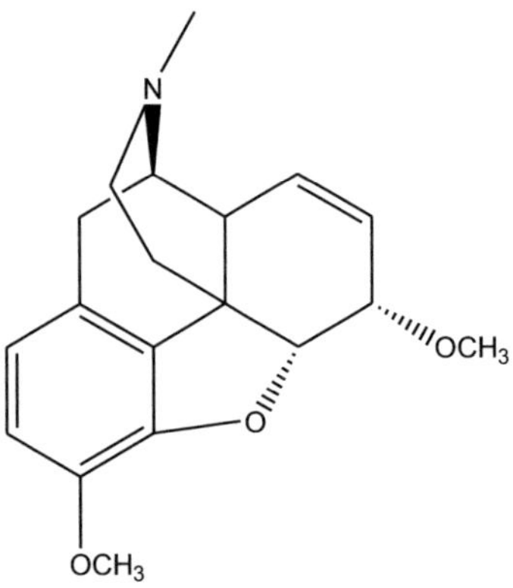

Thebaine (4)

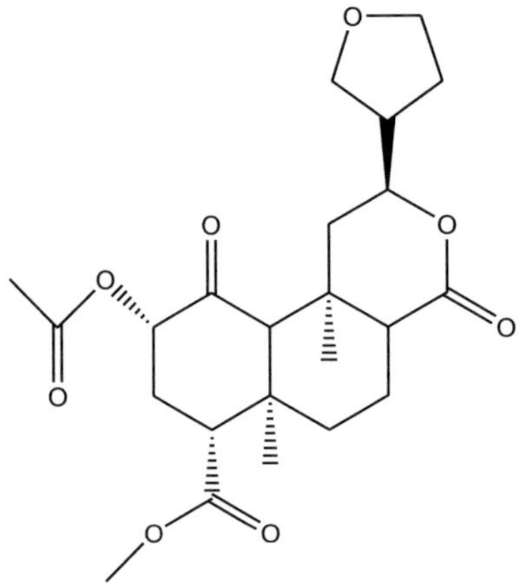

Salvinorin A (5)

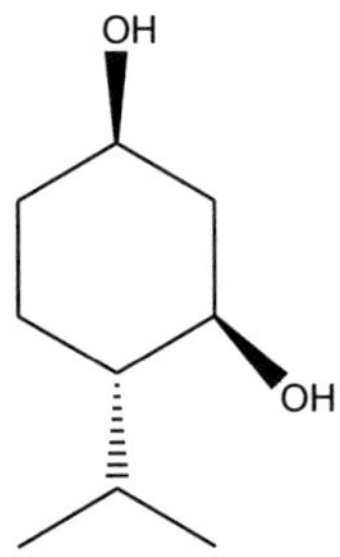

Menthol(6)

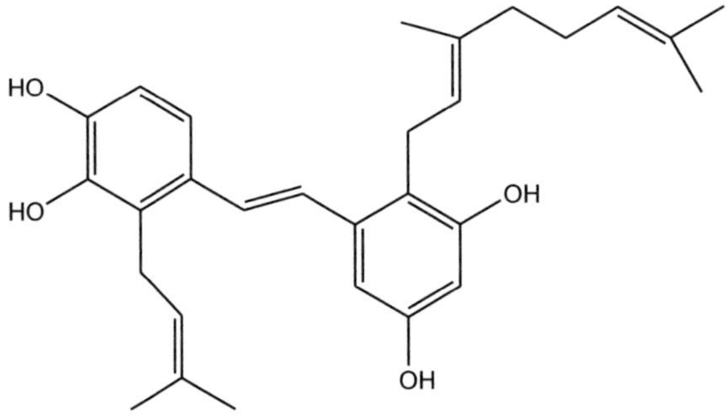

Pawhuskin (7)

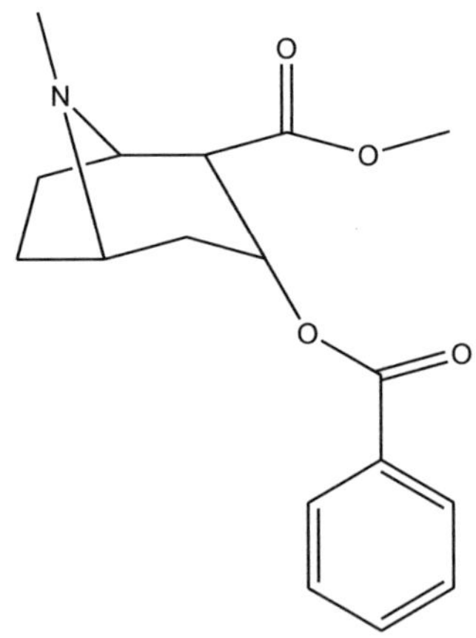

Cocaine (8)

Figure 1. Chemical structures of analgesic compounds from medicinal plants.

drugs on COX. These drugs act by blocking the COX-1 enzyme, which catalyzes the production of prostaglandins that are involved in numerous physiological functions, such as (a) maintenance of normal renal function in the kidneys, (b) mucosal protection in the gastrointestinal tract, and (c) proaggregatory thromboxane in the platelets. However, COX-2 expression can be induced by cytokines and other inflammatory mediators in a number of tissues, including endothelial cells, and is believed to have a role in the mediation of pain, inflammation, and fever. COX-2 agents only inhibit the COX-2 enzyme, whereas traditional NSAIDs block both versions in general [16].

After extensive acceptance of the cyclooxygenase enzyme (COX-2) inhibitors, it was revealed that many of the drugs in this class increase the risk of cardiovascular toxicity, which led to the removal of valdecoxib and rofecoxib, and others. On the other hand, etoricoxib appears comparatively safer to that of noncoxib NSAID diclofenac [17]. It is worth mentioning here that our research group has reported that pistagremic acid, a natural product isolated from *Pistacia integerrima*, can inhibit COX-2 enzyme owing to the hydrogen and hydrophobic contacts to significant active sites of molecule [17].

The key uses of NSAID medication are typically for joint- and spine-related pain. Its mechanism of action is through interaction with pro-inflammatory cytokines interleukin (IL-1a, IL-1b, IL-6) and tumor necrosis factor (TNF-α). Increased absorption of TNF-α is thought to produce the cardinal symptoms of inflammation. These pro-inflammatory cytokines result in chemo-attractants for neutrophils and help them to stick to the endothelial from migration. They also stimulate white cell phagocytosis and the production of inflammatory lipid prostaglandin E2 (PGE_2). The ability of NSAIDs to interfere with the production of prostaglandin during inflammatory cascade is the major mechanism cited for success of pain of medication. In normal pain, the archidonic pathway proceeds and results in the production of highly reactive mediators that are prostaglandin, prostacycline, histamines, and many others. These mediators cause the start of pain in the body.

2.7.2. Morphine

An additional distinguished example is *P. somniferum*, a flowering poppy that yields opium, which contains a potent narcotic alkaloid constituent called morphine that acts as an opioid receptor [52]. Morphine binds to opioid receptors; molecular signaling activates the receptors to mediate certain actions. μ (Mu) receptors exist in the brain stem as well as in thalamus activation, these receptors result in relief of pain and sedation. Kappa receptor is found in the limbic system, part of forebrain, spinal cord, and brain stem. Activation these receptors result in relief of pain and sedation. Delta receptor found in brain, spinal cord, and digestive tract, stimulation of delta receptor leads to analgesic.

2.7.3. Ziconotide

Ziconotide, also known as SNX-111, is a novel nonopioid analgesic drug. It is a synthetic version of ω-conotoxin MVIIA (ω-MVIIA), which is a peptide that is found in the venom of the fish-eating marine snail, *Conus magus*. It is a powerful analgesic drug that acts through a mechanism that involves selective block of N-type calcium channels. This action inhibits the discharge of pronociceptive neurochemicals such as glutamate, calcitonin gene-connected peptide, and material P in the brain and spinal cord, ensuing in pain relief. It has been approved for the treatment of severe chronic pain in patients only when administered by the intrathecal route. Importantly, prolonged administration of ziconotide does not lead to the development of addiction or tolerance [53].

2.7.4. Salvinorin

Salvinorin A is the main active psychotropic molecule in *Salvia divinorum*, a Mexican plant that has a long history of use as an entheogen by indigenous Mazatec shamans. Salvinorin A is considered a dissociative. It can produce psychoactive experiences in humans with a typical duration of action being several minutes to an hour [54, 55]. Furthermore, Salvinorin is a *trans*-neoclerodane diterpenoid, which acts as a κ-opioid receptor agonist. The mechanism of action of Salvinorin A on ileal tissue has been described as prejunctional, as it was able to adjust electrically made contraction, but not those of exogenous acetylcholine. A pharmacologically important feature of the contraction-reducing properties of ingested Salvinorin A on gut tissue is that it is only pharmacologically active on inflamed and not normal tissue, thus reducing possible side effects. Salvinorin produce a conditioned place aversion and decreases locomotors. It is able to modify dopaminergic pathway [55].

2.7.5. Pawhuskin A

Pawhuskin A is a bioactive naturally occurring stilbene reported from *Dalea purpurea*. Pawhuskin A has recognized to function as an opioid receptor antagonist, with special binding to the k receptor. Pawhuskin A is the most active natural compound making a small group of nonnitrogenous compounds with effect on the opiate receptor system [56].

3. Conclusions

This chapter has focused on information and relevant literature pertaining to analgesic plants and their explored chemical constituents. Furthermore, unexplored medicinal plants reported to be used in folk medicine have been highlighted. This chapter also provides references to research carried out on analgesic drugs. Additionally, this chapter describes the main mechanisms of action of natural products poisoning presenting analgesic properties.

Acknowledgements

The authors are grateful to the Higher Education Commission of Pakistan and the University of Swabi, KPK, for financial support.

Author details

Abdur Rauf[1]*, Noor Jehan[2], Zarka Ahmad[3] and Mohammad S. Mubarak[4]

*Address all correspondence to: mashaljcs@yahoo.com

1 Department of Chemistry, University of Swabi, Ambar, Khyber Pakhtunkhwa, Pakistan

2 Department of Geology, University of Swabi, Ambar, Khyber Pakhtunkhwa, Pakistan

3 Khyber Teaching Hospital, Peshawar, Peshawar, Khyber Pakhtunkhwa, Pakistan

4 Department of Chemistry, the University of Jordan, Amman, Jordan

References

[1] Uddin G, Rauf A, Siddiqui BS, Shah S. Preliminary comparative phytochemical screening of Diospyros lotus Stewart. Middle-East Journal of Scientific Research. 2011;**10**: 78–81

[2] Uddin G, Rauf A, Rehman T, Qaisar M. Phytochemical screening of Pistaciachinensis var. integerrima. Middle-East Journal of Scientific Research. 2011;**7**:707–711

[3] Kumar S, Shukla YN, Lavania UC, Sharma A, Singh AK. Journal of Medicinal and Aromatic Plants: Prospects for India. 1997;**19**:361–365

[4] Jain KN, Kulkarni KS, Singh A. Modulation of NSAID-induced antinociceptive and anti-inflammatory effects by alpha2-adrenoceptor agonists with gastroprotective effects. Life Sciences. 2002;**70**:2857–2869, 10. DOI: 1016/S0024-3205(02)01549-7

[5] Nowakowska Z. A review of anti-infective and anti-inflammatory chalcones. European Journal of Medicinal Chemistry. 2007;**42**:125–137. DOI: 10.1016/j.ejmech.2006.09.019

[6] Osadebe PO, Okoye FBC. Anti-inflammatory effects of crude methanolic extract and fractions of Alchorneacordifolia leaves. Journal of Ethnopharmacology. 2003;**89**:19–24. DOI: 10.1016/S0378-8741(03)00195-8

[7] Raza M, Shaheen F, Choudhary MI, Suria A, Rahman UA, Sompong S, Delorenzo RJ. Anticonvulsant activities of the FS-1 subfraction isolated from roots of Delphinium denudatum. Phytotherapy Research. 2001;**15**:426–430. DOI: 10.1002/ptr.792

[8] Efferth T, Kuete V. Cameroonian medicinal plants: Pharmacology and derived natural products. Frontiers in Pharmacology. 2010;**1**:123.

[9] Anonymous. Cancer pain relief and palliative care; report of a WHO expert committee. World Health Organization Technical Report Series, 804. Geneva, Switzerland: World Health Organization; 1990. pp. 1–75. ISBN: 92-4-120804-X.

[10] Dworkin RH, Backonja M, Rowbotham MC, Allen RR, Argoff CR, Bennett GJ, Bushnell MC, Farrar JT, Galer BS, Haythornthwaite JA, Hewitt DJ, Loeser JD, Max MB, Saltarelli M, Schmader KE, Stein C, Thompson D, Turk DC, Wallace MS, Watkins LR, Weinstein SM. Advances in neuropathic pain: Diagnosis, mechanisms, and treatment recommendations. Archives of Neurology. 2003;**60**(11):1524–1534

[11] Perrott D. A., Piira T., Goodenough B., & Champion G. D. (2004). Efficacy and safety of acetaminophen vs ibuprofen for treating children's pain or fever: a meta-analysis. Archives of pediatrics & adolescent medicine, **158**(6):521–526.

[12] Scottish Intercollegiate Guidelines Network (SIGN). 6.1 and 7.1.1. Guideline 106: Control of Pain in Adults with Cancer (PDF). Scotland: National Health Service (NHS); 2008. ISBN: 9781905813384

[13] Hochhauser D. Cancer and its Management. John Wiley & Sons; 2014. United States. p. 119. ISBN: 9781118468715

[14] Russell FM, Shann F, Curtis N, Mulholland K. Evidence on the use of paracetamol in febrile children. Bulletin of the World Health Organization. 2003;**81**(5):367–372

[15] Warden SJ. Prophylactic use of NSAIDs by athletes: A risk/benefit assessment. The Physician and Sports Medicine. 2010;**38**(1):132–138

[16] Rauf A, Uddin G, Siddiqui BS, Khan A, Khan H, Arfan M, Wadood A. In-vivo antinociceptive, anti-inflammatory and antipyretic activity of pistagremic acid isolated from *Pistacia integerrima*. Phytomedicine. 2014;**21:**1509–1515.

[17] Smith HS, Raffa RB, Pergolizzi JV, Taylor R, Tallarida RJ. Combining opioid and adrenergic mechanisms for chronic pain. Postgraduate Medicine. 2014;**126**(4):98–114.

[18] Driessen B, Reimann W. Interaction of the central analgesic, tramadol, with the uptake and release of 5-hydroxytryptamine in the rat brain in vitro. British Journal of Pharmacology. 1992;**105**(1):147–151

[19] Bamigbade TA, Davidson C, Langford RM, Stamford JA. Actions of tramadol, its enantiomers and principal metabolite, O-desmethyltramadol, on serotonin (5-HT) efflux and uptake in the rat dorsal raphe nucleus. British Journal of Anaesthesia. 1997;**79**(3):352–356

[20] Reimann W, Schneider F. Induction of 5-hydroxytryptamine release by tramadol, fenfluramine and reserpine. European Journal of Pharmacology. 1998;**349**(2-3)

[21] Gobbi M, Moia M, Pirona L, Ceglia I, Reyes-Parada M, Scorza C, Mennini T. p-Methylthioamphetamine and 1-(m-chlorophenyl)piperazine, two non-neurotoxic 5-HT releasers in vivo, differ from neurotoxic amphetamine derivatives in their mode of action at 5-HT nerve endings in vitro. Journal of Neurochemistry. 2002;**82**(6):1435–1443.

[22] Doyle D, Hanks G, Cherney I, Calman K, editors. Oxford Textbook of Palliative Medicine. 3rd ed. Oxford University Press; 2004;199–203.

[23] Zale EL, Maisto SA, Ditre JW. Interrelations between pain and alcohol: An integrative review. Clinical Psychology Review Oxford, England, U.K. 2015;**37**:57–71. DOI: 10.1016/j.cpr.2015.02.005; DOI: 10.1016%2Fj.cpr.2015.02.005. ISSN: 0272-7358

[24] Murnion B. Medicinal cannabis. Australian Prescriber. 2015;**38**(6):212–215. DOI: 10.18773/austprescr.2015.072; DOI: 10.18773%2Faustprescr.2015.072. PMC: 4674028. PMID: 26843715

[25] Wright, Stephen. "Cannabinoid-based medicines for neurological disorders—clinical evidence." Molecular neurobiology 36, no. 1 (2007): 129–136.

[26] Weathermon R, et al. Alcohol and Medication Interactions [Internet]. Available from: https:pubs.niaaa.nih.gov/publications/arh23-1/40-54

[27] Whiting PF, Wolff RF, Deshpande S, Di Nisio M, Duffy S, Hernandez AV, Keurentjes JC, Lang S, Misso K, Ryder S, Schmidlkofer S, Westwood M, Kleijnen J. Cannabinoids for medical use: A systematic review and meta-analysis. Journal of the American Medical Association. 2015;**313**(24):2456–2473. DOI: 10.1001/jama.2015.6358; DOI: 10.1001%2Fjama.2015.6358. PMID: 26103030

[28] Jensen B, Chen J, Furnish T, Wallace M. Medical marijuana and chronic pain: A review of basic science and clinical evidence. Current Pain and Headache Reports. 2015;**19**(10):50–54.

[29] Mehlisch DR. The efficacy of combination analgesic therapy in relieving dental pain. Journal of the American Dental Association. 2002;**133**(7):861–871

[30] Murnion B. P. (2010). Combination analgesics in adults. Aust Prescr, 33, 113–115.

[31] Thomas D-A, Maslin B, Legler A, Springer E, Asgerally A, Vadivelu N. Role of alternative therapies for chronic pain syndromes. Current Pain and Headache Reports. 2016;**20**(5):685–701

[32] Eardley I, Whelan P, Kirby R, Schaeffer A. Drugs used in the treatment of interstitial Cystitis. In: Drug Treatment in Urology United States. John Wiley & Sons; 2008. p. 65.

[33] Kornhuber J, Bleich S, Wiltfang J, Maler M, Parsons CG. Flupirtine shows functional NMDA receptor antagonism by enhancing Mg^{2+} block via activation of voltage independent potassium channels. Rapid communication. Journal of Neural Transmission. 1999;**106**(9-10):857–867. DOI: 10.1007/s007020050206; DOI: 10.1007%2Fs007020050206. PMID: 10599868

[34] Klawe C, Maschke M. Flupirtine: Pharmacology and clinical applications of a non-opioid analgesic and potentially neuroprotective compound. Expert Opinion on Pharmacotherapy. 2009;**10**(9):1495–1500

[35] Uddin G., Rauf A., Siddiqui B. S., Muhammad N., Khan A., & Shah S. U. A. (2014). Anti-nociceptive, anti-inflammatory and sedative activities of the extracts and chemical constituents of Diospyros lotus L. Phytomedicine, 21(7), 954–959.

[36] Brunton L, Chabner B, Knollman B. Goodman and Gilman's the Pharmacological Basis of Therapeutics. 12th ed. New York: McGraw-Hill Professional; 2010. ISBN: 978-0-07-162442-8

[37] Kliebenstein DJ. Secondary metabolites and plant/environment interactions: A view through *Arabidopsis thaliana* tinged glasses. Plant, Cell and Environment. 2004;**27**(6):675–684

[38] Karlovsky P. Secondary metabolites in soil ecology. Soil Biology. 2008;**14**:1–19. DOI: 10.1007/978-3-540-74543-3_1; DOI: 10.1007%2F978-3-540-74543-3_1. The current, generally accepted concept in line with Kossel's view is that primary metabolites are chemical components of living organisms that are vital for their normal functioning, while secondary metabolites are compounds which are dispensable

[39] Rogers K. The Components of Life: From Nucleic Acids to Carbohydrates. 1st ed. New York, NY: Britannica Educational Publishing in association with Rosen Educational Services; 2011. ISBN: 978-1-61530-324-3

[40] Cox DL, Nelson MM. Lehninger Principles of Biochemistry. 6th ed. New York, N.Y.: W.H. Freeman; 2013. ISBN: 978-1-4641-0962-1

[41] Boal D. Mechanics of the Cell. 4th printing ed. Cambridge, UK: Cambridge University Press; 2006. ISBN: 978-0-521-79681-1

[42] McCurdy CR, Scully SS. Analgesic substance derived from natural products (natureceutical). Life Sciences, 2005;**78**:476–484.

[43] Sitaramayya A. Introduction to Cellular Signal Transduction. Boston: Birkhäuser; 1999. ISBN: 978-0-8176-3982-2.

[44] Demain AL, Fang A. The natural functions of secondary metabolites. Advances in Biochemical Engineering/Biotechnology. 2000;**69**:1–39

[45] Williams DH, Stone MJ, Hauck PR, Rahman SK. Why are secondary metabolites (natural products) biosynthesized? Journal of Natural Products. 1989;**52**(6):1189–1208. DOI: 10.1021/np50066a001; DOI: 10.1021%2Fnp50066a001. PMID: 2693613.

[46] Firn RD, Jones CG. The evolution of secondary metabolism – A unifying model (PDF). Molecular Microbiology. 2000;**37**(5):989–994. DOI: 10.1046/j.1365-2958.2000.02098.x; DOI: 10.1046%2Fj.1365-2958.2000.02098.x. PMID: 10972818

[47] Strobel G, Daisy B. Bioprospecting for microbial endophytes and their natural products. Microbiology and Molecular Biology Reviews. 2003;**67**(4):491–502. DOI: 10.1128/MMBR.67.4.491-502.2003; DOI: 10.1128%2FMMBR.67.4.491-502.2003. PMC: 309047. PMID: 14665674

[48] Zaffiri L, Gardner J, Toledo-Pereyra LH. History of antibiotics. From salvarsan to cephalosporins. Journal of Investigative Surgery. 2012;**25**(2):67–77. DOI: 10.3109/08941939.2012.664099; DOI: 10.3109%2F08941939.2012.664099. PMID: 22439833

[49] Procópio RE, Silva IR, Martins MK, Azevedo JL, Araújo JM. Antibiotics produced by Streptomyces. The Brazilian Journal of Infectious Diseases. 2012;**16**(5):466–471. DOI: 10.1016/j.bjid.2012.08.014; DOI: 10.1016%2Fj.bjid.2012.08.014. PMID: 22975171

[50] Cochrane SA, Vederas JC. Lipopeptides from *Bacillus* and *Paenibacillus* spp.: A gold mine of antibiotic candidates. Medicinal Research Reviews. 2016;**36**(1):4–31. DOI: 10.1002/med.21321; DOI: 10.1002%2Fmed.21321. PMID: 24866700

[51] Saxena A, Kumari R, Mukherjee U, Singh P, Lal R. Draft genome sequence of the rifamycin producer amycolatopsisrifamycinica DSM 46095. Genome Announcements. 2014;**2**(4):e00662-14. DOI: 10.1128/genomeA.00662-14; DOI: 10.1128%2FgenomeA.00662-14. PMID: 24994803

[52] Hallett M, Albanese A, Dressler D, Segal KR, Simpson DM, Truong D, Jankovic J. Evidence-based review and assessment of botulinum neurotoxin for the treatment of movement disorders. Toxicon. 2013;**67**(June):94–114

[53] McGivern J. G. Ziconotide: A review of its pharmacology and use in the treatment of pain. Neuropsychiatric Disease and Treatment. 2007;**3**(1):69–85

[54] MacLean K, Johnson M, Reissig C, Prisinzano T, Griffiths R. Dose-related effects of salvinorin A in humans: Dissociative, hallucinogenic, and memory effects. Psychopharmacology. 2013;**226**(2):381–392. DOI: 10.1007/s00213-012-2912-9; DOI: 10.1007%2Fs00213-012-2912-9. PMC: 3581702. PMID: 23135605

[55] Roth BL, Baner K, Westkaemper R, Siebert D, Rice KC, Steinberg S, Ernsberger P, Rothman RB. Salvinorin A: A potent naturally occurring nonnitrogenous κ opioid selective agonist. Proceedings of the National Academy of Sciences of the United States of America. 2002;**99**(18):11934–11939. DOI: 10.1073/pnas.182234399; DOI: 10.1073%2Fpnas.182234399. PMC: 129372. PMID: 12192085

[56] Hartung AM, Beutler JA, Navarro HA, Wiemer DF, Neighbors JD. Stilbenes as κ-selective, non-nitrogenous opioid receptor antagonists. Journal of natural products. 2014;**77**(2);311–319